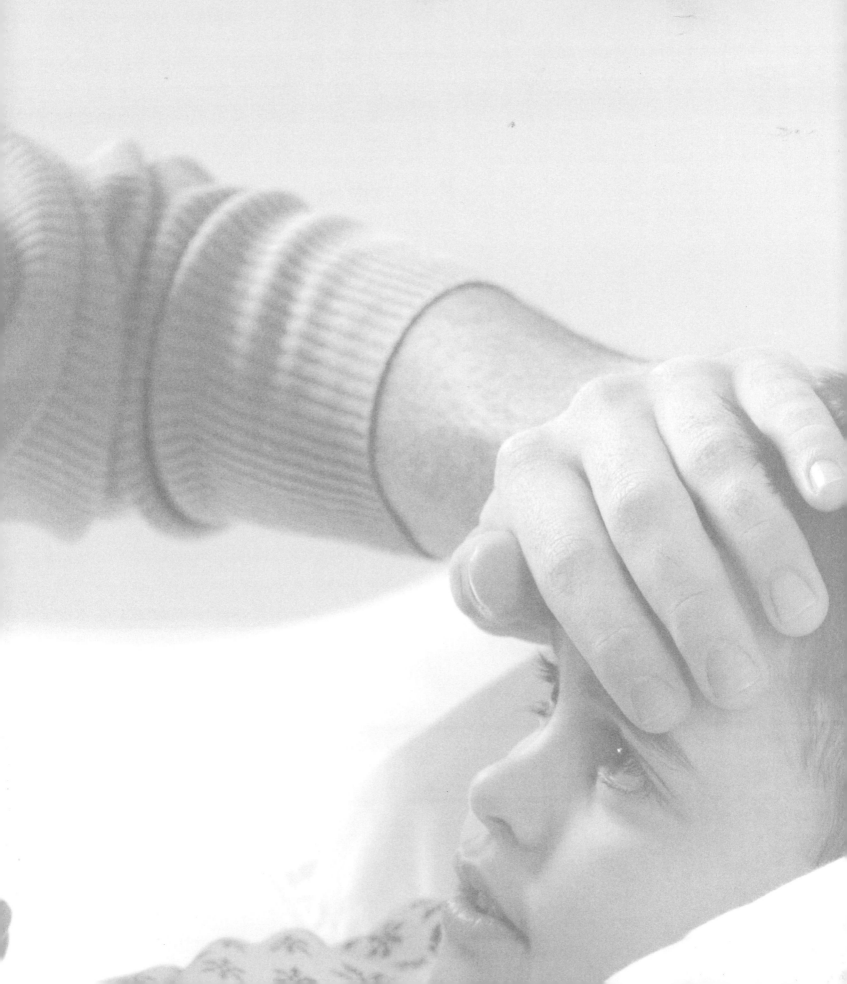

FAMILY HEALTH
ENCYCLOPEDIA

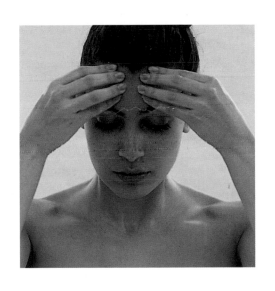

FAMILY HEALTH ENCYCLOPEDIA

The comprehensive guide to the whole family's health needs

Dr Peter Fermie MA, MB, BS, MRCGP, DCH, DRCOG

Dr Stephen Shepherd MB, ChB, MRCGP

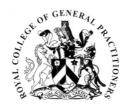

In Association with the Royal
College of General Practitioners

HERMES
HOUSE

This edition is published by Hermes House, an imprint of Anness Publishing Ltd,
Blaby Road, Wigston, Leicestershire LE18 4SE; info@anness.com

www.hermeshouse.com; www.annesspublishing.com

If you like the images in this book and would like to investigate using them for publishing, promotions or advertising, please visit
our website www.practicalpictures.com for more information.

Publisher: Joanna Lorenz
Managing Editor: Helen Sudell
Project Editors: Melanie Halton, Ann Kay
Text Editors: Sue Barraclough, Kim Davies, Cathy Meeus, Sonya Newland, Nikki Sims, Linda Sonntag
Designer: Nigel Partridge
Illustrations: Samantha Elmhurst
Editorial Reader: Jay Thundercliffe
Production Controller: Steve Lang

ETHICAL TRADING POLICY

At Anness Publishing we believe that business should be conducted in an ethical and ecologically sustainable way, with respect for
the environment and a proper regard to the replacement of the natural resources we employ.
As a publisher, we use a lot of wood pulp in high-quality paper for printing, and that wood commonly comes from spruce trees. We
are therefore currently growing more than 750,000 trees in three Scottish forest plantations: Berrymoss (130 hectares/320 acres),
West Touxhill (125 hectares/305 acres) and Deveron Forest (75 hectares/185 acres). The forests we manage contain more than 3.5
times the number of trees employed each year in making paper for the books we manufacture.
Because of this ongoing ecological investment programme, you, as our customer, can have the pleasure and reassurance of knowing
that a tree is being cultivated on your behalf to naturally replace the materials used to make the book you are holding.
Our forestry programme is run in accordance with the UK Woodland Assurance Scheme (UKWAS) and will be certified by the
internationally recognized Forest Stewardship Council (FSC). The FSC is a non-government organization dedicated to promoting
responsible management of the world's forests. Certification ensures forests are managed in an environmentally sustainable and
socially responsible way. For further information about this scheme, go to www.annesspublishing.com/trees

A CIP catalogue record for this book is available from the British Library.

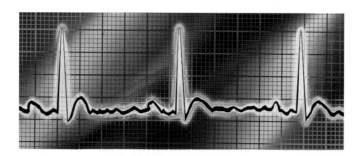

PUBLISHER'S NOTE

The *Family Health Encyclopedia* provides information on a wide range of health and medical matters, but is not
intended as a substitute for professional diagnosis. Any person with a condition or symptoms requiring medical attention
should consult a fully qualified practitioner or therapist. While the advice and information in this book are believed to be
accurate and true at the time of going to press, neither the authors nor the publisher can accept any legal responsibility or
liability for any errors or omissions that may be made, nor for any inaccuracies nor for any loss, harm or injury that comes
about from following instructions or advice in the book.

Foreword

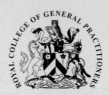

It's not easy taking good care of your health. If only each of us came with an instruction manual and a helpline number, then many of the inevitable worries that we all face would be so much easier to cope with. These days, we are constantly bombarded with health information and advice. TV and radio, magazines and the internet, all are full of the latest tips and theories. Some are good, some are dreadful. And it isn't always easy to tell which is which.

Finding help you can trust

Having someone you can really trust is essential, and this is where general practitioners and the health care team, including nurses and health visitors, can make such a difference. Local health practices form a vital part of our communities and each day finds millions of people consulting their doctor – often about their children's health or about problems related to the stresses of modern life.

The Royal College of General Practitioners is delighted to be associated with this invaluable book. You may not be able to keep your own GP on a shelf ready to answer your health queries, but this book comes close. The more you understand about health and illness, the better you will be able to help both yourself and those closest to you – and nothing can ever be more rewarding than helping loved ones in potentially difficult situations. If this book makes that task just a little easier, I will be delighted.

Professor David Haslam FRCGP

Chairman of Council, Royal College of General Practitioners

Contents

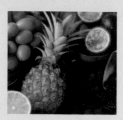
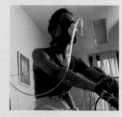
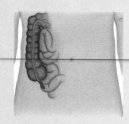
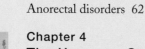
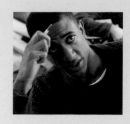
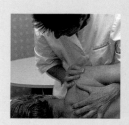
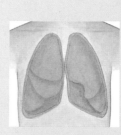
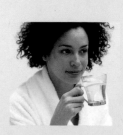

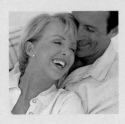

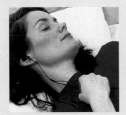

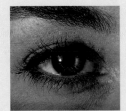

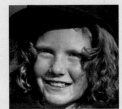

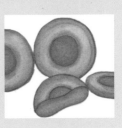

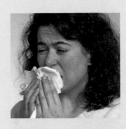

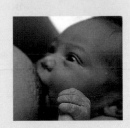

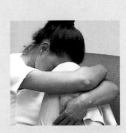

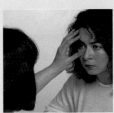

How to use this book

Clearly written text, special feature boxes, an explanatory glossary, a contacts listing and a detailed index all combine to make this invaluable health guide both accessible and easy to use.

The book begins with a general Healthy Living chapter that introduces you to all kinds of strategies for keeping yourself and your family fit and healthy. The chapters that follow are conveniently organized around each of the major systems of the body, from the heart and circulation to the blood and the immune system. The chapters begin with an introduction to that bodily system, which gives a valuable background context to what follows. The chapter then goes on to deal with the various conditions that commonly affect that particular part of the body.

Within an entry for a specific condition, you will find other features that help you to gain a concise and clear understanding of the main issues involved. These features are outlined below.

See Also boxes
These helpful cross-references point the way to other entries or features in the book that may provide useful extra information.

Specialist photographs
Hundreds of full-colour photographs help you to recognize problems and to see specific conditions and processes under the microscope.

Entry text
Each entry explains the most important issues in a clear, informed and non-technical way, offering readers the most up-to-date facts.

Asthma

SEE ALSO
- Anxiety, p000
- Eczema, p000
- Hayfever, p000

Asthma is a condition where intermittent narrowing of the airways results in breathing difficulties. In mild cases, the person may suffer only sporadic bouts of wheezing and shortness of breath, but some people can have disabling and potentially life-threatening attacks almost every day. Asthma has become much more common over the past two decades and cases are believed to have doubled in that time – although it is thought that this increase may be due to the fact that more people with mild symptoms are classified as asthmatics.

SIGNS AND SYMPTOMS
- Wheezing and coughing, which will often be more severe at night, in the early hours of the morning, and after exercise.
- Tightness in the chest.
- Shortness of breath.
- Panic and anxiety.
- Difficulty breathing out.

Asthma can develop at any age but generally it occurs first in childhood. The condition is often associated with allergies, which are becoming more prevalent. Common triggers for allergic asthma are house dust mites, pollen, mould and pet hair. Some of the more common food allergens (see box) can also trigger an asthmatic attack. Children who are affected by allergic asthma often also develop eczema or hay fever.

Most adults who suffer from asthma first developed the condition as children. However, asthma can also start in adulthood, usually after a respiratory infection. Smoking, polluted or cold air, and stress may all trigger asthma attacks.

HOW IS IT DIAGNOSED?
Some people suffer occasional attacks while others have frequent and severe attacks in response to a range of triggers. So it is not always easy for doctors to diagnose. The only clue that a child has asthma might be a cough that occurs at night or the fact that their breathing becomes wheezy during or after a bout of activity.

If your doctor suspects that you have asthma, you may be sent to hospital for further investigation. Tests that help with the diagnosis of asthma include spirometry and lung volume tests, which measure and monitor the rate and depth of your breathing. You may also be tested for allergic reactions to different substances, to pinpoint the likely trigger for your attacks. Blood tests may also be carried out, to check the level of oxygen in your blood.

CAUSES OF ASTHMA

Relaxed muscle layer / Normal airway / Mucus / Small blood vessels

Contracted muscle layer / Narrowed asthmatic airway / Excess mucus

△ In asthma, the muscles in the bronchi constrict, causing them to narrow. At the same time, the mucus that protects the airways from infection is produced in excess and the lining of the airways become inflamed. This means that very little air can get into or out of the lungs.

ASTHMA TRIGGERS
In any one individual, it is possible that there is more than one factor that initiates an asthmatic attack. Asthma may be triggered by:
- Upper respiratory tract infections, such as colds and flu.
- Lower respiratory tract infections, such as pneumonia and bronchitis.
- Allergy (allergens include housedust mites, pollen, hair and saliva from furry animals, such as cats and dogs).
- Exposure to cold air.
- Dampness and mould.
- Anxiety and stress.
- Air pollution.
- Cigarette smoke.

In rare cases, certain foods – such as milk, eggs, nuts and wheat – prompt an attack. Many people with asthma are sensitive to aspirin and taking tablets can initiate an attack.

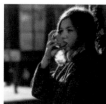
△ This picture shows a magnified image of flowering horse chestnut pollen. Pollen is a common trigger for attacks of allergic asthma.

MANAGEMENT OF ASTHMA
As yet, there is no cure for asthma. However, it can be managed extremely well with both drug therapy and by avoiding triggers – most people with asthma lead normal lives. In addition, many cases of childhood asthma become less of a problem with age and many cases disappear by the age of 20.

Doctors usually ask people with asthma to monitor their symptoms. Depending on the severity of your condition, you may be asked to perform self-assessment peak flow measurements every day in the morning and evening. This involves breathing into a peak-flow meter which measures the quantity of air you exhale per minute. Plotting these measurements on a graph helps to show whether you are on the correct dose of drugs and how effectively your asthma is controlled.

Almost all asthma drugs are inhaled in aerosolized form so that they are taken directly into the lungs where they can act instantly. A spacer device is used to make inhaling drugs easier for children.

There are two main kinds of inhalers – those that relieve an asthma attack and those that prevent future attacks:
- Reliever inhalers – These are normally blue in colour and contain drugs called bronchodilators, which widen the airways. They provide short-term relief for up to four hours.
- Preventer inhalers – These are usually low-dose corticosteroid devices and are normally brown in colour. They are used twice a day on a regular basis and have a protective effect upon the lungs by reducing any inflammation and the production of mucus.

Corticosteroids may also be prescribed as tablets, usually to relieve severe attacks or for people with long-term severe asthma.

SEVERE ASTHMA ATTACKS
A severe asthma attack can result in respiratory failure and coma. More than 5000 people a year in the US and nearly 2000 a year in the UK die as a result of an asthma attack. Most of these deaths could be prevented if the severity of the attack had been recognized and treatment had been sought. If an asthma attack becomes severe, you will have some of the following symptoms:
- Silent wheezing because breathing is very shallow.
- Severe breathlessness.
- Blue lips, fingers and toes – due to a lack of oxygen.
- Pale, clammy skin.
- Exhaustion and confusion.

If your inhaler is not providing any relief, try to keep calm and call for an ambulance. Sit upright in the most comfortable position you can find but do not lie down. Try to slow your breathing, if possible, until medical help arrives.

LIVING WITH ASTHMA
If you have asthma, you should always carry your medication with you in case of an attack. You should avoid known triggers, such as smoky or polluted atmospheres or exposure to cold air, and should not keep furry pets if you are allergic to them. Smoking is known to make the condition worse and therefore is not advisable. It is also a good idea to exercise regularly since this improves lung capacity and makes breathing easier. You may have to take preventive medicine from an inhaler to make this possible; if in doubt, discuss this with your doctor. Swimming is a particularly good exercise for people with asthma, because of the humid environment, but in theory any sport is possible.

If you find that your asthma is worse when you are stressed, try relaxation techniques or a form of yoga to control levels of stress, which will in turn cut down the risk of an asthma attack.

△ Asthma drugs act quickly to widen the airways and relieve symptoms. People with asthma should always carry their inhalers with them so that they can deal with a serious attack.

▽ People with asthma monitor their own condition from an early age. This young girl is breathing into a peak-flow meter, to measure her rate of exhalation.

Signs and Symptoms boxes
These blue boxes let you see the main symptoms of a condition at one quick glance, without having to hunt through the main text.

Full-colour artworks
Specially commissioned, fully annotated artworks are featured throughout the book, giving vital additional information.

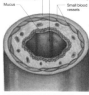
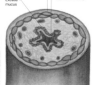

Information boxes
Beige-coloured boxes are there to provide all kinds of fascinating information, from prevention tips to related conditions.

HEALTHY LIVING

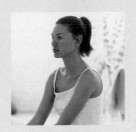

It is important to think carefully about lifestyle choices and their effect on your health. And it is never too late to take stock and discover how healthy (or unhealthy) your lifestyle really is. You can influence many areas of your life – and therefore health – whether in terms of dealing with stress more effectively, eating a more balanced diet, including more exercise in your daily routine or checking your alcohol consumption. A completely new lifestyle is not always necessary because small changes can be highly beneficial and gradual healthy choices are more likely to become an integral part of your life and so help you live more healthily for longer.

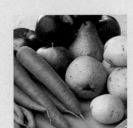

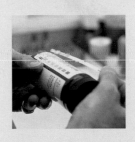

CONTENTS

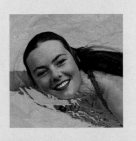

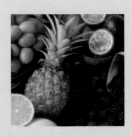

A healthy lifestyle

Your health is something that you can influence – for better or for worse – through the lifestyle choices you make every day. People today are generally much better informed than their parents' generation and the expectations of what medicine can do is also higher. It is possible to make small changes to the way you live which will lead to a healthier and longer life. Simple, realistic changes are by far the best – drastic measures usually prove difficult to sustain and tend to be followed for only a short time. Healthy choices are those that you make for life.

In the 21st century more people are living for longer – in fact, most of the world's population is living 20 years longer than their parents. What's the secret? Today, we have access to better food, sanitation and healthcare services.

CHANCE AND CHOICE FACTORS

Having a healthy lifestyle comes down to two factors – chance and choice. The chance factors are those you cannot change, such as your genetic make-up, which may protect you from or predispose you to illness throughout your life. But, if you find out

▽ Being self-aware means that you will notice abnormal symptoms earlier and so can alert your doctor to possible problems.

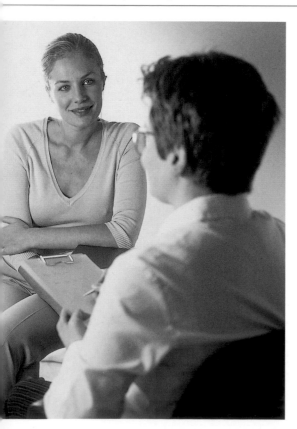

▷ Spending time doing things you enjoy can be invaluable to both your physical and your mental health. Gardening can be an active pursuit while giving your mind something to focus on during any stressful times.

that you are more likely to develop a condition, you can take positive steps to help you prevent the situation from arising. The choice factors are being aware of the foods you eat, whether you drink alcohol (and to what extent), whether you smoke, how much exercise you take and how you deal with day-to-day stress.

IT'S ALL IN THE BALANCE

As with most things in life, having a healthy lifestyle is all about a balanced approach. Occasional overindulgence won't, on the whole, damage your health irreparably but your body will need time to recover afterwards and some tender loving care.

Making changes to your life, say from having a cooked breakfast every morning to eating a bowl of yoghurt and muesli, can be a positive healthy choice but it's unlikely to be sustained if you just switch in one go. Start off with a change that you are more likely to sustain, such as switching half of your breakfasts to the more healthy option and then perhaps eventually just keep fried breakfasts for a weekend treat.

The same goes for exercise. It is a matter of deciding which activities you enjoy and which will fit in to your daily routine. The key is to increase the amount of exercise you do gradually. Whether it's a brisk 20-minute walk in the fresh air or a session at the gym, both will be beneficial to your heart, muscles, bones and lungs.

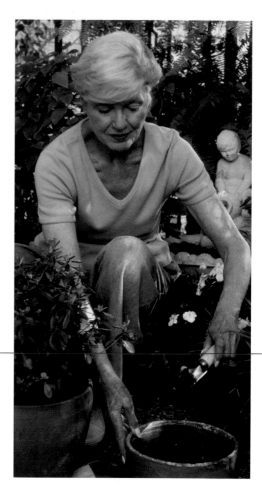

SELF-AWARENESS

Your doctor relies on information provided by you to diagnose a problem. So, make an effort to note what is normal for you on a regular basis – this could relate to functions such as eyesight and bowel movements, or the appearance of the skin, breasts and testicles for example. This means that you are much more likely to notice something out of the ordinary, which means you can mention it to your doctor at an earlier stage so that it can be treated more effectively.

START THEM OFF YOUNG

Healthy habits are best started in childhood because most bad habits are picked up then, too. If you have children, then one of the most effective ways to influence them is to lead by example – it won't do any harm to have a few hours in front of the television if it is balanced by something more active earlier or later in the day. But bad habits can soon become part of your child's normal life and changing these habits will become much more difficult later on.

Education on health-damaging habits, such as smoking, can also begin at a very early age and probably has the best effect when your children can see plainly that you yourself, for example, don't smoke.

Positive health influences can take many different forms, from promoting a healthy diet to making an effort to organize family-group activities on a regular basis. Bike rides or walks to the woods, for example, that allow you to spend time together as a family, will set a pattern for later in life.

▽ Involving children from an early age in fun and energetic activities can help to set the pattern for a healthy and active adult life.

POSITIVE THINKING

Keeping our lives happy and harmonious can very often be difficult and studies have shown that positive thinking can help us to deal more effectively with everyday stress as well as having a beneficial effect on our emotional health. Research has also demonstrated that a person's emotional wellbeing plays an important part in his or her physical health. It can be enormously beneficial, psychologically and physically, to make an effort to integrate positive thinking into every aspect of your life. You will reap the health rewards if you follow a few basic guidelines:

• Consider that it is often much easier to be negative and critical so make an effort to be positive and encouraging to yourself and to others.
• Keep crises in perspective and if possible try to see them simply as problems that you can solve.
• Focus on the good things in your life.
• When faced with a situation that you find stressful, try calming strategies such as taking deep breaths or visualizing tranquil scenes or images.

HEALTH SCREENING

Your doctor now has access to an ever-increasing array of sophisticated screening checks that can often detect potential diseases and conditions many years before they become apparent. By picking up such problems at an early stage, doctors hope that medical interventions will prevent disease progression or at least lead to more successful treatments.

▽ High blood pressure usually has no obvious symptoms so routine checks are vital to detect this condition.

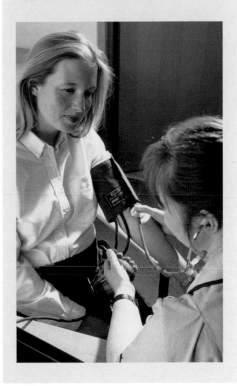

INFORMATION IS POWER

Health information has never before been so comprehensive and accessible, although some sources are not especially accurate or reliable. If your doctor suspects a particular condition, find out all you can about it by searching the Internet or by visiting your local library; there are plenty of patient groups and foundations for particular conditions, so you are very likely to find the facts you need. The more information you have the easier it will be to make decisions with your doctor about your healthcare. You will feel more confident and better able to ask questions, too.

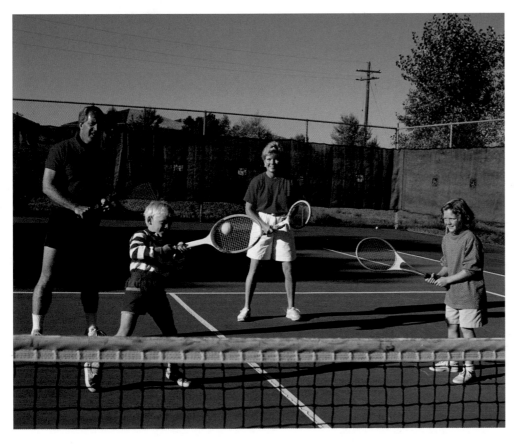

Learn to manage stress

SEE ALSO

➤ Exercise for life, p18

➤ Heart disease, p34

➤ Anxiety, p94

➤ Depression, p98

➤ Asthma, p130

Our lives seem to become increasingly stressful. We work harder than ever and our personal lives have become more complex. Family and community support systems are often not so readily available. So, stress is a major factor in most people's lives. Some stress may be beneficial: many people need a certain level of stress to perform at their best. It is when stress becomes excessive and unmanageable, with no apparent resolution, that problems start to arise. This is why it is very important to be able to recognize stress and know how to manage it.

SIGNS AND SYMPTOMS

Psychological symptoms of stress include:

➤ Mood fluctuations.

➤ Depression.

➤ Anxiety.

➤ Difficulty sleeping.

➤ Poor mental performance – difficulty concentrating and forgetfulness.

➤ Relationship problems.

Physical symptoms of stress include:

➤ Stomach acidity.

➤ Changing bowel habit, alternating bouts of diarrhoea and constipation.

➤ Breathing problems.

➤ Asthma.

➤ Palpitations.

➤ Migraines.

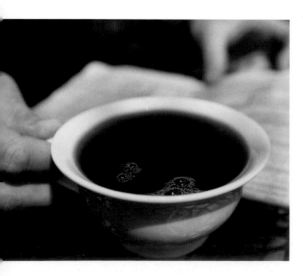

◁ Caffeine-containing drinks, such as coffee and hot chocolate, are useful stimulants but can also contribute to anxiety and insomnia.

It is usually possible to recognize when levels of stress become unmanageably high. Stress tends to manifest itself in either psychological or physical symptoms, but sometimes as both.

HOW TO DEAL WITH STRESS

As soon as you begin to feel that things are getting on top of you and your health is starting to suffer, try any or all of these approaches, first to identify, and then to deal with, stress in your everyday life.

• Work at identifying sources of stress in your life and consider whether or not you can make any changes that will leave you in greater overall control.

• Learn to manage your time better. Many people's stress is due to an overwhelming workload. To make work more manageable, write a list of goals for the day and list them in order of priority. Ticking off tasks as you complete them gives you a sense of achievement.

• Breathe deeply. A very effective and easy way to relieve stress is to focus on your breathing and make your breaths progressively deeper.

• A number of illicit drugs worsen feelings of stress and anxiety, including crack, cocaine and ecstasy.

• Look after your health. Eat healthily and drink alcohol and caffeine in moderation. By maintaining good overall health you reduce your tendency to illness and increase your ability to cope with whatever life throws at you.

• Try to avoid substances that might increase anxiety. A few cups of strong black coffee may wake you up in the morning but caffeine can increase levels of anxiety, especially in people already suffering from the effects of stress.

• Get into the exercise habit. Regular exercise helps to mobilize and utilize excessive amounts of adrenaline (caused by stress) and so helps to calm you down.

• Try to include some positive relaxation techniques on a daily basis. There is a range of alternative therapies that are all effective methods of relaxing and so reducing anxiety levels. These include yoga, massage, shiatsu, aromatherapy, reflexology and acupuncture.

WHAT IS YOUR STRESS SCORE?

Many life events can be a major source of stress; even when an event is a wholly desirable one, such as a wedding or house move. Read through the following stress "ratings" to see how they are linked to various major and minor life events. This will help you to focus on the factors that may be causing stress in your life and to establish if you can make any changes to alleviate the problem.

• Very high stress – Death of a spouse; divorce or marital separation; loss of job; house move; personal injury or illness.

• High stress – Retirement; pregnancy; change of job; death of close friend; serious family illness.

• Moderate stress – Large debts such as mortgage; trouble with parents-in-law; spouse starting or stopping work; trouble with boss; legal proceedings over debt.

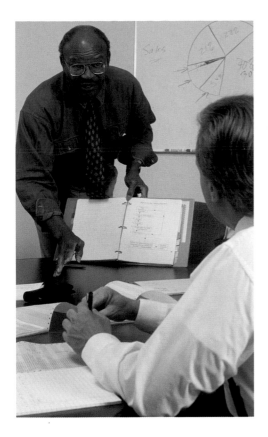

△ You will tackle challenges at work much more effectively if you have seven to eight hours of good-quality sleep every night. Arriving at work feeling refreshed means higher energy levels to handle stress.

• Low stress – Change in work conditions; change in schools; change in eating habits; small mortgage or debts; Christmas or other family holidays.

GET A GOOD NIGHT'S SLEEP

We spend approximately one-third of our lives asleep but many of the elements of this fundamental biological process – exactly why we sleep and how our bodies know when to sleep – still elude sleep science researchers.

An adequate period of sleep is necessary to allow the body and mind to rest properly and what is adequate will vary from person to person. Making sure that you have enough sleep is vital in terms of stress management so it is perhaps surprising then that many people do not allow themselves adequate periods of sleep.

An increasingly complex lifestyle that means you are continually struggling to deal with competing demands may lead you to feel that you cannot allow time for the luxury of a good night's sleep. But studies have shown that long-term sleep deprivation will eventually predispose a person to a range of physical and psychological problems.

PROBLEMS SLEEPING

If you are having difficulty sleeping or feel that you have poor-quality sleep, it may well be helpful to discuss the situation with your doctor. If you have already tried some of the self-help suggestions then it may be that you need a mild hypnotic drug to help you to re-establish a sleep pattern.

Overtiredness is a leading cause of reduced productivity at work as well as being a major cause of road accidents. Insomnia may also be a manifestation of anxiety and/or depression, both of which require specific treatment.

▽ Try to make a relaxation session part of your daily routine. Even if you have only 10 or 15 minutes to spare each day, you will benefit greatly from the calming influence of any relaxation technique.

SELF-HELP FOR A GOOD NIGHT'S SLEEP

If you have problems sleeping or feel that you don't get enough sleep, try out the following suggestions.

➤ Don't eat heavy meals late at night.

➤ Avoid caffeine-containing drinks late at night – remember that traditional bedtime drinks such as cocoa and hot chocolate contain caffeine.

➤ Don't drink too much alcohol.

➤ Tire yourself out physically by exercising during the day: physical activity has a calming effect on both mind and body. But, avoid exercising too late in the evening as it tends to be stimulating and keep you awake rather than promoting sleep.

➤ Practise meditation, yoga and/or relaxation exercises in the evening to create a relaxing mood, and a relaxing routine leading up to bedtime.

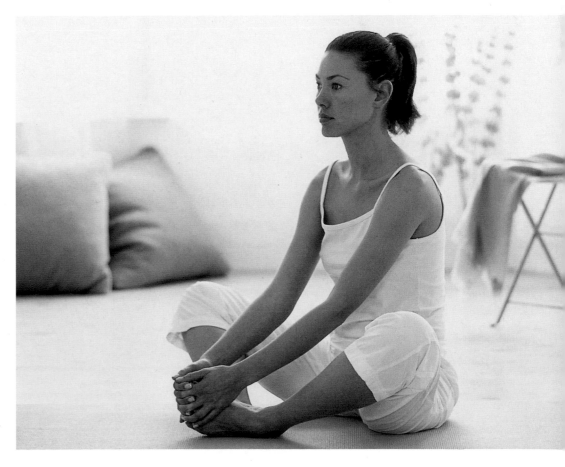

Eat healthily

SEE ALSO

➤ Atherosclerosis, p32

➤ Heart disease, p34

➤ Obesity, p48

➤ Coeliac disease, p56

➤ Anorectal disorders, p62

It may be a cliché to say "you are what you eat" but it is true. Your body requires a healthy combination of different foods and fluids in order to function properly and maintain good health. Balance is a key word in dietary matters. A healthy balanced diet comprises the three basic food types – protein, carbohydrate and fat – in the right proportions for optimum physical health. The foods your body needs will depend on how active your life is: if you have a demanding manual job your energy needs are higher than someone who works at a desk.

Eating patterns and diets vary around the world and studies have shown that this often bears a direct relation to the prevalence of certain diseases.

DIETS AROUND THE WORLD

The traditional British and American diets are often high in cholesterol and rich in calories. Such diets lead to an increase in obesity and heart disease. In contrast, a traditional Mediterranean diet, rich in fibre, olive oil, garlic, red wine and fish, lowers cholesterol and fat consumption. As a result, fewer people from Greece and Italy, for example, suffer from conditions such as obesity and heart disease.

The Japanese have always had a low incidence of heart disease because of the high quantities of fish that they eat. They also have low levels of colorectal cancer because their diet is generally high in fibre. These patterns are changing, however, because more Japanese people are adopting Western patterns of eating, and that includes higher fat consumption.

DIET-RELATED PROBLEMS

A range of digestive tract problems such as haemorrhoids, diverticular disease and constipation are related to the lack of fibre in Western diets.

Levels of obesity in the developed world are also increasing. Researchers believe this rise to be linked both to high levels of fat consumption and to diets that are increasingly rich in sugars.

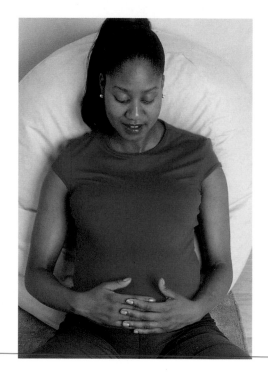

△ At certain times of life, such as during pregnancy, your body's demand for particular nutrients increases. Talk to your doctor about this to make sure you don't miss out.

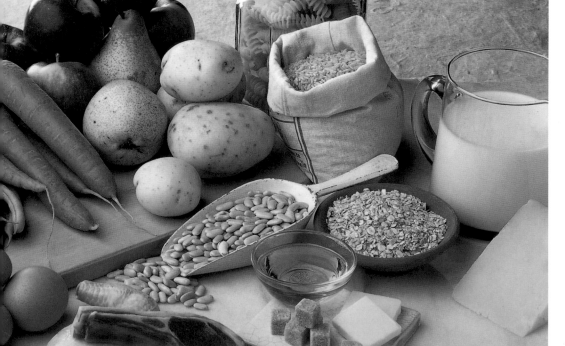

◁ It is important that you eat a variety of foods from the main food groups in order to provide your body with the balance of nutrients it needs to stay healthy.

THE RIGHT BALANCE

Try to ensure that you eat the correct combination of different food types every day. Current recommendations state that you should aim for:

➤ At least 40 per cent carbohydrate.

➤ About 30 per cent protein.

➤ No more than 30 per cent fat.

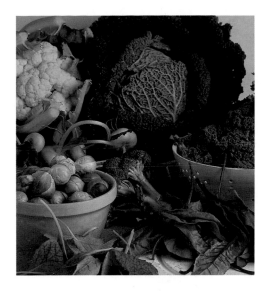

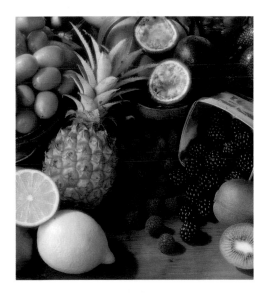

△ ▽ Fresh fruit and vegetables are a good source of carbohydrate (in the form of fibre), vitamins, minerals and natural sugars. To stay healthy aim for five portions of fruit and vegetables each day – this can include juices, dried fruit and tinned produce.

NOT JUST A COFFEE ISSUE
Caffeine is found in coffee, tea, hot chocolate, cocoa and a range of cola drinks, as well as in chocolate bars. Caffeine stimulates the brain and as a result is widely used to energize us in the morning and to help us stay awake at night if necessary. Too much caffeine, however, can irritate the digestive system and lead to a fast heart rate and raised blood pressure. Caffeine may also heighten feelings of anxiety and can be disruptive to sleep patterns.

WHAT IS A HEALTHY DIET?
A healthy diet needs to balance the consumption of the three basic nutrients – carbohydrate, protein and fat – and the micronutrients of minerals and vitamins. The healthiest diet relies heavily on sources of carbohydrate and protein and less on fat.

SOURCES OF CARBOHYDRATE
Carbohydrates – sugars and starches – are found abundantly in bread, potatoes, rice, cereals and pasta, most of which also provide rich sources of fibre. Wholegrain and unprocessed foods such as wholemeal pasta, brown rice and brown bread provide the healthiest carbohydrate sources but normal pasta, white rice and white bread also contain carbohydrate.

SOURCES OF PROTEIN
Meat and fish provide a rich source of protein and readily available energy. Furthermore, white meat from chicken and turkey contains a much lower proportion of fat than red meats such as beef and lamb. Eggs, fruits, nuts, beans, peas and lentils are sources of protein, and are particularly important foods for people following vegetarian and vegan diets.

SOURCES OF FAT
Fats are an important source of energy and supply the basic building blocks for your body's cells as well as helping you absorb certain vitamins. But the balance is important because too much fat, especially too much saturated fat, can lead to various health problems.

Try to choose most of your fat intake from the healthier unsaturated fats. These fats are believed to provide some protection against heart disease whereas saturated fats promote the clogging up of arteries in the body (atherosclerosis).

High levels of saturated fat are found in red meat, butter, some cheeses, some ice-creams and many biscuits, cakes and chocolate bars. Milk and dairy products can be high in fat but do supply rich sources of vitamins and minerals.

DEGREES OF SATURATION
The fats or oils you choose when cooking count in your fat consumption. Choose those from the unsaturated fats wherever possible to keep your intake of saturated fats to a minimum.

➤ Polyunsaturated fats:

Safflower oil.

Sunflower oil.

Corn oil.

➤ Monounsaturated fats:

Peanut oil.

Olive oil.

➤ Saturated fats:

Butter.

Coconut oil.

VITAMINS AND MINERALS
These micronutrients are found in abundance in fresh fruit and vegetables, nuts, beans, wholegrains, meat and fish. Most people can obtain enough vitamins and minerals from their diet and don't need to take daily supplements. (Although if you prefer to take a multivitamin then make sure it's a balanced one.) However, at certain times, such as during pregnancy or when breastfeeding, a person needs a higher supply of micronutrients, as do those with certain illnesses, such as the digestive condition coeliac disease.

▽ Choose your cooking oils wisely to increase the healthiness of a meal.

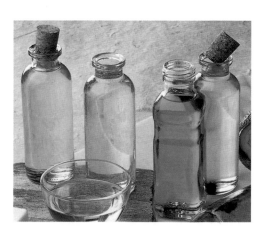

Weight control

A healthy weight is one where you are not too thin (light) or too fat (heavy) for your height. Being overweight or obese puts your health at risk, but so does being underweight. A healthy weight is one that you can maintain throughout life; fluctuating weight levels push up your risk of disease. Since the 1950s, increasing affluence, poor eating habits and more sedentary lifestyles have meant that obesity has become much more common in developed countries. Obesity affects both men and women, and recently is increasingly apparent among children.

Healthcare professionals use a particular method of working out whether a person is a healthy weight for his or her height. This method is known as the body mass index or BMI. The values differ for men and women but the calculation is exactly the same.

WORK OUT YOUR BMI

BMI = your weight in kilograms divided by (your height in metres) squared. (To convert your weight from pounds to kilograms multiply by 0.4536; to convert your height from feet to metres multiply by 0.3048.)

For example, Nikki weighs 65 kg and is 1.64 metres tall, so her BMI is
$65 \div (1.64)^2 = 24.17$

A healthy weight/height balance should give a BMI of between 18.5 and 25. If your BMI is under 18.5 then you are underweight. If your BMI is over 25 then you are overweight and if it exceeds 30 you are obese. However, some people feel more comfortable at a higher weight while others feel healthier carrying less weight around.

ARE YOU A HEALTHY WEIGHT?

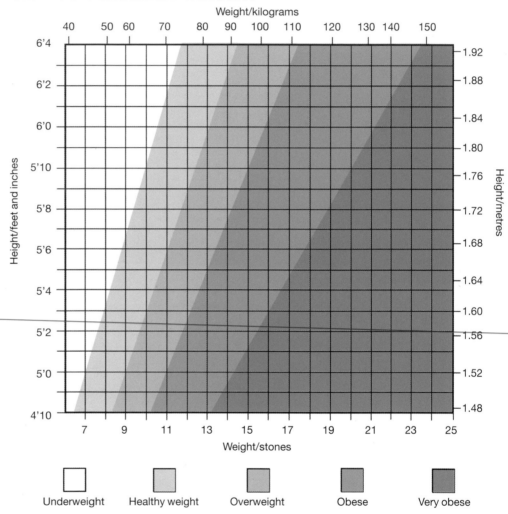

Underweight Healthy weight Overweight Obese Very obese

△ This chart shows at a glance whether your weight is healthy or unhealthy for your height. How does your weight score?

WEIGHTY ISSUES

Being overweight puts you at risk; obese people are more likely to suffer from:

➤ Heart disease.

➤ Stroke.

➤ Diabetes.

➤ Musculoskeletal problems, such as osteoarthritis.

WHAT ABOUT BODY FAT?

Sometimes the BMI reading alone is misleading and you may have to undergo a body fat measurement and waist–height ratio before your doctor decides if your weight is putting your health at risk.

Doctors also use waist size as another useful measurement of obesity and health risk. So whether you're an "apple" or a "pear" shape affects your heart's health. Fat around the waist indicates an increased risk of heart problems. A waist measurement of more than 89 cm (35 in) in women and 102 cm (40 in) in men indicates such a risk.

Although obesity is usually obvious, weightlifters or body builders, for example, have high BMIs but may well have a low proportion of body fat, which means that the risk of cardiovascular problems is low.

BURN CALORIES THROUGH EXERCISE

Exercise helps to use up calories and promote a higher level of health. If you are not used to exercising, simply taking a long, brisk walk two or three times a week will provide some benefit. But if you are able and motivated to exercise at a higher and more strenuous level, activities such as running, cycling and swimming are more effective at helping you to shed those unwanted pounds.

LOSING WEIGHT

If you have decided that you are overweight and wish to lose weight there are a number of important factors to consider:
• There are no short-term solutions.
• A short, sharp, shock diet is invariably followed by a gradual return to previous weight levels.
• Rapid weight loss is unhealthy.

It is probably a good idea to start out by assessing your diet and identifying high-fat and high-sugar foods that you eat. Try to calculate how many calories, on average, you usually consume; bear in mind that alcohol is high in calories – how often do you drink alcohol? If you do not eat much fat, you need to reduce your overall calorie intake or to increase your energy expenditure or both.

The recommended daily intake of calories is 2000 for women and 2500 for men but if you are unsure and want to discuss your requirements further visit your doctor or dietitian for advice.

APPORTIONING YOUR CALORIES

To achieve a steady, healthy weight loss, you should aim to reduce your daily intake of calories by about 600. For most women, this means a daily intake of between 1200 and 1500 kcal while the figure for men stands at about 1750–1950 kcal.

So that you never go hungry, try to spread your allowance throughout the day. Eating smaller meals more frequently will help to maintain steady blood sugar levels and make you less likely to feel the urge to binge on unhealthy foods.

MAKE A PLAN AND STICK TO IT

Follow this advice for a successful weight-loss programme.
• Set realistic and achievable goals.
• Alter your diet with a view to maintaining any changes for life.
• Reduce your consumption of high-calorie foods, such as fried foods, red meats, cakes, chocolates and sweets, cheese and dairy products.
• Cut down your consumption of alcohol and fizzy drinks.
• Choose low-calorie foods such as fruits, vegetables and lean meats.
• Drink 1.5 litres (2½ pints) of water a day;

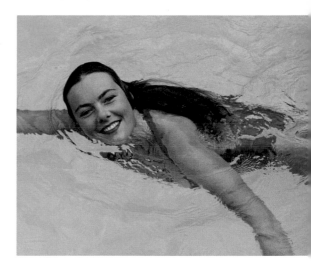

△ Swimming at least 20 lengths at your local pool can raise your metabolism, burn extra calories and help you to lose weight.

a good fluid balance improves health in general and assists the metabolic changes necessary to lose weight.

FIGHT MIDDLE-AGE SPREAD

Putting on weight as you get older is not inevitable. Although your body's metabolic rate slows down with age, the effect is modest. The best way to prevent weight gain during life is to remain physically active. Most people's middle-age spread is the result of becoming more sedentary but eating more or less as they did when they were active. This excess energy intake is stored in the body as fat.

▽ Your waist measurement can help your doctor to work out whether your weight is unhealthy for your height.

▽ If you are on a weight-loss diet check the scales once a week. Checking every day shows a negligible change and can be discouraging.

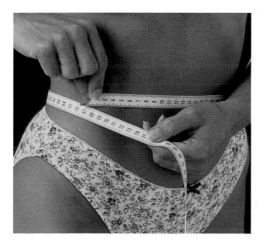

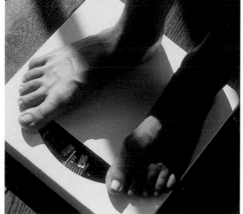

Exercise for life

Most people are aware that regular activity is a vital part of a healthy lifestyle. However, that doesn't make it any easier to find the energy and time for exercise in our busy lives. However, there are plenty of options for improving health besides a strenuous session at the gym and simply deciding to walk to work can have significant health benefits. Studies have shown that increasing levels of physical activity on a day-to-day basis is the key to long-term health. So, take a new look at how you can build activities into your life every day.

The amount of exercise that people take during their lives has dropped significantly over the past 50 years or so. An increasingly mechanized, automated and computerized world has reduced the amount of walking and heavy work that most of us need to do. There is therefore a greater potential role for regular physical activity, which should ideally be encouraged from a young age.

HEALTH BENEFITS OF EXERCISE

It's never too late to become more active. Just look at the many health benefits:

• Cardiovascular – Exercise that speeds up the rate of the heart and is taken for at least 30 minutes, three or more times per week, is an effective way of promoting cardiovascular health. Such exercise – known as aerobic exercise – strengthens the heart muscle so that it becomes more efficient at pumping blood around the body. As a result your heart rate (or pulse) slows down, showing that you are becoming fitter. Regular cardiovascular workouts also improve circulation, lower blood pressure and reduce blood cholesterol levels.

• Respiratory – People with lung conditions such as asthma and chronic obstructive lung disease often find that doing exercise that makes them slightly out of breath helps to improve their lung capacity and breathing patterns.

• Musculoskeletal – Regular exercise will help to keep muscles, tendons and ligaments strong and supple, reducing the tendency to problems such as lower back pain, particularly later in life. Building strong muscles requires working against a resistance, which is often provided by weights. Strength-building exercises also serve to stabilize joints and reduce the effects of diseases such as rheumatoid arthritis. Weight-bearing exercises, such as walking, dancing or skipping, can build strong bones and help to counteract the natural tendency of the bones to thin with age – a condition known as osteoporosis.

• Psychological – People who are active or exercise regularly enjoy a strong feel-good factor. Exercise also helps to relieve stress, channel aggression, lift depression and promote good sleep.

> **GET THE GO-AHEAD FROM YOUR DOCTOR**
>
> If you haven't exercised for some time or are starting a new sporting pursuit then it is a good idea to visit your doctor. He or she can give advice on exercise intensity, assess your current fitness level and discuss the implication of any conditions you may have. In this way, you and your doctor can agree a safe but effective plan of action for exercising regularly.

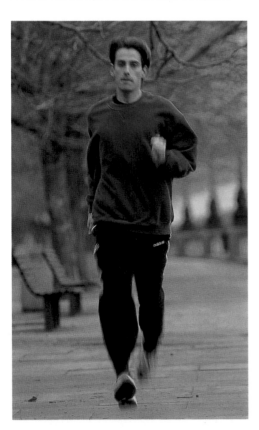

▽ Within four weeks of starting regular aerobic exercise, your heart and lungs will not need to work as hard so you will feel more energized.

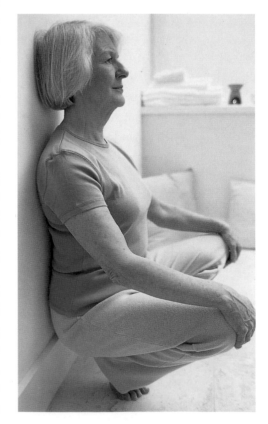

▽ Take time at the end of a workout to relax and stretch muscles. Cooling your body down in this way helps you to stay injury free.

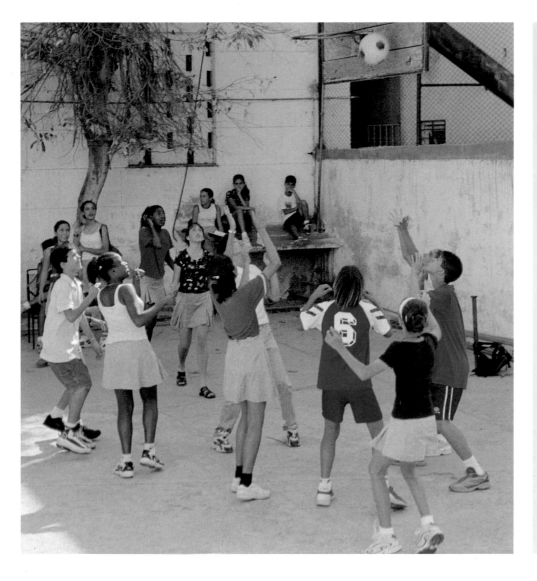

△ Taking part in team sports and games from an early age will help to develop physical and social skills that will be beneficial in adult life.

- Social – Many people enjoy playing as part of a team or in competitions. Such team activity expands your circle of friends and encourages feelings of mutual respect and shared responsibility while learning new skills.

WHICH ACTIVITY TO CHOOSE

This, of course, is a wholly personal choice. Some people naturally gravitate towards strenuous activities and thrive, while others never feel the need or desire to undertake such vigorous exercise.

The most important point to bear in mind is to choose an activity that you enjoy and is fun. Try to make time for regular periods of exercise (about three to five times a week). If you are not the gym-going type or running does not appeal to you, what about taking long walks, dancing or yoga?

As with all exercise and activity, it is important to have the proper equipment and any special training beforehand.

FITNESS PLANNING

When planning a structured exercise programme consider the following:

➤ Frequency – How often can you exercise?

➤ Intensity – How energetic do you want to be?

➤ Time – How long can you put aside for each exercise session?

➤ Type – What sort of activities do you enjoy doing?

WARM UP AND COOL DOWN

It can be easy to overexert yourself or pull a muscle when you start exercising so make sure that any bouts of activity are preceded by ten minutes or so of gentle "warm-up" exercises and stretches. Marching on the spot or cycling can raise your heart rate and the temperature of your muscles. Such aerobic activity should always be followed by some "cool-down" stretching exercises for the muscles and joints.

Never stop exercising so suddenly that you go straight from intense levels of activity to a complete standstill. Gradually step down the level of effort you put in towards the end of your session and then spend approximately 15 minutes stretching all the muscles you have worked. As well as improving your flexibility, such stretching will help reduce any stiffness in your muscles the next day.

Smoking and your health

In the Western world, almost 20 per cent of deaths are related to smoking. But despite such statistics, people continue to smoke and put their health at risk, mainly because they become addicted to the effects of nicotine in tobacco. This addiction puts the smoker in a vicious cycle or feeding his or her cravings. To be able to give up this disease-inducing habit, you must be motivated to do so and have a lot of willpower. Your doctor can discuss other strategies that can help you quit – it could well be the best health decision you ever make.

SMOKING HEALTH RISKS

There is overwhelming evidence to prove that smoking causes or is a contributory factor for a range of diseases, such as:

➤ Asthma.

➤ Bladder cancer.

➤ Chronic obstructive lung disease.

➤ Colorectal cancer.

➤ Excessive ageing of the skin.

➤ Heart disease.

➤ Lung cancer.

➤ Oesophageal cancer.

➤ Peptic ulcers.

➤ Stomach cancer.

➤ Stroke.

➤ Throat cancer.

Scientific studies have shown that smoking has various and wide-ranging effects (almost all harmful) on your body. There is also evidence that passive smoking increases the risk of disease.

SMOKE DAMAGE

• Cardiovascular system – Smoking encourages the development of atheroma, or fatty plaques, inside arteries around your body. Such furring up of arteries greatly increases the risk of heart attack and stroke. Smoking raises blood pressure and, by stimulating adrenaline production, it can cause disturbances to heart rhythms (arrhythmias). Smokers are more likely to develop clots in a blood vessel (thrombosis), which could prove fatal if part of the clot breaks off and travels to the lungs or the brain. Anyone who has smoking-induced lung disease will go on to develop smoking-related heart disease.

• Respiratory system – Toxic substances in cigarette smoke directly damage the protective linings of both the upper and the lower respiratory tracts. This makes it much easier for germs to invade and cause a respiratory tract infection, and it also increases the chances of developing asthma. Long-term smokers risk destroying their lungs, a condition known as chronic obstructive pulmonary disease. Smoking is the direct cause of 80 per cent of all cases of lung cancer.

• Digestive system – Nicotine acts on the digestive system in various ways via the bloodstream and by targeting the nerves supplying the digestive tract. Smoking promotes cancers of the oesophagus, stomach and colon/rectum. It also causes inflammation of the stomach and ulceration of its lining.

• Urinary system – Carcinogenic (cancer-causing) chemicals from inhaled tobacco smoke travel from the lungs in the bloodstream and promote cancer in other organs such as the bladder.

• Ears, nose and throat – The hundreds of harmful chemicals in tobacco smoke contribute to most cases of throat and laryngeal cancer.

• Skin – Smoking prematurely ages skin because, among other adverse effects, it is known to block blood vessels and limits the oxygen the skin needs to stay healthy.

• Pregnancy – Smoking is dangerous during pregnancy because the baby will be much smaller and its chances of survival are decreased. Children with parents who are smokers are more likely to suffer from asthma.

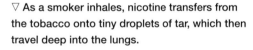

▽ As a smoker inhales, nicotine transfers from the tobacco onto tiny droplets of tar, which then travel deep into the lungs.

▽ This microscopic view of tissue taken from the lungs of a heavy smoker shows tar deposits clearly as black areas.

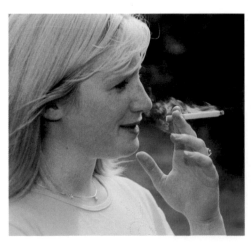

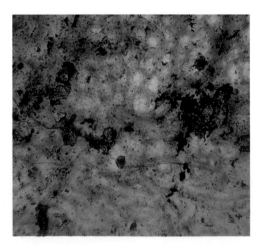

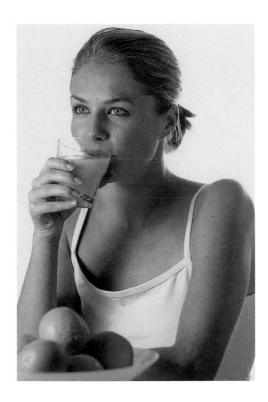

△ Orange juice accelerates the loss of nicotine from your body, which can help you fight your addiction more quickly.

PLAN TO GIVE UP

Once you have decided that you want to stop smoking, make a plan and tell people that you are going to stop and ask for their support. Try some of the following tips on quitting smoking for good.

- Make a list of all the health benefits of giving up and stick it to the fridge or in another prominent place.
- Keep low-calorie snacks to hand to snack on when you get the urge to smoke.
- Start your day off with a glass of freshly squeezed orange juice. Not only does it taste great, it also speeds removal of nicotine from your body.
- Make a note of how much money you save each week by not smoking and then work out how much money you will save over the next year.
- Cut down on caffeine. Some research shows that caffeine can make nicotine cravings worse so reduce the amount of tea or coffee you drink.
- Avoid bars and alcohol for a while. Many people want a cigarette when they have a drink and so the association between the two is often strong.
- Use your willpower to avoid giving in to temptation. Having a few puffs on a cigarette will just weaken your resolve so do not be tempted. If you do succumb, do not despair – many ex-smokers were successful only on their second or third time around.

ADVICE FROM YOUR DOCTOR

From time to time your motivation and willpower will need an extra boost so ask your doctor to provide you with details of any reputable, specialist clinics or self-help groups that are available in your area. It is often useful to talk to other people about what they have found helpful.

One of the most effective strategies against nicotine addiction is to adopt a three-pronged attack:

- Nicotine substitution – Whether as patches or chewing gum, using nicotine substitution therapy for a few months may help to break the ritual habit of smoking while at the same time gradually reducing the body's dependence on this powerful chemical.
- Medication – Drugs are now available to help to reduce nicotine dependency. These drugs need to be taken under medical supervision over a period of several months and so far have shown encouraging results.
- Complementary treatments – Some therapies, such as acupuncture and hypnotherapy, help people stop smoking. Many therapists offer a money-back guarantee if you start smoking again. Be sure to visit qualified professionals.

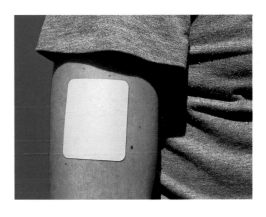

△ Nicotine patches deliver a continuous low dose of nicotine to the body. Some people find these helpful in the battle against smoking.

▽ Acupuncture – the placing of fine needles in specific "meridians" of the body – has helped many people to give up smoking.

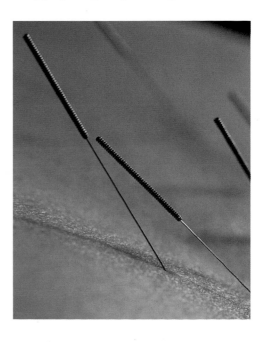

Sensible drinking

Alcohol is enjoyed by people around the world at all kinds of celebration and social occasion. It has a relaxing effect and complements the taste of many foods, but it can also cause considerable physical and psychological ill-health. A moderate intake of alcohol may protect against heart disease, but excessive binge drinking or sustained high intakes of alcohol can damage the liver irreparably and reduces life expectancy. Alcohol abuse and dependency can also cause or lead to serious physical, psychological and social problems.

When you drink alcohol, a small amount is absorbed in the stomach but the majority slips into your bloodstream via the small intestine. From here it goes to the liver, whose role it is to detoxify the blood and break down most of the alcohol. Excess alcohol then travels around the body, affecting different organs in various ways.

SHORT-TERM EFFECTS

Initially, alcohol depresses your central nervous system, leading to feelings of well-being and confidence and impaired judgement and thought processes. Your skin becomes redder as alcohol causes blood vessels in the skin to dilate. Alcohol also has a diuretic effect and so increases urine production, leaving you dehydrated.

Heavier drinking may result in further effects on the nervous system, which include slurred speech, memory loss, lack of coordination and control of your body's movements, and aggressive and antisocial behaviour patterns.

IN THE LONG TERM

When alcohol is drunk in excess over long periods, there are a number of detrimental side-effects and social consequences. The physical effects are:
• Liver damage.
• Heart muscle damage.
• Impotence.
• Reduced fertility.
• Brain damage.
• Increased risk of cancers of the mouth, throat and oesophagus.
• Pancreatitis, a condition where the pancreas becomes inflamed.

WHY SOME PEOPLE CAN'T TOLERATE ALCOHOL
Some people seem to be quite incapable of metabolizing alcohol and for such people alcohol can be a very dangerous substance. Even very small amounts of alcohol result in rapid drunkenness and may precipitate collapse. This problem arises when enzyme systems within the digestive system are incapable of breaking down and detoxifying alcohol. Such enzyme deficiencies are more common among Asian populations.

As well as damaging your physical health, alcoholism has far-reaching psychosocial consequences, including:
• Loss of employment.
• Family and marital breakdown.
• Loss of friends.

BENEFITS OF DRINKING
Moderate alcohol consumption appears to have beneficial effects on the circulation and research has shown that it may even have protective effects on your heart. Scientists are studying different alcoholic drinks for their beneficial properties and it is believed that red wine might offer significant cardioprotective benefits.

WHAT'S IN AN ALCOHOL UNIT?
If you are planning to drive or operate machinery then any alcoholic drink, no matter how small, will affect your ability. Alcohol intake is measured in units. Current recommendations state that men should not drink more than 3–4 units a day

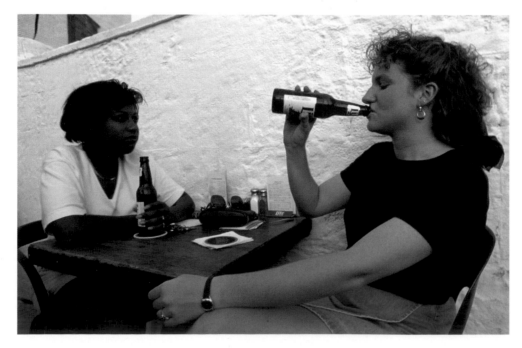

▽ Drinking with friends can help you to relax after a day at work, but it is always a good idea to stay within your limits.

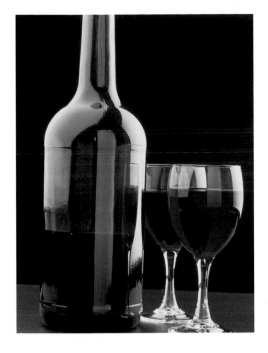

△ It is a good idea to be aware of the number of units you are drinking. For example, a small glass of wine counts as roughly one unit.

while for women the level is a maximum of 2–3 units. These recommendations were changed from weekly limits because there was a danger that people thought they could save up a week's worth of units and drink them all at the weekend.

One unit of alcohol is drunk in:
• Half a pint of beer (250 ml/8 fl oz).
• A small glass of wine (125 ml/4 fl oz).
• One measure of spirits (25 ml/⁴⁄₅ fl oz).

Beers, wine and spirits have very different strengths in terms of alcoholic content. Normal-strength beer, for example, may be 4 per cent alcohol whereas whisky is about 40 per cent; wine varies from 9 to 14 per cent (red wine is generally stronger than white wine).

ARE YOU DRINKING TOO MUCH ALCOHOL?

If you regularly drink more than the recommended safe limit of alcohol you could be putting your health at risk. Answer yes or no to the questions below (and be honest) to see if your drinking is affecting your lifestyle and whether it could soon become a habit that is controlling you.

1 Have you ever thought you should cut down on your drinking?
2 Have other people ever annoyed you by criticizing your drinking habits?
3 Have you ever felt guilty about your drinking?
4 Have you ever had an "eye opener" drink first thing in the morning?

If you said "yes" to two or more of the questions above, your drinking habits may be becoming problematic. Think about how you could reduce your alcohol consumption and perhaps make an appointment to visit your doctor for professional health advice.

WHEN DRINKING BECOMES A PROBLEM

Any of the following may indicate a potential problem with alcohol:
• Regular episodes of excessive consumption.
• Not being able to stop drinking once you have started.
• Days off work because of hangovers.
• Drinking in the morning.
• Not being able to remember what happened the previous night.
• Friends commenting on your drinking.
• Injury to yourself or someone else as a result of drinking alcohol.

WHERE TO GET HELP

Always consider consulting your doctor, who can help you assess the severity of your situation and consider appropriate strategies for dealing with the problem. Most countries have a range of specialist services available that can provide information, support and counselling. There are also centres that specialize in alcohol detoxification and rehabilitation. Certain drug treatments can also help people to stop drinking as well as reducing cravings for alcohol after stopping.

▽ Group therapy sessions at Alcoholics Anonymous have helped enormous numbers of people kick their addiction to alcohol.

METABOLIZING ALCOHOL

The rate at which alcohol is metabolized by the liver varies between individuals. It also depends on a person's weight, build, whether they are male or female and how regularly they drink alcohol (regular drinkers can metabolize it more quickly). On average, it takes 1 hour to eliminate 1 unit of alcohol from the body. But if you're having a heavy drinking session then your body can only deal with 1 unit per hour and so it takes a lot longer to metabolize the many units you've drunk during the evening. After a particularly drunken night out, you may still be intoxicated the next morning.

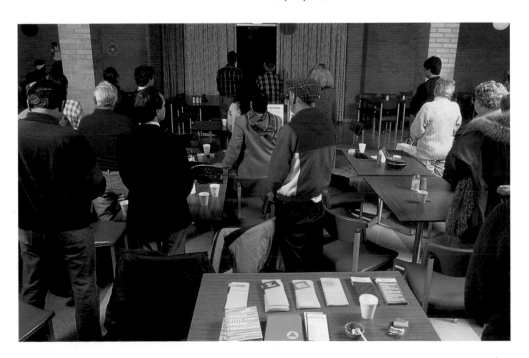

Routine health checks

There are a number of relatively simple interventions that can pick up potential medical problems before any symptoms or complications have developed. These are usually very simple tests that can be done or organized by your doctor. The number of these screening tests is gradually increasing. Many developed countries have national screening programmes for various types of cancer – breast cancer, cervical cancer, prostate cancer and colorectal cancer – while other vital checks monitor your hearing, sight, teeth, blood pressure and blood cholesterol.

Doctors now have a whole armoury of screening tests at their disposal to optimize their patients' health and to pick up any health problems as early as possible.

BLOOD PRESSURE MONITORING

Blood pressure rises gradually with age and this small increase is normal. Some people are more likely to develop high blood pressure as it may run in their family. High blood pressure increases the risk of several serious conditions but has no symptoms, which is why doctors often check your blood pressure as a matter of course. It is important that high blood pressure is picked up because most of the complications of this condition can be prevented by taking appropriate measures. This may involve lifestyle changes and/or taking regular medication.

It is recommended that you have your blood pressure checked on a regular basis, and ideally it should be checked by your doctor at least every two to three years from the age of 40 onwards.

BLOOD CHOLESTEROL TESTING

High levels of cholesterol have been linked to an increased risk of cardiovascular disease in general. A blood test measures cholesterol and other blood fats – what doctors refer to as your "lipid profile".

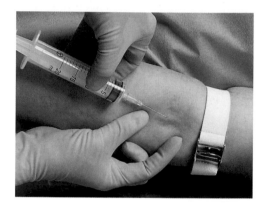

△ A sample of blood is taken from a vein in the arm. Several different tests can be carried out on one sample of blood.

Research has established healthy and "at risk" levels of blood cholesterol, but your age, blood pressure and whether or not you smoke must be taken into account. These levels are measured in millimoles per litre:
• More than 6.5 mmol/l means higher risk.
• Between 5.4 and 6.5 mmol/l means moderate risk.
• Less than 5.4 mmol/l means lower risk.

▽ In one test in the haematology laboratory blood is placed in a tiny tube in a centrifuge machine and spun at high speeds to separate the blood cells from the blood plasma.

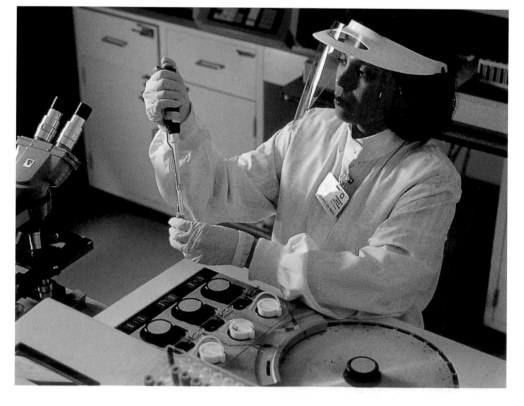

DENTAL CHECK-UPS

Regular trips to the dentist can help him or her spot the signs of gum disease early and give appropriate treatment. There may be some work needed, depending on how well you look after your teeth, to keep your oral hygiene to optimum standards. The gums are indicators of more general disease and your dentist may pick up early warning signs. Frequency of check-ups varies from dentist to dentist, but most recommend a six-monthly or annual check.

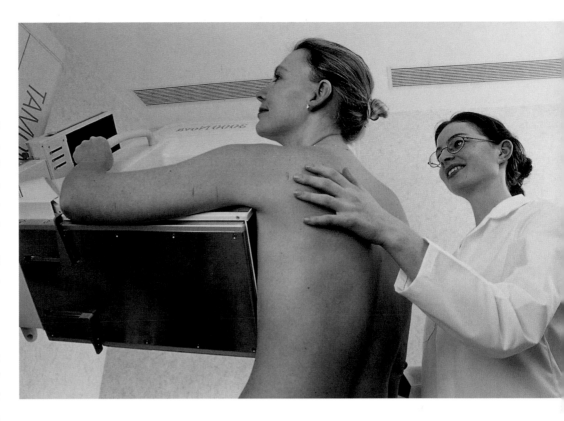

▷ Routine mammography screenings for breast cancer target older women, but many younger women also choose to be screened.

MAMMOGRAPHY

A mammogram is a simple X-ray of the breast to check for cancerous and precancerous tissue and hopefully catch the disease early on. It is routinely available in many developed countries for women between the ages of 50 and 65 and should be carried out every three to five years.

If your family has a history of breast cancer then routine screening from a much earlier age is very important.

CERVICAL SMEAR TESTS

A regular screening programme means that a cervical smear test can pick up on any cellular changes in the cervix so that further tests can be made and, if neccessary, treatment can begin before the development of cervical cancer.

A cervical smear test is a simple procedure that can take place at your doctor's surgery. The test will sometimes be done by your doctor but more often by the practice nurse. During an internal examination, a speculum is inserted in order to check the cervix. A spatula or small brush is then swept around the cervix to obtain a small sample of cervical cells. These samples are placed on a microscope slide and sent away to a hospital laboratory for analysis.

It is recommended that all women who are, or have been, sexually active have a smear test at least every three years.

PROSTATE TESTS

As a man ages, his prostate gland enlarges. In some men this is accompanied by cancerous changes. A blood test for prostate-specific antigen levels provides a non-specific indicator for prostate gland disease and the possibility of prostate cancer. This test is being increasingly used in men over the age of 50. It is hoped that this test will be done at regular and planned intervals in the future.

HEARING TESTS

Hearing becomes less acute with age. Over half of all people over the age of 70 have some degree of hearing loss, which is exacerbated when trying to hear above a background noise or music. Significant hearing loss may result in depression and loss of confidence.

It is not easy to monitor because it happens so gradually, but if you feel that you can't hear sounds well or clearly or if people have mentioned that you're not hearing what they say, ask your doctor to arrange a formal hearing test to see whether or not a hearing aid would correct the hearing deficiency.

EYESIGHT TESTS

It is normal for vision to diminish with age and this can often be corrected by an appropriate lens prescription for near and/or distant vision. As well as assessing your vision, ophthalmic practitioners can examine the eyes for evidence of cataracts and glaucoma, both of which become more common with age and which can be treated. Other diseases, such as diabetes or high blood pressure, can also be picked up because they affect your eyesight and your

optician may refer you to your doctor for further tests. It is a good idea to have a routine eye check once a year, even if you don't wear glasses, because you don't always notice deterioration in your eyesight.

DIABETES

Your doctor can carry out a quick test to check a sample of your urine for signs of diabetes. Where there is a strong family history of diabetes, tests may be carried out on a frequent basis.

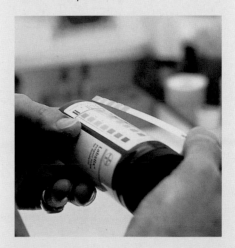

△ This simple dipstick test, to test urine for the presence of sugars, is over in under a minute or so.

Travel health and safety

Now that air travel is relatively inexpensive, more of us are travelling to exotic places. Whatever the destination, it is vital to know what precautions to take when travelling abroad – even for a two-week holiday. On the journey itself it is advisable to drink plenty of water, stretch your legs and avoid alcohol – to reduce the risk of deep vein thrombosis. Travel insurance comes high up the list of travel essentials, along with adequate planning in terms of prevention – via immunizations, malaria tablets and supplies of medicines.

PLANNING AHEAD

If you have a medical problem that requires attention from time to time, make sure you check out what medical facilities will be available at your destination. If you have a complex medical problem, visit your doctor or specialist so that they can write a medical summary for you to take with you.

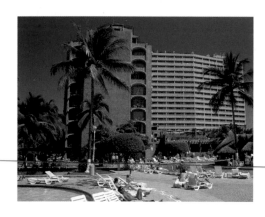

△ Even a short sun-and-sea package holiday will need some health preparation.

▽ Make sure you have sunscreen (minimum SPF15), and apply it often. Also remember that water intensifies the burning effects of the sun.

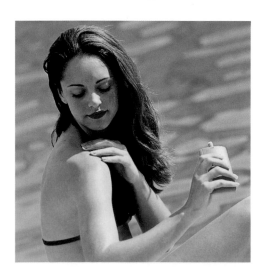

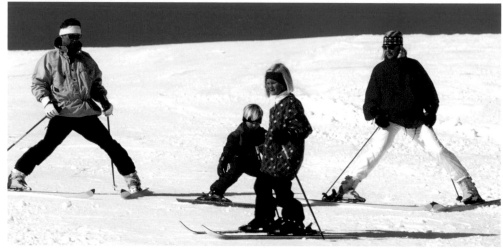

△ If you are going on a holiday that involves high-risk activities such as skiing, make sure that you have suitable medical cover.

ESSENTIAL COVER

It is essential to take out suitable travel insurance before any holiday. It is also a good idea to make sure that your insurance cover is appropriate to the activities that you intend to undertake on your holiday. So, bear this in mind if your holiday involves high-risk activities such as skiing, diving or hang-gliding.

STOCK UP ON MEDICINES

If you have to take medicines on a daily basis, make sure that you have more than enough to take away with you. It is a good idea to carry medication, stored in its original containers, in your hand luggage in case your suitcases go missing en route.

ARE YOU UP TO DATE?

A minimum of six weeks before you go on holiday, you should visit your doctor or practice nurse for advice on which immunizations are recommended or essential for your intended destination. It is also advisable to find out whether you need to take antimalarial tablets and if you do which of the many types available provide the right protection for your destination.

SAFE SEX

Many sexually transmitted infections are contracted on holidays or trips abroad. The best method of protection against such infections is using a condom. Be prepared and take a plentiful supply with you as they may not be quite so easy to come by once you are overseas.

AVOID STOMACH UPSETS

If there are any doubts about the safety of local water, drink bottled water and also use it for brushing your teeth and rinsing your mouth. In places where the water is unsafe it is a good idea to have drinks without ice and avoid foods that may have been washed in local water, such as salads, raw vegetables, shellfish and unpeeled fresh fruit.

THE HEART AND CIRCULATION

2

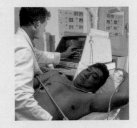

Your heart's beat is one of the most evocative sounds, symbolizing life itself. How you look after this amazing organ has great bearing on its health specifically and your health in general. Millions of people in the developed world suffer with disorders of the heart and circulation, many of which can be deadly. Because atherosclerosis and heart disease along with stroke are such major killers in the Western world, much medical research has already been done. Awareness of the major cardiovascular conditions, along with their symptoms, diagnosis, treatment and any preventative information, could help minimize your risk of such disorders.

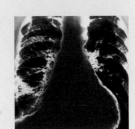

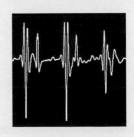

CONTENTS

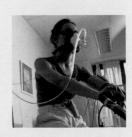

The cardiovascular system

Your heart and circulation are also known as the cardiovascular system (cardio means heart, vascular means blood vessels), and have developed to fulfil your body's constant need for oxygen and other nutrients dissolved in the blood. The driving force at the centre of this system is the heart, a powerful but simple pump. Every heartbeat pumps blood rich with oxygen and nutrients to every part of your body through a complex network of "pipes" – these are the blood vessels that carry the blood, and which make up the body's circulation system.

Your heart beats an amazing 100,000 times a day and has a pacemaker called the sinoatrial node, which sits in the right atrium. Electrical signals are generated from here and spread first to the atria, causing them to contract and push blood into the ventricles. After a short delay, which allows the ventricles to fill, the signals pass through the ventricles, which contract and pump blood out to the body and the lungs. Sometimes this pacemaker malfunctions and the heart beats more slowly or much faster than it should. In such cases, an artificial pacemaker can be installed to regulate its rate and rhythm.

MOVING BLOOD FORWARDS

To keep blood flowing in the right direction, there is a series of one-way valves. The mitral valve sits between the left atrium and ventricle, and the tricuspid valve sits where the right atrium and ventricle meet; these valves prevent backflow into the atria when the ventricles contract. Another pair of valves separate the ventricle from the arteries they pump into; these prevent blood flowing back into the heart when the ventricles relax. The aortic valve lies between the left ventricle and the aorta (the body's largest artery), and the pulmonary valve sits between the right ventricle and pulmonary artery.

When a doctor listens to your heart, he or she hears the familiar "lubb-dupp" sound; this sound is the snapping shut of the two pairs of valves. If the valves don't open or close properly, the blood can flow turbulently – like water down rapids – and cause extra sounds, known as a murmur.

THE HEART

▽ The heart is divided into a right and left side, and each side is divided further into an upper chamber (atrium) and a lower chamber (ventricle). The atria act as pre-filling chambers for the ventricles, which are the main pumping chambers. The left side pumps blood around the whole body so it is bigger and more powerful than the right side, which pumps blood around the shorter circuit to the lungs.

NOTE: Blue = deoxygenated (oxygen-depleted) blood; its oxygen has been used up by the body's cells. Red = oxygenated (oxygen-rich) blood. Blood vessels supplying the heart make sure that deoxygenated blood from the body is taken to and from the lungs to pick up oxygen and that oxygenated blood is pumped out to the body.

When the heart muscle contracts it is called systole (systolic pressure), and when the heart relaxes between contractions it is called diastole (diastolic pressure).

The difference in size between the two halves gives the heart its characteristic shape. Contrary to popular belief, the heart does not lie in the left side of the chest. It sits in the middle but the larger left side spreads to the left.

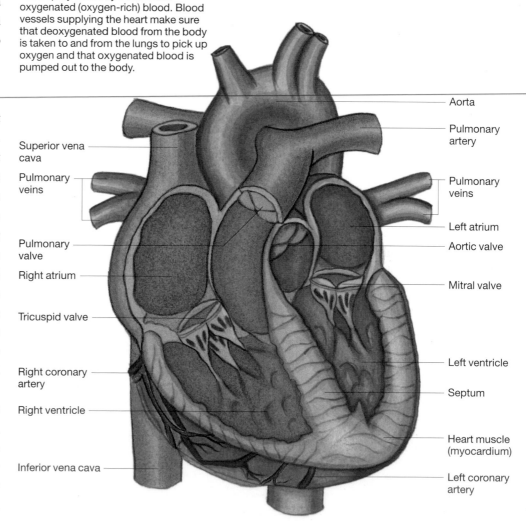

Superior vena cava

Pulmonary veins

Pulmonary valve

Right atrium

Tricuspid valve

Right coronary artery

Right ventricle

Inferior vena cava

Aorta

Pulmonary artery

Pulmonary veins

Left atrium

Aortic valve

Mitral valve

Left ventricle

Septum

Heart muscle (myocardium)

Left coronary artery

THE HEART AND CIRCULATION SYSTEM

▷ Mirroring the two sides of the heart, the circulation is made up of two separate systems – one supplying the body (systemic circulation) and one supplying the lungs (pulmonary circulation). The systemic circulation exits the heart from the left side and carries the blood to all parts of the body and returns to the right side of the heart. The pulmonary circuit carries blood from the right side of the heart to the lungs and then returns it to the left side, ready to be pumped around the body.

THE CIRCULATION SYSTEM

A journey around the body's circulation system begins in the heart's left ventricle. This contracting chamber forces a surge of blood into the aorta that passes through a network of ever-smaller arteries and capillaries. Blood then passes into bigger and bigger vessels until these form the vena cavae veins, which dump blood into the right atrium. From here, it passes into the right ventricle and is pumped into the pulmonary trunk and on to the lungs' capillaries. Here, oxygen dissolves into the blood and carbon dioxide is removed. Oxygen-rich blood travels through the pulmonary veins, into the left atrium and on to the left ventricle, ready to start the journey again.

THE BLOOD VESSEL "FAMILY"

There are five types of blood vessel – artery, arteriole, capillary, venule and vein. Arteries and arterioles carry blood away from the heart to the capillaries, which nourish the tissues, while venules and veins deliver blood back to the heart. The blood pressure in arteries is high and, because their walls are muscular and elastic, they pulse with the pressure wave of each heartbeat. By the time blood reaches the veins, blood pressure is very low. Veins have valves that snap shut to stop backflow and keep the blood flowing in the right direction as it travels back to the heart. If the leg valves deform and become blocked, they appear as purple "cords" of varicose veins.

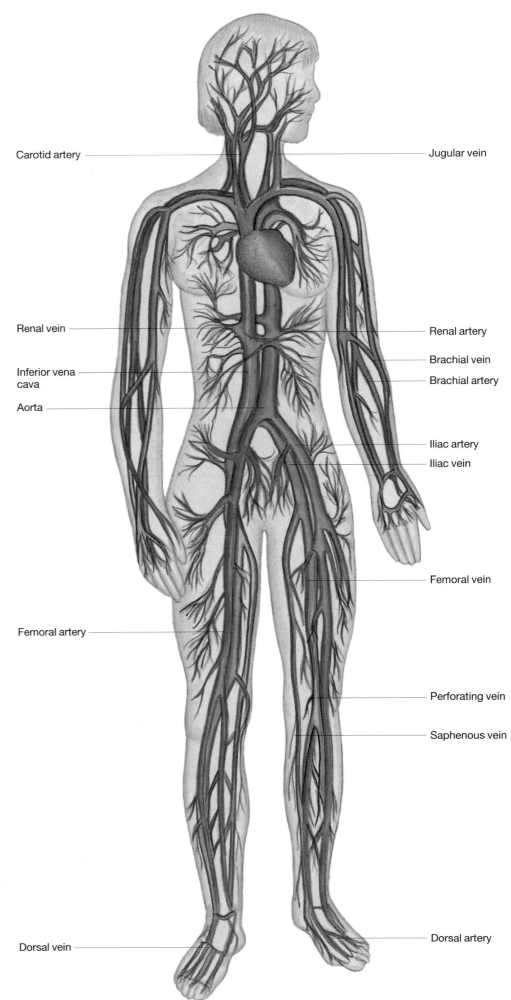

Carotid artery

Jugular vein

Renal vein

Renal artery

Brachial vein

Inferior vena cava

Brachial artery

Aorta

Iliac artery

Iliac vein

Femoral vein

Femoral artery

Perforating vein

Saphenous vein

Dorsal vein

Dorsal artery

High blood pressure

Persistently high blood pressure, also known as hypertension, can damage arteries and body organs, including the kidneys and the heart itself. This insidious disease is a major factor for heart disease, heart attacks and strokes. In fact, high blood pressure increases the risk of stroke six times and the risk of a heart attack threefold. Health education and screening programmes aid the early detection of high blood pressure and, together with improved treatments, have helped to significantly reduce the incidence of strokes and heart attacks.

Persistently high blood pressure is a common problem and it is important to treat it when it occurs because it significantly increases the risk of a stroke.

There are times when everyone's blood pressure is high. Your blood pressure fluctuates throughout the day, being lowest during sleep then rising on getting up, and reaching its higher value sometime mid-morning. On top of your normal values are times of stress, nervousness, excitement and physical activity – all of which raise your blood pressure.

Although people's blood pressure has a range of values that are acceptable, doctors will consider 120/80 mmHg as a "normal" reading. The first number of the reading relates to the blood pressure when the heart muscle contracts – systole – and the second number relates to pressure during its relaxation phase – diastole.

SIGNS AND SYMPTOMS

The difficulty with high blood pressure (hypertension) is that it usually occurs without any obvious symptoms. So, it is advisable to have regular health checks and to have your blood pressure checked at least every 4 to 5 years.

WHAT COUNTS AS HIGH BLOOD PRESSURE?

Most doctors agree that blood pressure is high if the reading is more than 150/95 mmHg (or 130/80 mmHg in people with diabetes). However, as blood pressure varies, it is important to take at least three consecutive high readings before a diagnosis can be made.

For some people, the very act of going to see a doctor or nurse makes their blood pressure shoot up – a phenomena known as "white coat hypertension". To obtain an accurate blood pressure reading, these patients may wear a small machine, that takes readings over a 24-hour period.

DIFFERENT TYPES OF HIGH BLOOD PRESSURE

There are three basic types of high blood pressure or hypertension:

1 Essential or primary hypertension – Nine out of ten people with high blood pressure have this type and the exact cause is unknown, although it involves many risk factors.
2 Secondary hypertension – About 10 per cent of people have high blood pressure due to another disease, such as kidney disease, rare endocrine disorders or heart valve problems, or in rare cases it is due to interactions with a drug.

MEASURING BLOOD PRESSURE

Doctors usually use a device called a sphygmomanometer to measure blood pressure, although some doctors now have electronic machines instead. This device has an inflatable cuff linked to a column of mercury or sprung dial. The blood pressure values are given in millimetres of mercury (written as mmHg for short).

A blood pressure reading is shown as two numbers, for example, 140/90 mmHg. The first number on the reading is the systolic pressure – the pressure when the heart contracts and when the pressure is at its highest. The second number is the diastolic pressure and corresponds to the resting and therefore the lower pressure between the heartbeats.

The cuff is placed around the upper arm over the main artery – the brachial artery – and inflated to block the blood flow. The doctor places a stethoscope just below the cuff on the inside of the elbow. As the cuff is gradually deflated, blood rushes through the artery and this turbulent flow can be heard via the stethoscope (or microphone in electronic devices). The doctor can monitor the changes in the sounds and identify the point at which the blood is flowing smoothly (through the unsquashed brachial artery), this is the diastolic pressure.

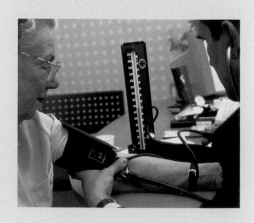

▽ Routine blood pressure tests are vital for at-risk groups such as the elderly because hypertension may show no symptoms.

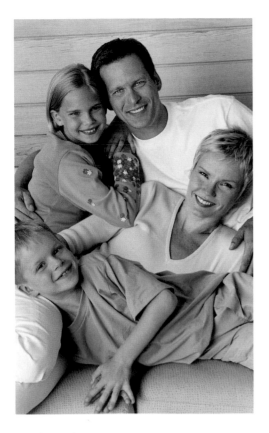

△ High blood pressure can run in families, so if this is the case in your family make an appointment for a check with your doctor.

3 Malignant hypertension – In this rare type, blood pressure can soar to dangerous levels, requiring urgent hospital treatment.

KNOW THE RISK FACTORS

High blood pressure can run in families, but doctors have identified other factors that can put you at risk of high blood pressure; some are similar to those for heart disease.
• Increasing age (as you get older, your arteries become stiffer and push your blood pressure up).
• Being overweight.
• Excessive alcohol consumption.
• Smoking.
• High-salt diet.

DIAGNOSING HIGH BLOOD PRESSURE

If your doctor measures your blood pressure and it is consistently high, they will also want to do a few extra tests. Tests include using a dipstick to check a sample of urine for the presence of protein (which would

indicate kidney damage) or glucose (which would indicate diabetes) as well as taking a blood sample to send to a laboratory to assess your kidneys' function. Your doctor may also examine the back of your eye using an ophthalmoscope as high blood pressure can cause damage to the light-sensitive layer of the retina. Other tests can be done to check for any underlying disorder and include a chest X-ray and electrocardiogram (ECG).

TREATMENT OPTIONS

The first line of treatment is not medication. Your doctor will recommend lifestyle changes to reduce high blood pressure. These changes include losing weight if overweight, reducing alcohol intake, cutting down salt consumption, taking regular exercise and, most importantly, giving up smoking.

Some doctors advocate biofeedback training. In biofeedback, you learn how to enter a relaxed state at will. Specialized equipment feeds back information about your heart rate, muscle tension and stress levels. You receive a continuous stream of this information as you practise certain relaxation techniques. In time, you learn to control your body's responses and help to reduce your high blood pressure.

If such measures fail, the next line of attack is drug therapy, which is a lifelong strategy. There are many antihypertensive drugs available; the common groups are:
• Thiazide diuretics.
• Beta-blockers.
• ACE inhibitors.
• Calcium antagonists.
• Alpha-blockers.

Many doctors use a thiazide or beta-blocker as first-line treatment; although ACE inhibitors work better for people with diabetes. Many antihypertensive drugs can cause side-effects, making people reluctant

▷ If the heart works against high pressure over a long period of time, the heart muscle becomes thicker – indicated in red on this coloured chest X-ray image.

to continue taking their medicine. It is important to bear in mind that the benefits of treatment include significantly reducing the risk of a heart attack or stroke. This is particularly pertinent for people with diabetes, who are more susceptible to the effects of high blood pressure.

It is quite usual to have to take two or more drugs. Furthermore, you may have to try several combinations until you find the one that works for you.

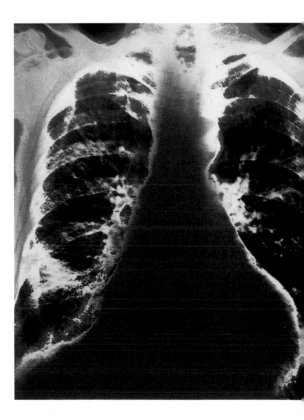

Atherosclerosis

Atherosclerosis is the furring up of arteries by the formation of fatty plaques called atheroma. Such narrowing of the arteries restricts blood flow and oxygen supply to the body's tissues. Atherosclerosis can affect arteries in any part of the body, the most serious, being when it blocks up the heart arteries or those that supply the brain. There are often no symptoms – the first sign could be a heart attack. It is vital, therefore, that you recognize the risk factors and do all you can to minimize your risk of atherosclerosis and any associated conditions.

The word "atherosclerosis" comes from Greek – *athere* meaning porridge and *skleros* meaning hardening. This word derivation conjures up an image of exactly what happens as atherosclerosis develops.

The plaques that form and fur up arteries are made of atheroma – this is a mixture of cholesterol, dead muscle cells, fibrous tissue, clumps of platelets and sometimes calcium.

NO ARTERY IS SAFE

Atherosclerosis can silt up arteries in any part of the body and may affect:

- The heart, causing heart disease (the coronary vessels are easily blocked).
- The brain, causing a stroke.
- The legs, causing poor circulation (see box on peripheral vascular disease) or even gangrene.
- The intestine, causing parts to die.

PERIPHERAL VASCULAR DISEASE

If the fatty deposits of atherosclerosis form in arteries taking blood to the legs, most commonly in the arteries of the pelvis and the artery just above the knee, they will cause the leg muscles to become cramped and painful with exertion. This pain usually occurs in the calf muscle and subsides with rest. Doctors refer to this condition as intermittent claudication. As the blockage gets worse, the exercise needed to produce the pain gets less until pain may be present even at rest. In this situation the leg barely has enough blood to survive and, if left untreated, gangrene will develop, possibly requiring an amputation.

As with all effects of atherosclerosis, you can help to prevent such a condition developing by giving up smoking and exercising regularly. The exercise will prevent the claudication from worsening and in many cases will improve it. If the condition is very severe, surgeons can bypass the blocked vessel using a patient's own vein or an artificial artery.

RECOGNIZE THE RISK

There are a number of well-recognized risk factors for atherosclerosis, and of these many can be changed for the better. Making changes to these risk factors where possible saves lives.

These factors fall into two categories: those you can change and those you cannot. Because some of these risk factors are unchangeable, it is all the more important that you reduce those that you do have the power to change.

HOW ATHEROSCLEROSIS DEVELOPS

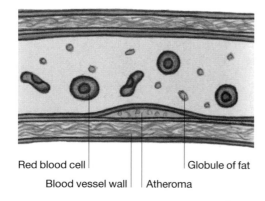

Red blood cell | Globule of fat

Blood vessel wall | Atheroma

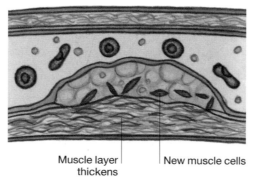

Muscle layer thickens | New muscle cells

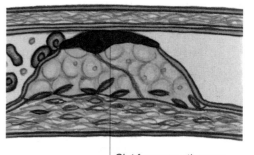

Clot forms on atheroma and blocks the artery

1 The underlying process of atherosclerosis can start even before you are born. A tiny deposit, or plaque, mainly of fats – called an atheroma – develops on the inside of a blood vessel wall.

2 Over years this plaque grows, furring up the artery and reducing the blood flow. If the flow of blood in the arteries in the legs is reduced, for example, it can cause pain on walking, known as claudication.

3 As the plaque grows it can split and rupture. If this happens, the body forms a clot on the plaque. This clot and plaque can permanently block the blood vessel, starving the tissue of vital oxygen.

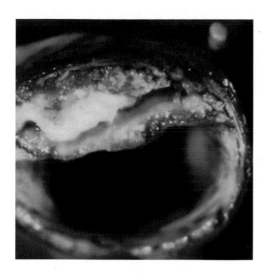

△ This magnified view of a slice through an artery shows a thick deposit of atheroma caused by atherosclerosis.

CHANCE FACTORS

The non-modifiable risk factors include:

- Age – The older you are, the greater the risk of developing this condition.
- Ethnicity – Studies have shown that some ethnic groups are more likely to suffer from atherosclerosis.

ANEURYSMS

Another result of atherosclerosis is a weakening of the blood vessel wall caused by the fatty deposits. A weak spot in the wall can balloon and form an aneurysm. Aneurysms most commonly affect the aorta, especially as it passes through the abdomen. As an aneurysm gets larger it becomes increasingly likely to burst, which can cause sudden and massive blood loss and is usually fatal.

Aortic aneurysms are usually detected by chance when a doctor examines your abdomen or an investigation is done for another reason. If they are detected they can be repaired surgically. This is a major operation, but has a very good success rate. Sometimes an aneurysm may leak before it bursts, resulting in severe sudden back pain that radiates to the thighs. In this case, surgeons can try to repair the aneurysm before it bursts and prevent future ruptures.

- Genetic inheritance – Heredity plays a part in the health of the cardiovascular system and atherosclerosis often runs in families. The inherited condition hyperlipidaemia, which causes high levels of fat in the blood, also increases the risk of atherosclerosis.
- Gender – Men are more likely to suffer from atherosclerosis because it seems that the production of oestrogen protects women against the development of atheroma but it is not clear if this protection continues after menopause for those taking hormone replacement therapy. The risks even out once women stop producing oestrogen.
- Diabetes – People with diabetes are at high risk of developing atherosclerosis because it can be associated with high cholesterol levels. In diabetes, the fatty plaques form much faster. Well-controlled glucose levels lessen the risk but it is especially important to control other factors, such as high blood pressure and high blood cholesterol levels.

CHOICE FACTORS

Factors you can influence for the better include the following:

- Smoking – Cigarette smoking promotes atheroma formation within the arteries.
- High blood pressure – Hypertension increases your risk of atherosclerosis.
- High blood cholesterol levels – Recent studies have shown that high levels of cholesterol in the blood increase the risk of atherosclerosis.
- Obesity – Being overweight or obese is linked both to poor cardiovascular health in general and to a higher risk of atherosclerosis.
- Inactivity – Regular physical exercise lowers the risk of atherosclerosis.

It would be a mistake to think you are too young to worry about atherosclerosis because it can be present for years before it causes symptoms. The first signs can start in adolescence – or even in childhood – so the earlier you make changes the better.

ASPIRIN – A WONDER HEART DRUG

The humble aspirin in small doses is the most useful drug doctors have for treating heart disease. It thins the blood, thereby preventing clots forming on fatty plaques, and also slows the growth of the plaques themselves. In cases of heart disease, angina or after a heart attack, doctors will prescribe a daily dose of aspirin (75 mg, one quarter-strength aspirin tablet).

PREVENTING ATHEROSCLEROSIS

Your doctor will discuss your risk factors and recommend lifestyle changes you can make. You may have a cholesterol test, where a sample of your blood is analysed in a laboratory. Your doctor will check your "lipid profile" for values of HDL and LDL cholesterol (high- and low-density lipoproteins). HDLs give some protection against arterial disease but LDLs do not.

Cholesterol levels can be kept low by eating plenty of fresh fruit and vegetables and cuttting down on animal fats, such as full-fat milk, cheese, eggs and red meat. However, someone with high cholesterol levels will probably take cholesterol-lowering drugs as well as eating a low-fat diet. Recent studies have shown that these drugs improve the long-term risk of developing heart disease.

▽ Regular activity from an early age can help prevent the development of tiny plaques of atheroma within the arteries.

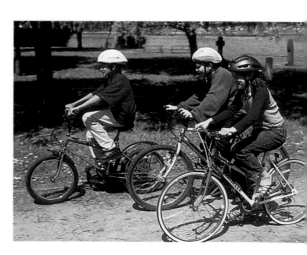

Heart disease

Heart disease is inextricably linked with atherosclerosis and the two are responsible for the biggest cause of death in the Western world. When atherosclerosis furs up the heart's arteries it is known as coronary artery disease or heart disease. As with atherosclerosis, it is vital to know if any risk factors for heart disease apply to you and then take steps to minimize these. Heart disease may develop insidiously and the first symptom could be a heart attack. It is never too early to start looking after your heart and visiting your doctor for a check-up if necessary.

When one or both of the heart's coronary arteries is blocked by deposits of atheroma, the tissue beyond the blockage no longer receives a blood supply and so the heart muscle dies due to oxygen starvation.

KNOW THE RISK FACTORS

There are well-recognized risk factors for heart disease and these mirror those for atherosclerosis. In order to assess your risk factors, your doctor will probably ask you questions about your state of health, diet, exercise habits and smoking as well as checking your blood pressure.

SIGNS AND SYMPTOMS

In the early stages of heart disease there may be no symptoms. In later stages, the first symptom is usually chest pain (angina) on physical exertion or a heart attack. Some people develop arrhythmias (see box) and suffer from associated palpitations and dizziness.

Some risk factors you can change and some you cannot. So it is vital to reduce any choice factors that apply to you.

CHANCE FACTORS

The non-modifiable risk factors include the following:

• Genetic inheritance – Heart disease often runs in families and is more common in people from northern Europe.

• Gender – Statistically women under 65 are less likely to suffer heart disease than men under 65; oestrogen offers women protection until menopause but then the risk rises to equal that of men.

• Ethnicity – Some ethnic groups have been shown to be at higher risk of suffering from heart disease.

HEART ARRHYTHMIAS

You may have felt at times that your heart is pounding, thumping or racing, especially when you are feeling anxious. Such palpitations can be explained by the fact that you have suddenly become aware of the beating of your heart (something you may not normally notice). However, such abnormal heart rhythms – also known as arrhythmias – can occur due to clogging of the heart's arteries by heart disease.

➤ Atrial fibrillation – In this common abnormal rhythm, the atria of the heart fail to contract properly, causing the heart to beat irregularly and sometimes to beat incredibly fast. The person may become short of breath and faint. It can be controlled or corrected with drugs. A small electric current (defibrillation) may be passed through the heart to restore normal atrial rhythm.

➤ Ventricular fibrillation/tachycardia – If the heart's ventricles enter one of these rhythms the heart stops and the person collapses and loses consciousness. No blood flows to the brain and death can occur quickly. Cardiopulmonary resuscitation (CPR, or mouth-to-mouth) keeps blood flowing to the brain and allows time for medical or paramedical staff to attempt to restart the heart.

➤ Bradycardia – In this condition the heart beats abnormally slowly, causing a person to feel very unwell, short of breath and faint. It can occur as a side-effect of certain heart drugs but may also result from a heart disorder. If this condition persists, a person may have to undergo surgery to have a temporary or permanent artificial pacemaker fitted which will restore a normal rhythm to the heartbeat.

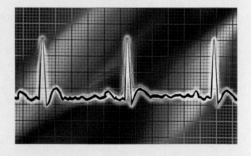

△ This electrocardiogram (ECG) shows the electrical activity in a normal heart.

▽ This ECG shows abnormal activity within the heart's electrical system, in this case causing a fast heartbeat (tachycardia).

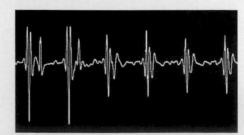

HEART MURMURS

When blood flows through the heart it usually does so silently and smoothly. Sometimes the blood may become turbulent – like water rushing down river rapids. This turbulent flow causes a heart murmur. The commonest murmur is a flow murmur. It is completely normal and shows that a healthy heart is beating vigorously enough to cause turbulent blood flow. The exact nature of a murmur is best confirmed using the diagnostic technique of ultrasound scanning of the heart – known as echocardiography.

In children, abnormal murmurs are most often due to "holes in the heart". In most cases this causes no problems, but the condition can be corrected surgically if necessary.

In adults, an abnormal murmur may be the result of a heart attack or it can be due to a heart valve that was damaged by rheumatic fever as a child. Most adult murmurs need no treatment apart from antibiotic protection during any invasive procedure, such as operations or dental extractions. Artificial or pig heart valves can be used to replace severely damaged valves.

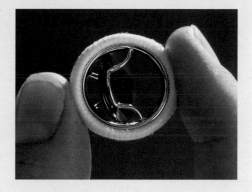

△ Surgeons can replace faulty valves that may cause a murmur with artificial ones.

- Age – In general, heart disease is more common with increasing age.
- Diabetes – People with diabetes are at high risk of developing heart disease and stroke. Well-controlled glucose levels lessen the risk but it is especially important to control other risk factors.

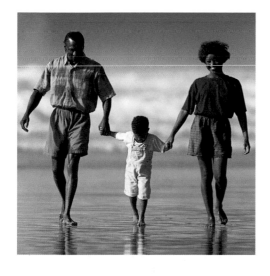

△ Studies have shown that African-Americans are more at risk from heart disease. Take care of your heart to ensure that it is as healthy as it can be and visit your doctor regularly.

CHOICE FACTORS

If the following factors apply to you it is important to remember that you have the power to change them.

- Smoking – Between 30 and 40 per cent of deaths from coronary artery disease can be attributed to smoking. The more you smoke, the higher the risk – there is

▷ This coloured angiogram shows a blockage in one of the heart's coronary arteries. Such a blockage could cause a heart attack.

no safe level. Even one cigarette a day increases the risk of heart disease. After quitting the level of risk decreases rapidly, although it can take up to 20 years to dwindle to that of a non-smoker.
- High blood pressure – Hypertension increases your risk of heart disease threefold. If you manage your high blood pressure, your risk is reduced, although it is still higher than someone with normal blood pressure.
- High cholesterol levels – Doctors now know that there is a direct link between high levels of cholesterol in the blood and the risk of heart disease.
- Obesity – Being overweight is linked to poor heart health and the risk of heart disease can be easily three times more than a person of healthy weight.
- Inactivity – Regular physical exercise can dramatically reduce the risk of developing heart disease.

TREATING HEART DISEASE

The treatment options for heart disease are covered on the next pages when we look at the commonest symptom of heart disease – angina. Symptoms can be controlled with drugs but in severe cases or after a heart attack surgery may be the only option.

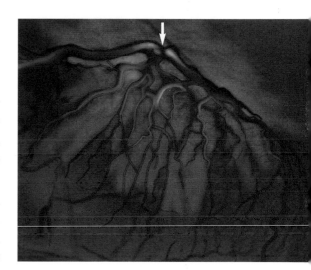

HEART INFECTIONS

Infections of the heart, particularly of the heart valves (rheumatic fever and endocarditis) used to be quite common, but occur less and less in the developed world. Pericarditis, an inflammation of the tough fibrous sac around the heart (the pericardium), is quite common and may be due to infection by viruses, bacteria or fungi. Symptoms include crushing pain in the centre of the chest and shortness of breath. Fortunately this condition is most often caused by a virus and will settle, leaving no long-term damage. Occasionally fluid may build up around the heart, which can interfere with its beating and so doctors will operate to drain this in order to restore normal heart function.

Angina

Angina is chest pain that originates in the heart muscle itself. The blood vessels taking blood to the heart – the coronary arteries – can become partially blocked with the fatty plaques caused by atherosclerosis (in this case also known as heart disease). There may be enough blood for the heart at rest, but during activity – when the heartbeat can increase from 75 to 190 beats per minute – the muscle cannot get enough blood and it "hurts". This is reflected by the fact that angina is brought on by exercise but subsides when activity is stopped and the person rests.

SIGNS AND SYMPTOMS

Angina can be mild or severe. The pain, which is heavy or crushing, is typically in the centre of the chest and can radiate up the neck and down the arms, most commonly the left arm. You may also feel short of breath and sweaty.

Angina is not easy to diagnose from physical symptoms, particularly as the symptoms of other conditions, such as indigestion, are similar.

HOW IS IT DIAGNOSED?

Testing usually begins with an exercise electrocardiogram (ECG) – where you walk on a treadmill (or cycle on an exercise bike) while hooked up to a machine that records the heart's electrical activity. The level of exercise is slowly increased until the patient feels pain and the electrocardiogram pattern changes.

Further tests include a coronary angiogram, in which you lie flat on a table and a doctor inserts a fine tube into your heart via an artery in your groin. A special dye is injected into the arteries and X-ray pictures are taken. Any narrowed arteries are clearly visible on the X-ray images.

TREATMENT OPTIONS

Angina usually responds well to drug treatment. The most common drugs used in treating angina are the following:
• Nitrates – These drugs come as fast-acting sprays or tablets that go under the tongue and ease the pain during an angina attack. Daily long-acting tablets reduce the need for the sprays.
• Beta-blockers – These tablets reduce the workload of the heart, prevent pain and slow the gradual worsening of angina.
• Calcium antagonists – These drugs ease the heart's workload to help prevent pain.

A standard treatment is a low, daily dose of aspirin to prevent more atheroma from building up within the heart's arteries.

LIFESTYLE ISSUES

Once angina is diagnosed, your doctor will assess your risk factors for heart disease and probably suggest lifestyle changes, such as quitting smoking or a low-fat diet.

▽ During an exercise ECG electrodes attached to the chest relay information about the heart's electrical activity while a cuff on the arm monitors blood pressure.

UNSTABLE ANGINA

Angina gets worse over time and less and less activity will provoke the pain. If your angina suddenly worsens or you are experiencing pain at rest, it could be due to a blocked coronary artery causing a heart attack. If this happens, you should see a doctor urgently.

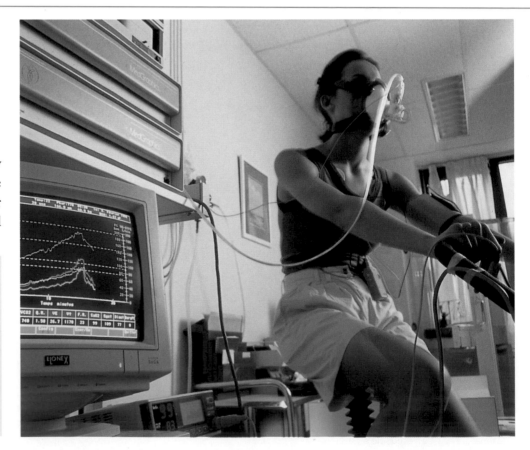

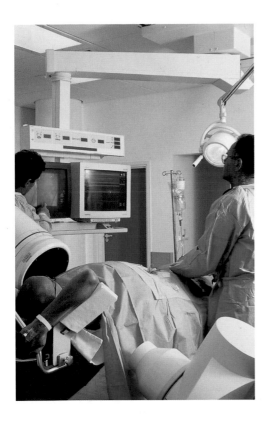

◁ This surgeon is carrying out an angioplasty. A balloon catheter is inserted into the patient's groin and advanced slowly up an artery into the heart. Once in the partially blocked coronary artery, the balloon is inflated and deflated to widen the artery and increase blood flow.

MEDICAL INTERVENTIONS TO TREAT BLOCKED ARTERIES

There are two levels of intervention for reinstating blood supply to the heart muscle once a coronary artery has become blocked or narrowed by plaques of atheroma. The intervention chosen will depend on how badly the arteries are narrowed. As with any operation, these carry certain risks.

1 Angioplasty – During this procedure for narrowed but not completely blocked arteries, a fine hollow tube (catheter) is inserted into your heart and a tiny balloon at the catheter's tip is inflated and deflated a few times to squash the plaque and widen the artery. Such a procedure is carried out on an outpatient basis and is performed using local anaesthetic

2 Bypass surgery – If coronary arteries are very narrow or completely blocked, a new route for the blood supply is made using what is known as a bypass graft. Surgeons have two options for the bypass graft – they either use an artery that already lies within your chest or they remove a piece of a vein from your leg. Sometimes a person may have two, three or four blockages to bypass. In these cases the procedure would be called a double, triple or quadruple bypass. Bypass surgery is done under general anaesthetic and takes between three and five hours. It is now one of the most frequently performed surgical procedures.

BYPASS SURGERY OPTIONS FOR BLOCKED CORONARY ARTERIES

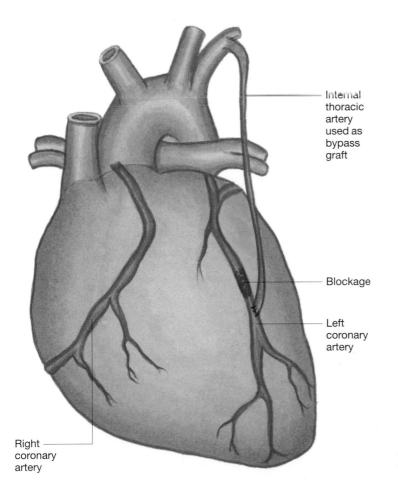

Internal thoracic artery used as bypass graft

Blockage

Left coronary artery

Right coronary artery

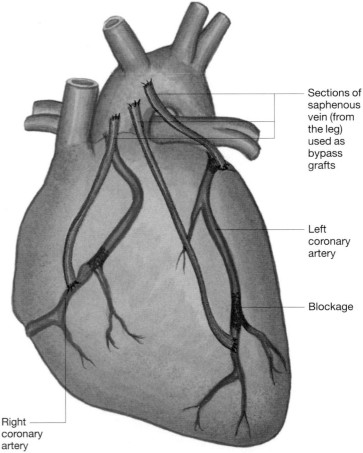

Sections of saphenous vein (from the leg) used as bypass grafts

Left coronary artery

Blockage

Right coronary artery

△ In the first option, heart surgeons detach an artery – the internal thoracic artery – from the chest wall and re-attach it beyond the blockage to reinstate the heart muscle's continuous blood supply.

△ Alternatively, pieces of a vein in the inside of the leg – the saphenous vein – are removed and cut into sections, which can then be used to re-route the blood supply around any number of blockages.

Heart attack

A heart attack, or myocardial infarction, occurs when a blood vessel has become blocked. When a part of the heart muscle loses its blood supply in this way it can suffer irreversible damage and die. Having a heart attack can be a very frightening experience but a large proportion of heart attack sufferers return to normal life after a recovery period. A heart attack can also damage the heart's pacemaker and cause arrhythmias. Studies have shown that one in four heart attacks goes unnoticed – these "silent" heart attacks only become apparent on ECGs.

SIGNS AND SYMPTOMS

The pain of a heart attack is similar to angina but may be more severe. It also lasts longer than angina pain, is not eased by rest and is not relieved by nitrate sprays or tablets. Symptoms include shortness of breath, sweating, nausea and dizziness. An angina sufferer who has chest pain for more than 20 or 30 minutes may be having a heart attack and should seek urgent medical help.

The key to a good outcome in treating a heart attack is speed in clearing the blockage in the artery so that there is less likely to be permanent damage to the heart.

ACTION AT THE HOSPITAL

• On arrival, an ECG test or blood tests confirm a diagnosis instantly.

▽ Speed is key to the successful treatment of a heart attack. Ambulance paramedics can start treatment on the way to hospital.

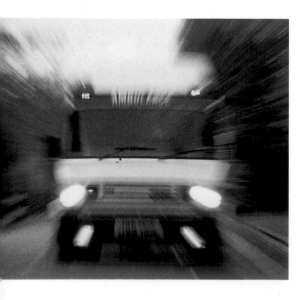

• The first treatment is aspirin, which will be given by the ambulance crew or your doctor to prevent further clot formation.
• Oxygen given via a mask will also help limit the damage.
• Morphine or another strong opiate may be given to lessen the pain.
• Doctors will try to dissolve the clot causing the blockage using drugs or may have to perform an angioplasty.

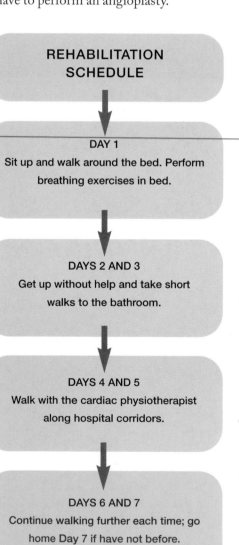

REHABILITATION SCHEDULE

⬇

DAY 1
Sit up and walk around the bed. Perform breathing exercises in bed.

⬇

DAYS 2 AND 3
Get up without help and take short walks to the bathroom.

⬇

DAYS 4 AND 5
Walk with the cardiac physiotherapist along hospital corridors.

⬇

DAYS 6 AND 7
Continue walking further each time; go home Day 7 if have not before.

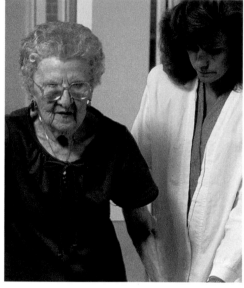

△ A rehabilitation schedule means that, with expert help, a patient can make as fast a recovery as possible after a heart attack.

LIFE AFTER A HEART ATTACK

The first step to recovery is to build up the heart again to cope with everyday life. So, during your week's hospital stay you won't just rest in bed, you will start special exercises, usually with a physiotherapist or cardiac nurse. Risk factors for heart disease have to be identified and changes made to prevent future heart attacks.

Many people recover completely from a heart attack, and it is largely due to a structured rehabilitation programme. Positive thinking also plays an important part in the recovery. It is easy to become depressed after such a life-threatening event – many people fear another attack and that can be enormously stressful. Studies have shown that a positive attitude speeds up the recovery process and return to a normal life.

Heart failure

Heart failure does not mean that the heart has stopped working; it indicates that it has become less efficient at pumping blood around the body and so cannot meet the body's constant demand for oxygen-rich blood. This condition tends to be most common in those over the age of 80 and is afflicting increasing numbers of people in developed countries every year. The degree to which someone is affected by their heart failure varies: some individuals have no symptoms at all while others may be severely disabled by the restricted mobility it confers.

The heart has two sides and either side or both can be affected by heart failure. In left heart failure, the left ventricle is unable to pump oxygen-rich blood out to the body and so fluid accumulates in the lungs, known as pulmonary oedema. Right-side heart failure causes fluid to build up in the body tissues – the legs, ankles and feet being the most obvious places. Initially, only one side may be affected but in time both sides usually fail.

CAUSES OF HEART FAILURE

Any disorder that affects the heart's ability to pump blood effectively can cause heart failure. About 70–80 per cent of cases are due to damaged heart muscle from heart disease and/or a heart attack. High blood pressure is another common cause: a heart that has pumped against high pressure for years on end suffers from the strain put on the muscle tissue. Other conditions that can also lead to heart failure are leaking or stiff heart valves, and, rarely, anaemia, extreme obesity and hyperthyroidism.

MAKING LIFESTYLE CHANGES

Once a diagnosis of heart failure has been made, your doctor will talk to you about how making simple changes to your everyday life can also help your condition. You should avoid strenuous exercise, although gentle exercise can actually help your condition. Smoking should definitely be given up and being overweight puts unnecessary strain on your heart. Avoiding salty foods is also a good idea.

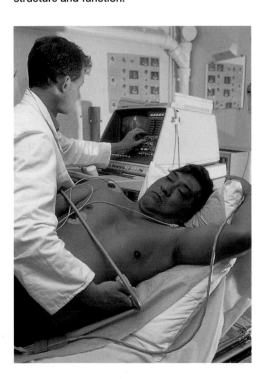

▽ Ultrasound scanning of the heart, known as echocardiography, is used to assess the heart's structure and function.

HOW IS IT DIAGNOSED?

Your doctor may make a diagnosis after asking you about your symptoms and an examination. He or she may want to carry out a few confirmatory tests, such as:

➤ ECG – This test assesses the electrical activity within the heart.

➤ Chest X-ray – This imaging technique checks the size of the heart and whether there is fluid on the lungs.

➤ Echocardiography – This investigation looks at the heart's internal structure and function.

SIGNS AND SYMPTOMS

Many people suffer heart failure without any symptoms whatsoever, especially in the early stages of the disease. When symptoms do eventually become apparent, they may include:

➤ Muscle weakness and fatigue.

➤ Loss of appetite.

➤ Cold hands and feet.

➤ Swollen ankles.

➤ Breathing difficulties (typically in left-sided heart failure) such as shortness of breath, which often becomes worse when lying flat and on exertion.

TREATMENT OPTIONS

Although heart failure is a progressive disease, current drug treatments are powerful and have been shown to improve the length and quality of life for people suffering from the condition. Heart failure cannot be cured but it can be controlled, and your doctor may prescribe the following drugs as part of a long-term treatment:

• Diuretics – These drugs eliminate excess fluids via the kidneys. This reduces the amount of blood to be pumped and decreases the strain on the heart.

• ACE inhibitors – These drugs work by widening the blood vessels, thereby reducing the workload of the heart.

Drug therapy is usually successful at treating symptoms and improving quality of life. Unfortunately, heart failure is a progressive disease and so tends to become more severe over time.

Thrombosis and embolism

In thrombosis, a blood clot (or thrombus) forms in a blood vessel and blocks the blood flow. Occasionally clots form spontaneously, most commonly in the veins of the legs. Clots below the knee are very common and don't usually cause problems; if the clot sits above the knee, the affected leg can become hot, swollen and painful, indicating a deep vein thrombosis. If a fragment of clot – called an embolus – breaks off, it travels through the heart and circulation until it becomes stuck in a blood vessel. An embolus lodged in the lung is potentially fatal.

Blood clotting is a vital survival mechanism, but when the blood clots for no reason it can be very dangerous. A clot can form in any artery or vein in the body, but most commonly in the veins in the legs, due to a lack of movement of the blood flow. If such a clot forms in a deep vein, in the leg or in an artery, it can be serious and needs prompt medical diagnosis and treatment.

If a clot, or a clot fragment, blocks an artery, blood cannot reach the tissues. If a blockage occurs in an artery supplying the brain, lungs or heart, it could be fatal.

KNOW THE RISK FACTORS

Many factors increase the chance of developing a deep vein thrombosis:
• Family history.
• Obesity.
• Smoking.
• Immobility, such as sitting for long periods during a long journey or while recovering from surgery.
• Dehydration.
• Drugs, such as the contraceptive pill.
• Surgical procedures.

SIGNS AND SYMPTOMS OF THROMBOSIS AND DVT

The symptoms of thrombosis depend on the location of the clot. Symptoms of a deep vein thrombosis include:

➤ Pain in the legs, even at rest.

➤ Enlarged veins beneath the skin.

➤ The area becomes hot, swollen and red.

MINIMIZING THE RISK OF DEEP VEIN THROMBOSIS

If you are going on a long journey (by car, train, bus or plane), take a few simple steps to avoid a DVT.

➤ Wear special support socks just before and during the journey.

➤ Get up and stretch your legs every now and then.

➤ Drink plenty of water and avoid drinking alcohol.

➤ Point and flex your toes, to help return the blood in your legs to your heart.

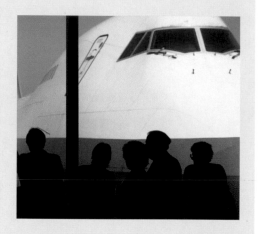

△ Long-distance travel increases the risk of a DVT developing so take note of the precautionary measures to minimize the risk.

HOW CLOTS ARE DIAGNOSED

Your doctor may suspect you have a clot in a deep vein after taking your medical history and after examining you. To confirm any clinical suspicions, the doctor may then arrange for you to have an ultrasound or Doppler ultrasound scan of the affected area. This imaging technique enables doctors to assess the blood flow and to establish if the vessel is blocked and, if so, how badly.

If the test results show the signs of a possible pulmonary embolism, then an urgent hospital appointment for a specialized test called a ventilation-perfusion scan will be arranged. Doctors will probably take a blood sample to check the levels of blood gases – oxygen and carbon dioxide – which will give them more information on your condition and confirm how the treatment should proceed.

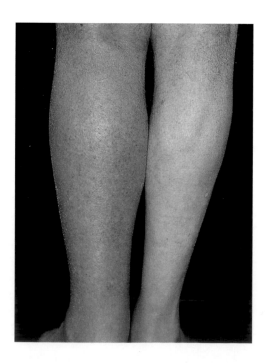

▽ This back view clearly shows redness and swelling in the lower half of the left leg – caused by clotting in a vein deep within the leg muscle.

DISSOLVING CLOTS

If you are at high risk of thrombosis, such as after surgery, you'll be given special support stockings to improve the circulation in your legs. Furthermore, doctors may administer a blood-thinning (anticoagulant) drug to prevent clots from forming and those that already exist from enlarging.

If a clot has already developed, doctors will want to thin the blood with bigger doses of anticoagulants – initially this is done by injection (heparin) and afterwards by mouth (warfarin). A clot in a deep vein may need such anticoagulant treatment for six weeks or so, whereas a pulmonary embolism would be treated for at least three months. Some people are prone to clots in their deep leg veins and so have to take anticoagulant drugs for life.

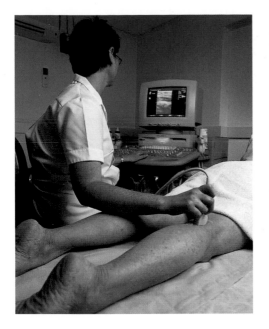

△ This patient is undergoing a Doppler scan, which is used to check for evidence of deep vein thrombosis.

Raynaud's disease and phenomenon

SEE ALSO

➤ Autoimmune diseases, p211

Having painfully cold hands on a frosty winter's day, if you are not wearing gloves, is a perfectly normal response. Your body is conserving heat by taking blood away from the skin. However, in those suffering from Raynaud's disease this response sends the arteries into spasm.

Raynaud's disease is most commonly seen in young women. It usually affects the fingers and toes but can affect the ears, nose and lips. Some diseases, such as systemic sclerosis, and certain drugs can cause symptoms that appear identical to those of Raynaud's disease but in these cases it is referred to as Raynaud's phenomenon.

▽ This Raynaud's sufferer has abnormal blood flow due to arterial spasms.

SIGNS AND SYMPTOMS

Usually both hands or feet are affected, and attacks may last minutes or hours. The changes follow a certain pattern:

➤ The small blood vessels go into spasm, reduce the blood flow and cause a dramatic colour change. The skin may turn white or dark purple.

➤ There may also be a "pins and needles" sensation.

➤ As the skin begins to warm up, the affected area changes to blue as the blood starts to flow more normally again. Finally the skin becomes red as the arteries open up once more. This red phase can be very painful.

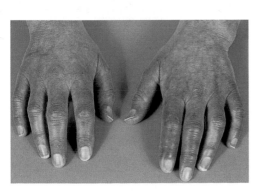

TREATMENT OPTIONS

One of the most effective treatments is keeping the hands and feet as warm as possible, and mild cases can be remedied by wearing extra-thick gloves and socks in cold weather. Smoking constricts the arteries and worsens the symptoms of Raynaud's disease so giving up smoking will also be helpful.

During an attack, exercises that stimulate circulation may speed up recovery.

In severe cases, your doctor can prescribe calcium channel blockers. These drugs promote the relaxation of the muscle in the artery wall, which goes into spasm in Raynaud's disease, and so keeps the arteries open and blood flowing to the area.

Varicose veins

SEE ALSO

➤ Weight control, p16
➤ Exercise for life, p18
➤ The cardiovascular
   system, p28

Varicose veins are a very common problem that often runs in families. They occur when the small superficial veins in the skin of the legs become distorted and dilated, and appear on the surface as lumpy, purple cords. Faulty valves in superficial or deep veins mean that blood can flow backwards, from deep to superficial, and overfill the small veins. Some people mistakenly believe varicose veins are due to jobs which involve a lot of standing, such as hairdressing or working in a shop. Standing will aggravate an existing problem but not actually cause it.

Women are more susceptible to varicose veins than men, and being overweight increases the pressure on the superficial veins, which can lead to varicose veins.

SIGNS AND SYMPTOMS

Varicose veins can ache, occasionally bleed and most seriously lead to ulcers around the ankle, which can be very difficult to treat. For some reason varicose veins can cause the skin at the ankle to change, causing, first, an itchy rash and, second, a brown pigmentation that can easily break down into an ulcer.

SIMPLE SELF-HELP MEASURES

If you have varicose veins, the following suggestions may help you feel more comfortable:

• Avoid standing for long periods of time.
• Exercise or walk about during the day to keep the blood flowing in your legs.
• Put your feet up when you can.
• Wear elasticated support stockings if your doctor has recommended these.
• Lose some weight if you are overweight.

TREATMENT OPTIONS

Although varicose veins can be unsightly and painful, surgery is most commonly carried out if there is thought to be a danger of leg ulcers developing. However, some people have varicose veins removed for cosmetic reasons.

There are four basic treatment options:
1 People with mildly problematic varicose veins may find that wearing support stockings is helpful.
2 Painful veins may subside after injection with a sclerosing agent, a substance that shrivels up the vein and closes it off.
3 Tying off the superficial veins so that no blood flows into them (see below).
4 The last option is to remove the vein completely. Two small incisions are made at the top and bottom of the vein, and the surgeon literally strips the vein out.

TYING OFF VARICOSE VEINS

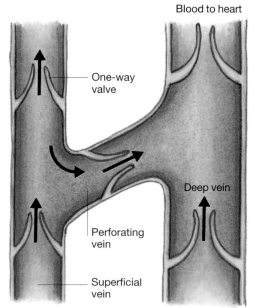

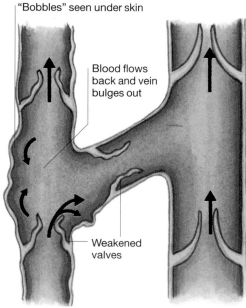

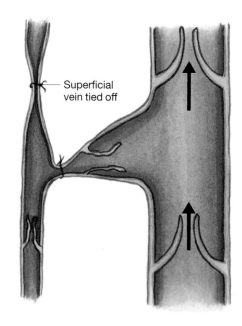

△ In healthy veins there are one-way valves to make sure that the blood flows in the right direction – from superficial to deep veins and then to the heart.

△ A weak valve in a superficial vein, or in a vein connecting superficial to deep veins, allows blood to flow back and overfill the superficial vein, causing the vein to bulge.

△ Tying off problem veins is an effective technique to prevent blood from flowing into them. The blood flow is diverted via the deep vein on its trip back to the heart.

THE DIGESTIVE SYSTEM

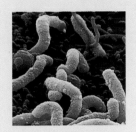

The digestive system is the body's power source. It breaks down food so that sugars, fats, proteins, vitamins, minerals and water can be absorbed into the blood, and used to provide energy for growth and repair. Anything the body cannot use is expelled as faeces. Fibre in food is not used by the body for fuel but is essential to the passage of faeces – and may help to protect against disease. Keeping to a healthy weight, following a balanced diet and eating regularly helps to keep the digestive system functioning.

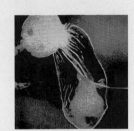

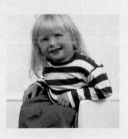

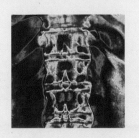

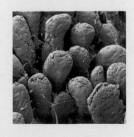

The process of digestion

SEE ALSO
➤ Eat healthily, p14
➤ Digestive disorders, p46
➤ Colorectal cancer, p58

Your digestive system comprises the digestive tract and the accessory organs of the liver, pancreas and gallbladder. The digestive tract is a tube about 8 metres (26 feet) long. It is divided into various sections, each with a specialized function. The aim of the system is to provide your body with energy and the raw materials for growth and repair, and to get rid of any waste. To work efficiently, your body needs sugars, fats and proteins. Special proteins called enzymes help break down the foods you eat into simple components for your body to use.

The process of digestion starts in the mouth. Here the teeth work with the muscular tongue and with saliva to cut, crush and mix food to a mush, ready to be swallowed. The chewing and grinding increases the surface area of the food so that a special enzyme found in saliva can start to break down the food's sugars. Once a ball of food is swallowed it travels down the throat into the oesophagus; to prevent food entering the respiratory system via the other "tube" in the throat (the trachea), a small flap called the epiglottis closes over it.

ON THE WAY TO THE STOMACH

Food travels down the length of the oesphagus to the stomach by a process of muscular contraction and relaxation called peristalsis. You are unaware of this, as with other movements within the digestive tract. At the end of the oesophagus, a ring of

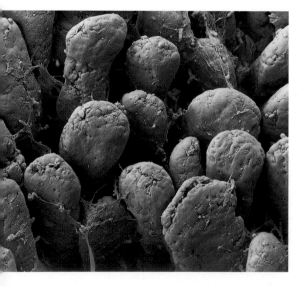

▽ Projections called villi cover the small intestine's surface. Nutrients are absorbed into the bloodstream through capillaries in the villi.

muscle (sphincter) opens to allow food into the stomach. The food changes very little as it passes through the oesophagus.

AN ACTIVE ENVIRONMENT

The stomach's many muscle layers twist and turn to grind, churn and mix the food with a germ-killing acid and a host of enzymes that have various functions. The stomach is a J-shaped muscular bag that acts like a water system header tank – it stores food after a meal and then allows it bit by bit into the next part of the digestive tract, the small intestine. Another ring of muscle called the pyloric sphincter controls how much food squirts into the duodenum, the first part of the small intestine.

HOW FOOD IS ABSORBED

Part of the way along the duodenum, substances from the gallbladder (in the form of bile to help fat digestion) and the pancreas (enzymes and an alkaline substance to neutralize the stomach's acid) are released. They are then mixed with the mush that was once food. Digestion continues within the small intestine but its main function is one of absorption – about 80 per cent of food molecules are absorbed through the walls of the small intestine. These walls are covered in tiny, finger-like projections called villi, which increase the surface area available for the absorption of food molecules into the bloodstream.

GUT FLORA

Your body houses trillions of bacteria and a huge proportion of these live in your large intestine – your gut flora. These "friendly"

THE FIBRE FACTOR

Your diet comprises three food types – carbohydrates, fats and proteins. An important sub-type of carbohydrate is fibre, which has a major effect on the health of your digestive tract. Fibre exists as water-insoluble fibre (found mainly in cereals, fruit, vegetables and pulses) and water-soluble fibre (found in oats, bran, beans and pulses). Insoluble fibre absorbs water on its passage through the large intestine, making larger, softer faeces; it also reduces the transit time in the colon, which it is thought may help to prevent cancer of the colon. Soluble fibre, on the other hand, forms the main food for your gut flora.

bacteria feed off the material that passes through and in return they produce a range of vitamins, help to break down bile pigments and keep harmful bacteria at bay by competing with them for food.

IN THE LARGE INTESTINE

The large intestine has three parts: the caecum, colon and rectum. This is where water, vitamins and minerals are absorbed from our food, through the large intestine's walls. Food material is also gradually compacted in the large intestine, a process that starts at the caecum.

The dehydrated food remains finally finish their journey through the colon at the rectum, where they are stored (now known as faeces), ready for excretion. Strong anus sphincters control when the faeces are excreted.

THE DIGESTIVE ORGANS

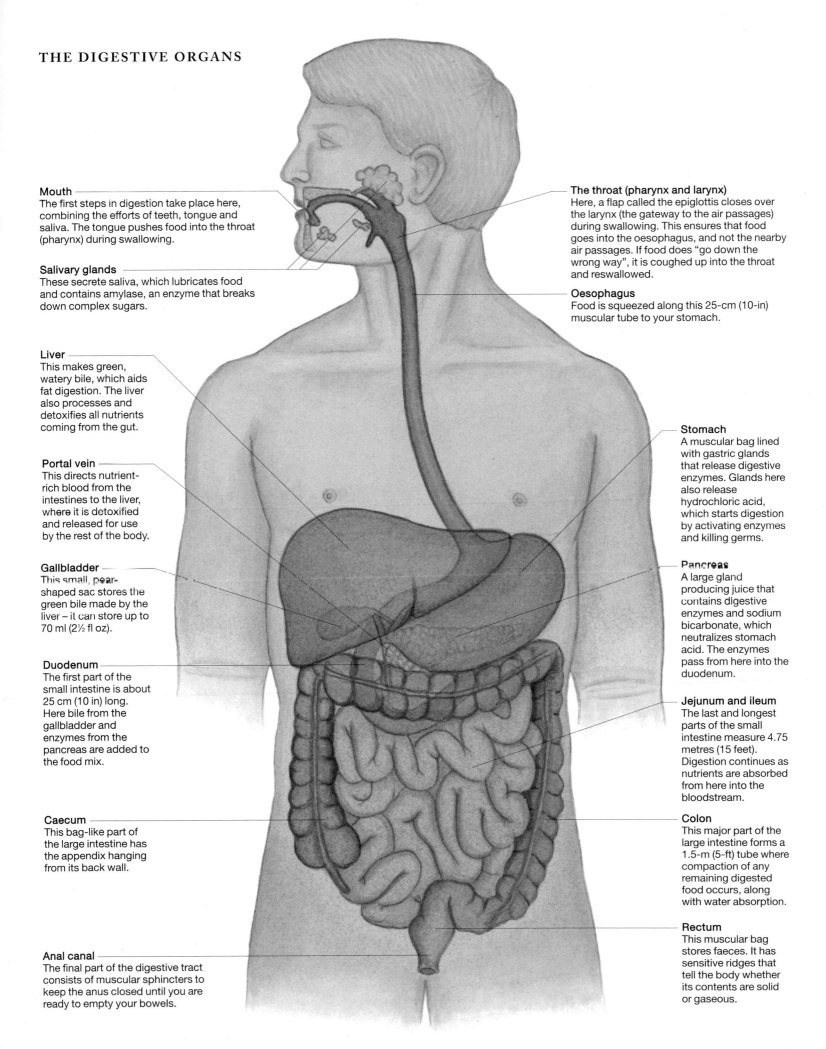

Mouth
The first steps in digestion take place here, combining the efforts of teeth, tongue and saliva. The tongue pushes food into the throat (pharynx) during swallowing.

Salivary glands
These secrete saliva, which lubricates food and contains amylase, an enzyme that breaks down complex sugars.

Liver
This makes green, watery bile, which aids fat digestion. The liver also processes and detoxifies all nutrients coming from the gut.

Portal vein
This directs nutrient-rich blood from the intestines to the liver, where it is detoxified and released for use by the rest of the body.

Gallbladder
This small, pear-shaped sac stores the green bile made by the liver – it can store up to 70 ml (2½ fl oz).

Duodenum
The first part of the small intestine is about 25 cm (10 in) long. Here bile from the gallbladder and enzymes from the pancreas are added to the food mix.

Caecum
This bag-like part of the large intestine has the appendix hanging from its back wall.

Anal canal
The final part of the digestive tract consists of muscular sphincters to keep the anus closed until you are ready to empty your bowels.

The throat (pharynx and larynx)
Here, a flap called the epiglottis closes over the larynx (the gateway to the air passages) during swallowing. This ensures that food goes into the oesophagus, and not the nearby air passages. If food does "go down the wrong way", it is coughed up into the throat and reswallowed.

Oesophagus
Food is squeezed along this 25-cm (10-in) muscular tube to your stomach.

Stomach
A muscular bag lined with gastric glands that release digestive enzymes. Glands here also release hydrochloric acid, which starts digestion by activating enzymes and killing germs.

Pancreas
A large gland producing juice that contains digestive enzymes and sodium bicarbonate, which neutralizes stomach acid. The enzymes pass from here into the duodenum.

Jejunum and ileum
The last and longest parts of the small intestine measure 4.75 metres (15 feet). Digestion continues as nutrients are absorbed from here into the bloodstream.

Colon
This major part of the large intestine forms a 1.5-m (5-ft) tube where compaction of any remaining digested food occurs, along with water absorption.

Rectum
This muscular bag stores faeces. It has sensitive ridges that tell the body whether its contents are solid or gaseous.

Digestive disorders

SEE ALSO

➤ Eat healthily, p14
➤ The process of digestion, p44
➤ Diarrhoea, vomiting and constipation, p228

Your bowel habit is probably the best indicator of how well your digestive system is functioning. And when it comes to your bowel habit, you are unique. Everyone's digestive system functions slightly differently – so "normal" can be seen as anything from bowel movements three times a day to just three times a week. The most important aspect of monitoring your digestive health is that you are aware of what is normal for you. That way, you will be able to spot anything out of the ordinary and bring it to the attention of your doctor if necessary.

The digestive system copes very well with a wide range of substances – but it can react violently if you take in contaminated food or drink, poisons, some drugs or other irritants. Some digestive symptoms, such as vomiting and diarrhoea, can be the body's straightforward and relatively brief response to a harmful substance – enabling it to expel the substance as quickly as possible. Others, such as constipation or bloating, may be the result of eating the wrong things over a longer period of time – causing the digestive system to work less efficiently. Minor symptoms such as indigestion can

▽ Young children are unembarrassed about going to the toilet, but as we grow older we find it difficult even to discuss our bowel habits.

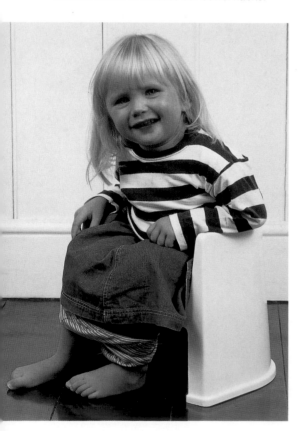

often be a result of the person eating in the wrong way – for example, when they are in a hurry or stressed or when they are sitting in an awkward position that impedes the digestive process.

Although most digestive symptoms are the result of a short-term problem, they can also indicate several serious disorders that need prompt medical treatment. A pain in the abdomen, for example, could be the result of cancer, or a less serious but still uncomfortable condition such as peptic ulcers, or of a temporary complaint such as a mild attack of gastroenteritis.

It is often difficult to determine the cause of a digestive symptom – peptic ulcers and stomach cancer cause pain in the same area of the abdomen, for example. Because of this it is important to see a doctor for a proper investigation if a symptom continues for longer than a few days – or if it is particularly violent.

DIGESTIVE SYMPTOMS

Most people experience bouts of vomiting, diarrhoea, abdominal pain, constipation, flatulence and bloating from time to time. These episodes are usually few and far between and often settle within a day or so. Only if these symptoms are severe or if they persist should you be concerned and visit your doctor. These are some of the commonest digestive symptoms – and how you should act if you notice them.

• Blood – Whether it is in vomit or in the stools, the presence of blood is never normal. There may be a simple reason for the blood – such as haemorrhoids (piles) or an anal fissure (tear) – but it could

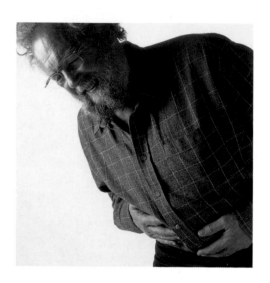

△ Abdominal pain is very common. Often the cause is a minor problem that passes quickly, but regular or very severe pain should be investigated by a doctor.

also indicate a more serious problem. It is therefore essential that you see your doctor for a diagnosis.

• Abdominal pain – Abdominal pain can be the result of a wide range of conditions – from over-eating and menstruation to serious disorders. If you suffer regularly from pain in your abdomen or if the pain changes, consult your doctor.

• Constipation or diarrhoea – Everyone suffers from occasional bouts of these. However, if your bowel habit changes suddenly and remains changed, it could indicate a serious condition and you should visit your doctor without delay.

• Vomiting – Vomiting is a common symptom of many diseases related to digestion, but it also occurs in other disorders. Bouts of vomiting can cause dehydration, so it is important that you drink plenty of fluids. If vomiting persists or if there is blood in your vomit, contact your doctor.

- Tenesmus – This word describes the feeling that you have not completely emptied your bowel after defecation. It can be a sign of serious disease, so it is wise to see your doctor.
- Weight loss – Any unexplained weight loss needs further medical investigation.
- Loss of appetite – Appetite tends to decrease naturally with age, but a sudden loss of appetite can be a sign of certain diseases and needs evaluation by a doctor.
- Bloating and flatulence – These are common symptoms which can produce discomfort and even pain. However, they rarely indicate serious disease.

INVESTIGATING DISORDERS

After asking you a series of questions about your state of health and your specific symptoms, your doctor may perform an

---

DON'T BE SHY

Many people are embarrassed when they have to discuss any digestive problems. They may either delay going to their doctor or feel unable to tell the whole story when they are there. Never feel embarrassed when talking about anything with doctors – they are used to dealing with such information and it is very important that your doctor has all the information you can give on your symptoms to be able to make an accurate diagnosis.

Your doctor will probably ask the following questions.

➤ How often do you empty your bowels? (A normal range is anything from three times a day to three times a week.)

➤ Is the stool loose and watery, hard and pellet-like, pale or foul smelling?

➤ Is there any blood or mucus in the stool? Is there fresh blood on the toilet tissue after wiping?

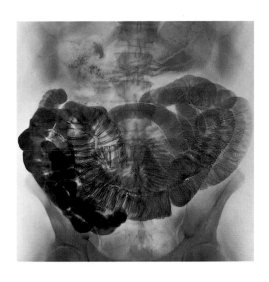

▷ X-rays such as this, taken after the patient was given a barium enema, clearly reveal any abnormalities in the small intestine.

examination of your rectum and will use a gloved finger to do so. This should not hurt but it will probably feel undignified and uncomfortable. However, it is important that the doctor is able to carry out a complete examination. Serious digestive diseases are best treated as quickly as possible so it is vital that you are honest with your doctor about any symptoms you are suffering even if you feel embarrassed about discussing them.

FURTHER TESTS

If your doctor feels that further investigation is required, you may be referred to a hospital for any or all of the following tests:

- Contrast X-rays – X-rays of the digestive tract can be very useful in detecting disease, especially if they are combined with a contrast dye or other medium that shows up white on an X-ray image. Barium sulphate is often used for this purpose. It may be mixed with water and drunk (called a barium meal) or injected into the rectum (a barium enema), before a series of X-rays are then taken. The barium makes it possible to see an outline of the inside of the digestive tract on the X-ray that enables a doctor to identify any potential problems.
- Endoscopy – This investigation involves looking inside your digestive tract via a flexible telescopic instrument. A flexible endoscope, which may be passed through the mouth or through the anus and rectum, makes it possible for a specialist to examine almost all sections of the digestive tract. Small instruments can be fed down into special channels within the endoscope to take samples of tissue (biopsies) or even to treat some conditions without surgery.
- Ultrasound scanning – Solid organs of the digestive system such as the liver are usually investigated using the non-invasive method of ultrasound.

PROCEDURE FOR AN ENDOSCOPY OF THE UPPER DIGESTIVE TRACT

⬇

You may be given an intravenous sedative or anaesthetic before the procedure. A local anaesthetic may be sprayed on the back of the mouth, and a mouth guard will be used to protect your lips and teeth.

⬇

A flexible tube with a small camera at its tip is inserted through the mouth, oesophagus and into the stomach and duodenum. A steering control enables the specialist to guide the endoscope.

⬇

Images from the endoscope camera appear on a screen, allowing the specialist to see any ulcers or other abnormalities.

⬇

The specialist may take small samples of abnormal tissue (a biopsy) using a tiny surgical instrument attached to the endoscope. The biopsy is then sent to a laboratory for analysis.

Obesity

Obesity is a condition in which there is excess accumulation of fat. Obesity is growing more common in the developed world, due to modern habits of eating unhealthy "junk" foods and an increasingly sedentary lifestyle. It is not necessarily that obese people eat more than the average person, but that they all eat more than their bodies actually need. However, people do tend to put on weight as they get older, due to metabolic changes. Rarely, obesity is due to an underactive thyroid gland, Cushing's syndrome or to corticosteroid drugs.

Being very overweight puts your health at risk – obese people are at high risk of dying prematurely due to heart disease, diabetes and stroke, and are also more likely to suffer back pain and other complaints because of the extra strain placed on their bodies. However, being moderately overweight will not usually have an adverse effect on your health – especially if you eat a balanced diet and exercise regularly.

COMPLICATIONS OF OBESITY

Obesity can result in the development of many different complaints and more serious diseases including:

➤ Arthritis of the hips and knees.

➤ Back pain.

➤ Breathlessness.

➤ Gallstones.

➤ Heart disease.

➤ Hiatus hernia.

➤ High blood pressure.

➤ High cholesterol levels.

➤ Menstrual problems.

➤ Post-operative problems, such as chest infection or deep vein thrombosis.

➤ Stroke.

➤ Type II diabetes.

➤ Varicose veins.

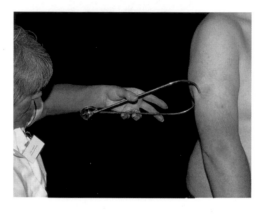

△ Weight-management clinics use various methods to determine the amount of body fat. This specialist is measuring fat with calipers.

Health education programmes aimed at children and adults seek to prevent obesity by emphasizing the importance of a healthy, balanced diet and active lifestyle.

DEFINING OBESITY

Healthcare professionals use the body mass index (BMI) to measure whether or not someone is a healthy weight for their height. The BMI uses a simple calculation (body weight in kilograms divided by height in metres squared). A person is described as obese if their BMI is above 30 if they are male and above 28 if they are female. The BMI serves as a guide only and your doctor will take many other factors into consideration. Waist size, for example, is often significant because extra weight around the waist is linked to cardiac risk.

TREATING OBESITY

The only sure way to lose weight is to eat less and exercise more. Losing weight gradually, and slowly increasing the amount of exercise that you do, is the healthiest and most effective way to reach and maintain a healthy weight. There are also medical options for treating obesity, including drug therapy and, as a last resort, surgery.

• Drugs – A number of drugs have been tried out for obesity with limited success and often with serious side-effects. New drugs, which block the absorption of fat or act on the brain to reduce the appetite, have become available. However, drugs can only do so much, and even people taking obesity drugs need to have, and maintain, willpower.

• Surgery – This is an extreme solution and is used only for the very obese when all diets have failed. The two commonest procedures are wiring the jaws so that only liquid food can be taken, and an operation called a gastroplasty, in which most of the stomach is stapled shut so that only smaller meals can be eaten.

▽ This X-ray shows a hiatus hernia, where part of the stomach protrudes through the diaphragm. Obesity puts extra pressure on the stomach, increasing the risk of a hernia.

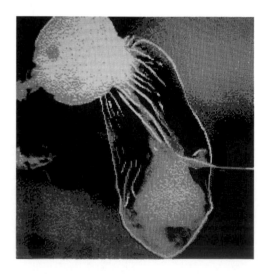

Oesophagitis

SEE ALSO
➤ Eat healthily, p18
➤ Smoking and your
   health, p20
➤ Endoscopy, p47

Food travels through the mouth and throat to the stomach via a thin, muscular tube called the oesophagus. Food then travels into the stomach in a one-way system in order that the stomach acid does not flow back in to the oesophagus. A number of conditions, however, can cause acid to flow back, or reflux, into the oesophagus, causing the lining to become inflamed and painful. The condition can usually be brought under control by avoiding provoking factors such as fatty foods or alcohol and by taking antacids or other drugs.

FACTORS THAT MAY PROVOKE OESOPHAGITIS

The reflux of acid into the oesophagus can be a result of:

➤ Eating too many fatty foods, chocolate, coffee and alcohol.

➤ Eating large meals.

➤ Smoking.

➤ Pregnancy or obesity.

➤ A hiatus hernia, in which part of the stomach forces through the diaphragm and affects the valve that prevents acid from flowing backwards.

The swelling and inflammation of the lining of the oesophagus causes chest pain, known as heartburn or dyspepsia, which is made worse by lying down or bending forward. Other factors, such as eating spicy foods or drinking hot liquids or alcohol, can also aggravate the burning sensation. In severe cases, the oesophagus may bleed.

WHAT MIGHT YOUR DOCTOR DO?

Your doctor may suspect oesophagitis from your symptoms. Contrast X-rays or an endoscopy may be carried out if it is not a straightforward case.

The first line of treatment is to avoid or reduce the provoking factors. Acid suppressants are usually the first line of defence and various drugs can be used to reduce stomach acid secretion. In severe cases, surgeons can form a new valve at the top of the stomach to prevent reflux.

FURTHER COMPLICATIONS

In rare instances, severe inflammation causes a narrowing, or stricture, in the oesophagus. If continually exposed to acid, the oesophageal lining can transform itself to resemble that of the stomach. This is known as Barrett's oesophagus and is a precancerous condition. Regular monitoring and lifelong drug treatment is needed in order to suppress the production of acid.

Cancer of the oesophagus

SEE ALSO
➤ Endoscopy, p47

This is the eighth most common cancer in the world. There is a particularly high incidence in Iran, which may be due to the widespread use of stoneground flour and the silicates it contains. The main risk factors in developed countries are smoking and a high alcohol consumption.

One of the main symptoms of oesophageal cancer is difficulty swallowing, which occurs first with solids and eventually even fluids cause pain. The pain is usually only apparent once the cancer has spread.

WHAT MIGHT YOUR DOCTOR DO?

After a history and examination, your doctor may refer you for an endoscopy or contrast X-ray to diagnose the cancer. The only cure is to remove the cancer surgically.

Unfortunately this form of cancer is fast-growing and it is often diagnosed when surgery is no longer an option. Chemotherapy and radiotherapy can be given to slow the disease's development, and other treatments focus on keeping the oesophagus open so that the person can continue to eat and drink.

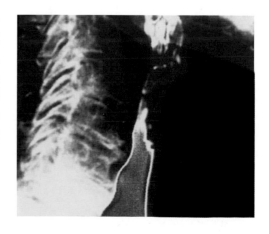

▷ Contrast X-rays are useful diagnostic tools, and allow doctors to see abnormalities such as tumours or ulcers in the oesophagus.

Peptic ulcers

Stomach acid is hydrochloric acid, one of the strongest acids that exists. Its function is to destroy anything unpleasant that may be ingested with food and drink and to activate one of the main stomach digestive enzymes. Despite the mucus coating of the stomach and duodenum, their linings can come under attack from this powerful acid. An ulcer is an area of tissue that has been damaged by acid. Peptic ulcers occur in the duodenum (duodenal ulcers) and the stomach (gastric ulcers). Fortunately, treatment is successful in 90 per cent of cases.

Duodenal ulcers are three times more common than gastric ulcers and the 20 to 45 age group are most likely to be affected. On the other hand, people with gastric ulcers are likely to be over 50.

SIGNS OF PEPTIC ULCERS

Many people affected by ulcers do not have any symptoms – or they may experience only minor discomfort that they put down to indigestion. However, ulcers can cause severe pain in the upper abdomen. With duodenal ulcers, the pain worsens when the stomach is empty – it may be relieved by eating but recurs later. Gastric ulcer pain is usually made worse by eating. The pain caused by either type of ulcer is similar to the pain that occurs as a result of stomach cancer, so prompt investigation is essential.

WHY PEPTIC ULCERS OCCUR

The vast majority of peptic ulcers are caused by infection with *Helicobacter pylori* bacteria. People living in unhygienic living

AREAS AFFECTED BY PEPTIC ULCERS

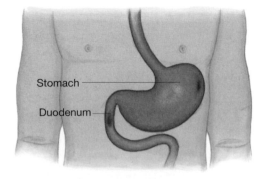

Stomach

Duodenum

△ Peptic ulcers are most likely to develop in the duodenum – the first section of the small intestine – but can also occur in the stomach.

SIGNS AND SYMPTOMS
➤ The main symptom of peptic ulcers is pain in the upper abdomen. Sometimes the pain is so severe it wakes sufferers at night.

➤ Nausea and vomiting.

➤ Loss of appetite and weight loss.

conditions are particularly at risk from this infection. Other causes include:
- The long-term use of aspirin or non-steroidal anti-inflammatory drugs.
- Excessive alcohol or, possibly, caffeine consumption.
- Smoking.

Stress is a contributory factor, for those suffering from dyspepsia, because it increases acid production. There may be a genetic factor since there often seems to be a family history of the condition.

WHAT MIGHT YOUR DOCTOR DO?

Your doctor may suspect ulcers from your symptoms, but will probably refer you to a hospital for tests. The tests may include a blood test, to establish if there are antibodies against the bacteria in your blood. Your doctor may also recommend an endoscopy where biopsy samples of the ulcer can be taken. These biopsies can be tested in a laboratory, both for the presence of *H. pylori* and to rule out the possibility of stomach cancer. If an endoscopy is not appropriate a urea breath test can be done to confirm the presence of *H. pylori*.

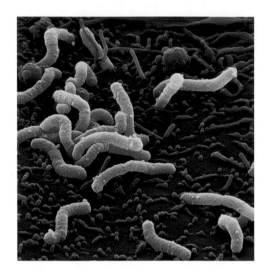

△ *Helicobacter pylori* bacteria, shown here on a human gastric cell, are the commonest cause of stomach ulcers and can also cause gastritis. The infection can be cleared with a simple course of antibiotics.

A NEW DISCOVERY

Doctors used to think that ulcers were caused primarily by stress. However, a revolution in understanding ulcers happened in the 1980s when researchers discovered that a tiny, innocent-looking bacterium, often seen on biopsies of stomach ulcers, was in fact the culprit. The precise mechanism of how *H. pylori* does this is still unclear but it seems to interfere with the mucus layer, making it more vulnerable to attack by the stomach's acid. *H. pylori* plays a role in the development of stomach cancer.

H. pylori can now be detected with blood and/or breath tests. It is also detected by a quick test done on samples of ulcerated tissue taken during an upper digestive tract endoscopy.

GASTRITIS

This inflammation of the stomach lining demonstrates similar symptoms to ulcers, and can be easily treated by taking antacids for the pain and implementing preventive measures such as reducing alcohol intake and giving up smoking. Gastritis can develop suddenly (acute gastritis) or develop gradually over many months or years (chronic gastritis). The acute form is commonly caused by excessive alcohol consumption or taking anti-inflammatory drugs, such as aspirin.

Chronic gastritis may cause no symptoms other than a vague feeling of ill health. However, it can result in significant damage to the stomach lining, causing bleeding and ulceration. It is also a risk factor for stomach cancer. In the past, the causes of long-term gastritis were not known and so there was no effective treatment available. Now that *H. pylori* has been identified as a major cause of the disease, a course of antibiotics usually clears it up. Chronic gastritis is sometimes caused by sustained, excessive alcohol consumption or smoking.

▽ The classic duodenal ulcer sufferer has long been seen as a 20–45-year-old man with a highly stressful job. However, although stress, along with alcohol and smoking, can exacerbate duodenal ulcers, recent studies show that bacteria may be the main cause.

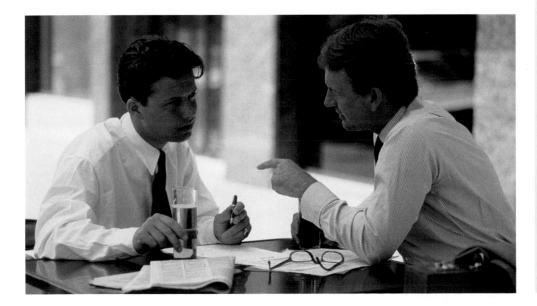

▷ This surgeon is studying screen images of a digestive tract he is exploring with an endoscope. He is able to guide the endoscope to explore any area he wishes to examine.

TREATMENT OPTIONS

Treatment of ulcers is more straightforward now that we know that *H. pylori* is often the cause. *H. pylori* eradication relies on the administration of two antibiotics and a PPI (proton pump inhibitor) for seven days, with six weeks' worth of acid-suppressing drugs to help heal the affected areas. If *H. pylori* is present, 90 per cent of ulcers can be healed with one course of treatment. A second course of treatment usually settles the majority of the remaining ulcers.

Those ulcers caused by aspirin or non-steroidal anti-inflammatory drugs usually settle if the drug is stopped. However, in cases of osteoarthritis, for example, such anti-inflammatories are essential. In these cases, your doctor will prescribe a drug to be taken with the anti-inflammatory to protect your stomach and duodenum from ulceration. Recently, Cox 2 inhibitors have been used as an alternative to anti-inflammatories because they have minimal gastrointestinal side effects.

To prevent ulcers from recurring, your doctor may advise you to make long-term lifestyle changes, such as reducing high levels of stress at work, giving up smoking or drinking less alcohol, as appropriate.

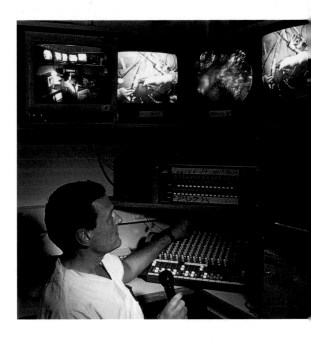

COMPLICATIONS OF PEPTIC ULCERS

Surgery was commonly used to remove ulcers before *H. pylori* was found to be the main cause. Today, surgery is used to treat complications of peptic ulcers.

➤ Haemorrhage – Duodenal ulcers tend to occur directly over a large blood vessel and can damage it, causing copious bleeding. This bleeding can usually be stopped with injections via an endoscope, but some cases still need a surgeon to tie off the vessel to halt the bleeding.

➤ Perforation – A hole in the stomach can form at the site of a peptic ulcer and the stomach contents can spill into the abdominal cavity, causing a life-threatening inflammation called peritonitis. It may be necessary for a surgeon to sew up the cavity; this is followed by ulcer drug therapy.

➤ Pyloric stenosis – Peptic ulcers can lead to scarring and narrowing (stenosis) of the exit valve from the stomach (the pyloric sphincter). A bad stenosis stops most food leaving the stomach and results in copious vomiting. Most patients need surgery to repair the pylorus.

Stomach cancer

Stomach cancer is the second most common cancer worldwide, after lung cancer. It is particularly common in Japan and China, probably due to dietary factors. Unfortunately, the incidence of this cancerous tumour of the stomach lining is increasing in the Western world. Stomach cancer tends to spread rapidly, so treatment is often focused on slowing the disease's progression rather than curing it. In Japan, where there is extensive screening, the disease is diagnosed at an earlier stage and about 90 per cent of those affected are cured.

KNOW THE RISKS

There are several risk factors for stomach cancer. Chronic gastritis (inflammation of the stomach lining) caused by long-term infection by *Helicobacter pylori* is the main factor. Other risk factors include:

➤ Smoking.

➤ A diet that is low in fibre.

➤ Diets rich in salty, pickled and smoked foods.

➤ High alcohol consumption.

Diets that are high in fibre promote general digestive health, and can help to reduce the risk of stomach cancer. Peptic ulcers are not a risk factor for stomach cancer, but it can often be difficult for doctors to distinguish between a peptic ulcer and early stomach cancer.

Stomach cancer usually develops in the lining of the stomach, but may spread rapidly to other sites in the body. Most of those affected are over the age of 50, and men are twice as likely to develop the disease as women.

WHAT MIGHT YOUR DOCTOR DO?

After listening to your symptoms, your doctor may examine you to check for evidence of a mass in the upper abdomen. Your doctor may then refer you to hospital for an endoscopy, in which the stomach will be examined through a thin viewing instrument. Biopsy specimens will be taken during an endoscopy, and then sent for analysis. You may also be sent for a contrast X-ray, which clearly shows the structure of the stomach and any abnormalities.

The stomach is a large "bag" so there is plenty of room for a cancer to grow before it causes any symptoms. Once symptoms start they are usually only mild and are not distinctive – they include abdominal pain, nausea and weight loss. Because of this, stomach cancer is often not diagnosed until the cancer has already spread to other parts of the body.

If diagnosed early in its development, it is usually possible to remove the tumour surgically – this is the procedure in about 20 per cent of cases. The surgery involves the partial or complete removal of the stomach, and removal of the surrounding lymph nodes to which the cancer can spread. Surgery may also be performed to

SIGNS AND SYMPTOMS

➤ Upper abdominal pain, which is indistinguishable from that caused by a peptic ulcer.

➤ Pain in the stomach after eating.

➤ Nausea and vomiting.

➤ Loss of appetite.

➤ Weight loss.

relieve symptoms where the cancer has spread to other areas of the body. Patients are usually given a course of chemotherapy and radiotherapy to control the growth of the tumour and to delay the development of the disease. Strong pain relief may also be necessary.

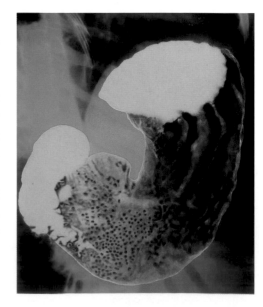

▽ A contrast X-ray shows up the structure of the stomach and can reveal the presence of a tumour – this image shows a healthy stomach.

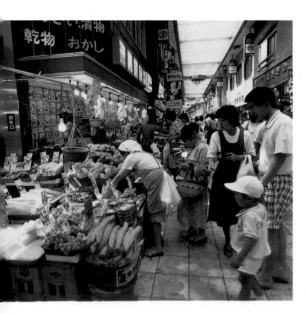

◁ Dietary habits may explain the high levels of stomach cancer in China and Japan – specifically raw fish and smoked, salty and pickled foods.

Pancreatitis

SEE ALSO
➤ Sensible drinking, p22
➤ Disorders of the liver, p54
➤ Diabetes, p66

Inflammation of the pancreas is an uncommon disorder which may occur suddenly (acute pancreatitis) or develop over a long period of time (chronic pancreatitis). Once it has become inflamed, the pancreas releases its digestive enzymes into the abdominal cavity, rather than into the small intestine. These powerful chemicals then start to digest nearby tissues, causing severe pain, fever and vomiting. The condition can be fatal – in the very worst cases, one in five patients dies – but most people recover with time and treatment.

Acute pancreatitis may be caused by gallstones, alcohol abuse, certain drugs (such as diuretic drugs) and, rarely, viruses. In most cases no obvious cause can be found. The progressive loss of function seen in chronic inflammation of the pancreas is usually a consequence of the long-term abuse of alcohol.

WHAT MIGHT YOUR DOCTOR DO?

Your doctor may suspect pancreatitis from hearing your symptoms and may take a sample of blood for testing. Occasionally, as needed, you will be referred for an abdominal ultrasound or a CT scan. Blood tests to determine blood sugar levels may be carried out.

Treatment focuses on relieving pain and other symptoms. You may need to be treated in hospital and given intravenous fluids and antibiotics to fight infections. Once the acute attack has settled, the underlying cause can be treated. For example, if a gallstone was the cause, you will usually need to have your gallbladder removed, and you may have to abstain from drinking alcohol.

Repeated attacks can seriously damage the pancreas, which ultimately affects both its digestive functions (leading to poor digestion of food) and its hormonal functions (resulting in diabetes). You may need to take enzyme supplements, and will require insulin treatment if diabetes occurs.

SIGNS AND SYMPTOMS
➤ Severe pain in the upper abdomen, which is often more severe when the patient moves.

➤ Fever.

➤ Nausea and vomiting.

➤ Bruised appearance of the skin of the abdomen.

In cases of acute pancreatitis, symptoms appear suddenly and may be severe. Symptoms of chronic pancreatitis develop gradually. In many cases people only notice their symptoms in the later stages of the disease.

Cancer of the pancreas

SEE ALSO
➤ Eat healthily, p14

Pancreatic cancer is a rare cancer that often produces no symptoms until it is well advanced. Doctors do not know the exact cause but it has been linked with diet, particularly diets high in fatty foods and low in fibre. Smoking may also be a contributory factor.

If your doctor suspects pancreatic cancer, from taking a medical history and an abdominal examination, he or she will refer you for a CT scan to check if there is a tumour. Pancreatic cancer spreads rapidly. Surgery to remove the whole tumour is rarely possible and other treatments tend not to be successful.

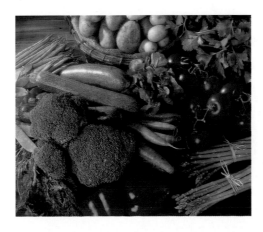

▷ A high-fibre diet that is rich in fruits and vegetables helps to protect against the risk of many cancers, including pancreatic cancer.

SIGNS AND SYMPTOMS
➤ Abdominal pain.

➤ Weight loss.

➤ Yellowing of the skin and the whites of the eyes (jaundice), which is caused by the fact that a cancer in the pancreas can block the bile duct and the flow of bile.

Disorders of the liver

The liver is an amazing organ that performs a wide variety of biochemical functions. It is the body's chemical factory and it has a great ability to heal itself when damaged. The liver must be severely damaged before its function is affected but when it does fail, there are serious and life-threatening consequences. This organ responds to most damage in the same way: initially there are signs of jaundice, then the liver becomes inflamed (a condition known as hepatitis) and, if the damage persists, scar tissue forms in the liver (cirrhosis).

WHAT DOES THE LIVER DO?

The liver has a range of vital biochemical functions which include:

➤ Producing blood proteins and controlling blood sugar levels.

➤ Regulating the transport of fat around the body.

➤ Manufacturing bile.

➤ Removing hormones, drugs and toxins from the blood

➤ Playing a part in the immune system.

HEPATITIS

Hepatitis, or inflammation of the liver, is usually caused by bacteria, viruses and parasites. Hepatitis viruses A, B, C, D and E – are often responsible. These viruses have features in common but vary in the ways they are spread and in their long-term effects. Hepatitis A is the most common cause of hepatitis, followed by hepatitis B.

• Hepatitis A – This is often an epidemic that is spread by mouth, usually by eating contaminated food. The virus causes fever, jaundice, abdominal discomfort and tiredness, which subside over a period of three to six weeks. Long-term effects are rare and no treatment is needed. A vaccine is available for those going to affected areas.

• Hepatitis B – This virus causes a more serious infection and it is transmitted via contaminated blood or needles and by sexual intercourse, particularly among homosexual men. Symptoms may be similar to hepatitis A but many cases show no symptoms. Most people recover, but a few die from acute liver failure. The disease can persist and the patient can become a carrier and infect other people.

• Hepatitis C, and particularly D and E viruses are rarer causes of hepatitis.

THE STRUCTURE OF THE LIVER

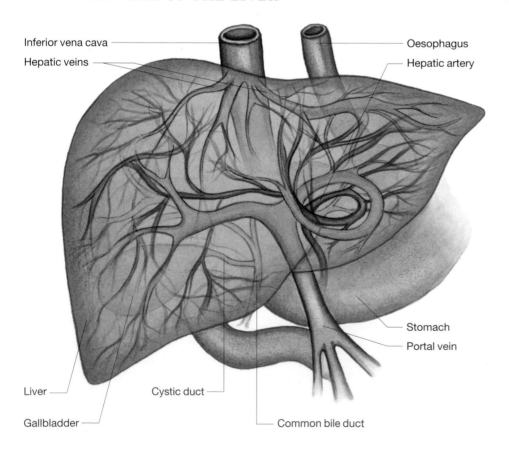

Inferior vena cava
Hepatic veins
Oesophagus
Hepatic artery
Stomach
Portal vein
Liver
Cystic duct
Gallbladder
Common bile duct

◁ The liver acts as a detoxification unit. Blood is sent from the aorta for cleansing via the hepatic artery. It is released into the hepatic veins, which drain into a central vein (inferior vena cava). The liver receives nutrient-rich blood from the small intestine (via the portal vein). The liver also makes bile, which is stored in the gallbladder. When needed for digestion bile is sent via the cystic and common bile ducts to the duodenum.

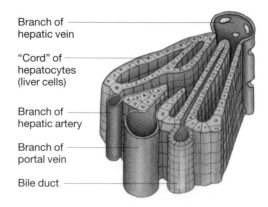

Branch of hepatic vein
"Cord" of hepatocytes (liver cells)
Branch of hepatic artery
Branch of portal vein
Bile duct

△ A section of the liver, served by a branch of the portal vein, hepatic artery and bile duct.

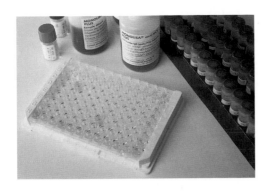

△ In this test for hepatitis C, blood has been added to substances produced by the virus. Infected blood contains antibodies that react with these viral substances – an enzyme has been added so that the sample turns yellow if such a reaction occurs. This test is positive.

A blood test will confirm which type of hepatitis virus is present, and specific antiviral agents are then given to treat the different forms. There are excellent vaccines available for hepatitis A and B that are used both to prevent infection if a person is exposed to the virus and to give lifelong protection to at-risk groups, such as healthcare workers.

ALCOHOLIC LIVER DISEASE

The commonest cause of long-term liver disease in the developed world is excessive alcohol consumption. Excess alcohol can cause permanent damage to body organs.

The liver rapidly removes alcohol from the bloodstream, but if there is too much alcohol the liver cells can become damaged and die. Excess alcohol leads to hepatitis at first, followed by scarring or cirrhosis and

PARACETAMOL OVERDOSE

Many drugs may adversely affect the liver, but one of the most dangerous is paracetamol. Even a small overdose of as little as 15 paracetomol tablets can be fatal. There is an antidote, but it must be administered within eight hours of the overdose to be most effective. If treatment fails, liver failure can occur, leading to coma and death.

eventually to liver failure and death. This process can take many years, even in very heavy drinkers, and if the alcohol abuse stops the liver can recover to some extent. Damage is more likely to occur in those people who drink to excess on a regular basis rather than occasional binge drinkers. It is also more common in men.

A doctor can diagnose alcoholic liver disease based on a person's medical history and liver function blood tests. The only treatment is to abstain from alcohol.

GALLSTONES

Bile is produced in the liver and then stored and made more concentrated in the gallbladder. The gallbladder contracts in response to a fatty meal and releases bile to break up fats during digestion. Bile pigments give faeces their brown colour.

Stones formed from cholesterol and bile can develop in the gallbladder. Up to 20 per cent of the population have gallstones, which most commonly affect those over 40. Often a person will have more than one stone at a time.

In most cases, gallstones cause few problems, but in severe cases they can block the exit of the gallbladder or the bile duct (a tube that carries bile to the small intestine) and stop the flow of bile. Bile can cause the gallbladder to become inflamed and infected – a condition known as

▽ Many gallstones are very small and cause no symptoms, but some are as large as golfballs. This stone is about 2 cm (¾ in) in diameter.

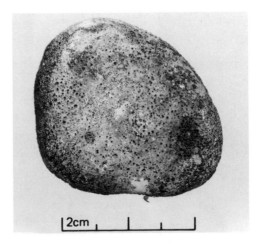

2cm

CAUSES OF JAUNDICE

In jaundice, there are high levels of bilirubin (the breakdown product of red blood cells), and this is what causes the skin and whites of the eyes to turn yellow. High bilirubin levels can be due to a number of factors:

➤ Excessive red blood cell destruction, such as in haemolytic anaemia.

➤ Liver damage, such as cirrhosis.

➤ Bile duct obstruction, such as from gallstones or pancreatic cancer.

▽ Damage to the liver can lead to jaundice, where the whites of the eyes turn yellow.

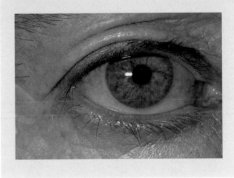

cholecystitis – which causes pain under the ribs on the right-hand side, particularly after a fatty meal.

If a gallstone is forced into the bile duct, it can cause great spasms of pain. A blocked duct may also cause pancreatitis (inflammation of the pancreas). If the stone blocks the flow of bile it can cause jaundice. The stools may also become very pale and hard to flush away, due to undigested fat.

If gallstones start causing problems and the gallbladder stops working properly, the removal of the gallbladder and its stones is the only treatment. A gallbladder cannot recover once it stops functioning correctly, and you can manage without one. Removal of the gallbladder, a procedure known as cholecystectomy, is usually carried out via keyhole techniques and involves only a short stay in hospital. The bile duct usually expands after the operation to form a new storage area for bile.

Coeliac disease

SEE ALSO
➤ The process of
   digestion, p44
➤ Diabetes, p66

People with coeliac disease have an allergy to a protein found in gluten. Gluten is present in wheat, rye, barley and oats and their products. In those affected, the lining of the small intestine becomes inflamed and flattened as the finger-like projections (villi) responsible for absorbing nutrients are destroyed. Exactly how the damage is caused is not known, but the only real solution is to avoid gluten by following a strict diet. Most people find that their symptoms improve rapidly and may disappear altogether if they continue with a gluten-free diet.

SIGNS AND SYMPTOMS
➤ Abdominal bloating.

➤ Weight loss.

➤ Loose, foul-smelling stools.

➤ Sometimes, a skin rash.

➤ In children, normal growth patterns are affected.

It may be difficult for a doctor to diagnose the disease because the symptoms are vague.

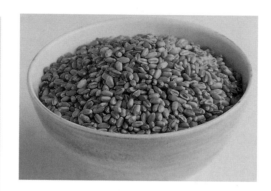

The symptoms of coeliac disease can often be vague and similar to other conditions and so doctors often find it difficult to diagnose the disorder.

◁ Wheat is one of the main foodstuffs to avoid on a gluten-free diet, but other cereals such as oats, corn, rice and millet contain gluten too.

WHAT MIGHT YOUR DOCTOR DO?
Your doctor can confirm a diagnosis by taking a sample of blood and sending it for tests, and by taking a biopsy sample from the jejunum (the middle section of the small intestine) for investigation.

If coeliac disease remains untreated, a range of related conditions can develop and there is also thought to be a higher risk of diabetes and cancer.

Appendicitis

SEE ALSO
➤ The process of
   digestion, p44

The appendix is a thin sac at the end of the first part of the large intestine, the caecum. In appendicitis, it becomes inflamed and infected. If it is left untreated, it could burst and can be life-threatening. The cause is not always obvious, but it can result from a blockage.

If your doctor suspects appendicitis, you will be referred immediately for hospital treatment. The appendix is removed in an operation called an appendicectomy, which can be performed by keyhole surgery.

There are a range of other conditions that have symptoms similar to those of early appendicitis. To avoid the risk of unnecessary surgery, most surgeons will often observe the patient for a few hours. If the signs and symptoms worsen, then the appendix is swiftly removed. If the patient remains stable or improves, an operation is not thought to be necessary.

POSITION OF THE APPENDIX

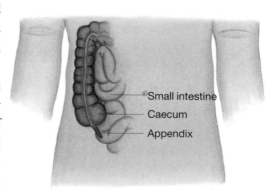

Small intestine

Caecum

Appendix

△ The actual function of the appendix is not clear. In rabbits it is used to store bacteria to digest cellulose, but in humans it is redundant.

SIGNS AND SYMPTOMS
➤ Nausea and vomiting.

➤ Diarrhoea.

➤ A mild fever.

➤ Loss of appetite.

➤ Initially, the pain will be around the navel area.

➤ Later, tenderness will develop on the right-hand side of the abdomen.

Irritable bowel syndrome

SEE ALSO
➤ Eat healthily, p14
➤ Digestive disorders, p46
➤ Endoscopy, p47

Irritable bowel syndrome, or IBS, is a common and poorly understood condition. It is twice as likely to affect women as men, and usually develops between the ages of 20 and 30. It has been given different names, including spastic colon, over the years and is probably the result of abnormal functioning of the large intestine. The large intestine regularly contracts along its length to empty itself during defecation. If this contraction occurs at other times in an uncoordinated manner, it may cause abdominal pain and other symptoms of IBS.

SIGNS AND SYMPTOMS
➤ Colicky abdominal pain, which is often eased by defecation.

➤ Abdominal bloating, also eased by defecation.

➤ Alternating hard and very soft motions.

➤ Flatulence.

Irritable bowel syndrome symptoms tend to come and go and will usually persist for many years.

The symptoms of IBS are often made much worse by stress or depression. There is also evidence that if you suffered from abdominal pain as a child you are more likely to develop IBS in adulthood.

INVESTIGATING IBS
Unfortunately, there is no definitive test for diagnosing IBS and any investigations tend to be aimed at ruling out other more serious conditions that share similar symptoms. The number of tests you are given will depend on your symptoms and your age. The tests may range from simple blood tests to a comprehensive examination of the large intestine with the help of contrast X-rays and endoscopy.

TREATMENT OPTIONS
Many people with IBS respond well if they are put on to high-fibre diets that include plenty of wholemeal bread, cereals and vegetables. Other treatments include antispasmodic drugs to reduce the spasm of the large intestine. Psychological treatment may also help some people. In the most severe cases, the debilitating symptoms of IBS can cause depression and may be treated with appropriate antidepressant medicines.

Diverticular disease

SEE ALSO
➤ Colonscopy, p59

In diverticular disease, diverticula (small, blind-ended sacs or pouches) form at the side of the large intestine. These develop when part of the intestinal wall bulges outwards through a weakened area. This condition affects one-third of people in the West by the time they are 50.

SIGNS AND SYMPTOMS
➤ Bright red blood from the rectum.

➤ Bouts of diarrhoea and constipation.

➤ Pain on the left-hand side of the abdomen, which is relieved by a bowel movement.

➤ If the diverticula become inflamed – diverticulitis – there will be severe pain and tenderness in the lower abdomen.

Diverticula are associated with a low-fibre diet. Most diverticula cause no problems and three-quarters of those with the condition do not realize that they have it. Occasionally the diverticula become blocked and infected – a condition known as diverticulitis. If they perforate or burst, they lead to a severe form of peritonitis.

DIAGNOSING DIVERTICULAR DISEASE
The diagnosis may be obvious from the symptoms but is often confirmed by a barium enema. Your doctor may also refer you for a colonoscopy, in which the colon is examined by means of a flexible tube with a camera attached. CT or ultrasound scanning are also sometimes used.

TREATMENT OPTIONS
A high-fibre diet can minimize the symptoms. Antispasmodic drugs may be prescribed to relieve abdominal pain. Most attacks of diverticulitis settle with antibiotics and a fluid-only diet to rest the intestines. But if you have more than three or four attacks in a year, surgery to remove a section of intestine may be necessary.

Colorectal cancer

Doctors do not know why the colon and rectum are affected so much by cancer – colorectal cancer is one of the most common tumours in the developed world. It rarely affects people under the age of 40, but the incidence increases with age and most people with this condition are over 60. Most large intestinal cancers occur in the very end of the colon (the sigmoid colon) or in the rectum, which is why a rectal examination is so important. Although they can run in families, 90 per cent of colorectal cancers occur in people without a strong family history.

Medical researchers have identified a number of risk factors in connection with colorectal cancers, which include:

• Diet – Diets high in animal fat and low in fibre increase the risk of colorectal cancer. The disease is rare in countries where a high-fibre diet is the norm.

• Ulcerative colitis – People affected by this inflammatory bowel disease have an increased risk of colorectal cancer.

• Familial polyposis coli – This inherited

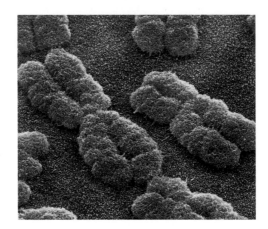

◁ Human chromosones hold the key to one in ten cases of colorectal cancers. Tests may soon be available to pinpoint those at risk.

condition causes the formation of fleshy growths called polyps in the large intestine. These polyps tend to become cancerous and people with this condition have regular examinations by endoscopy to check their intestinal health.

• Genetics – The genetic changes in DNA that lead to colorectal cancer are now well understood. For tissue to transform from normal to cancerous, a chain of events has to occur. Some links in the chain are inherited, making members of some families more prone to colorectal cancer. Tests are being developed to pick up these genetic changes and find out who is most at risk. Aspirin and other anti-inflammatory drugs may offer some protection from colorectal cancer.

THE STRUCTURE OF THE COLON

▽ The colon is a tube that absorbs water from food remains and compacts faeces. It divides into four parts: ascending (moving up the right of the abdomen), transverse (crossing to the left), descending (moving down the body) and the sigmoid colon (which meets the rectum). Doctors can examine the colon with tubes called sigmoidoscopes and colonoscopes.

WHEN TO SEE YOUR DOCTOR

If you notice a sudden and persistent change in your bowel habit, blood or mucus in the stools and/or regular abdominal pain,

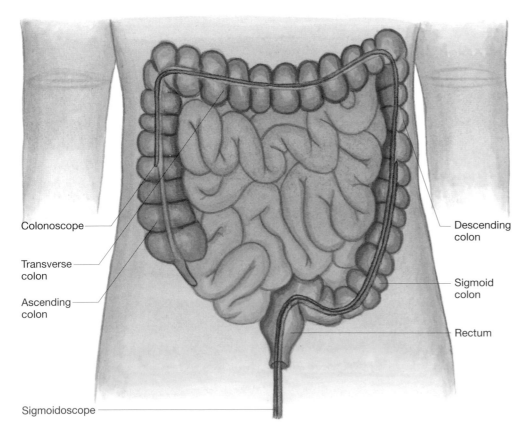

Colonoscope

Transverse colon

Ascending colon

Sigmoidoscope

Descending colon

Sigmoid colon

Rectum

SIGNS AND SYMPTOMS

➤ Abdominal pain.

➤ Change of bowel habit.

➤ Passage of blood or slime with the stool.

➤ Loss of appetite.

➤ Rectal discomfort or a feeling of fullness after defecation.

you should make an appointment to see your doctor. Another symptom is the feeling that the rectum has not emptied properly after defecation.

Like many cancers, colorectal cancer is curable if it is diagnosed early enough, so prompt investigation of any symptoms is very important.

INVESTIGATING COLORECTAL CANCER

Colorectal cancer can be picked up before any symptoms appear by screening. If you visit your doctor with symptoms, you will probably have an abdominal examination where your doctor will examine your rectum using a gloved finger. You will be asked for a stool sample, which will be tested for the presence of blood.

Your doctor is likely to refer you to a hospital for a series of tests such as a sigmoidoscopy (which involves a flexible tube being passed through the rectum to allow examination of the sigmoid colon) together with a contrast X-ray, or a colonoscopy (which involves a flexible endoscope being passed around the entire length of the colon). In both of these cases, the whole of the large intestine can be examined for evidence of tumours.

During an endoscopy, a biopsy sample of tissue can be taken and tested in a

▽ This coloured contrast X-ray shows a cancer in the colon, highlighted in red.

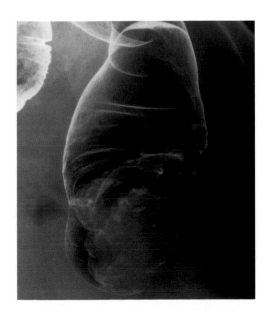

SCREENING FOR COLORECTAL CANCER

Colorectal cancer can be picked up early using specific screening tests. Testing for blood in the faeces (known as a faecal occult blood test) is now done routinely (over the age of 50) in the United States and Australia. The opinion of doctors is divided over this test because it has a high false-positive rate – that is, blood in the faeces is very often an indication of a non-cancerous condition. It is therefore recommended that people with a strong family history or other known risk factors for the disease undergo regular colonoscopy to survey the large intestine from an earlier age.

laboratory for signs of cancer. If cancer is confirmed, a CT scan will usually be performed to check how far the cancer extends and whether it has already spread to other parts of the body.

PROCEDURE FOR A COLONOSCOPY

↓

The day before the procedure, you will be given laxatives to empty the bowels. A sedative or anaesthetic may also be given intravenously just before the procedure.

↓

The colonoscope, a narrow, flexible tube with a camera attached to its tip, is then inserted into the rectum and guided around the colon.

↓

Images from the camera are displayed on a monitor, allowing a specialist to guide the instrument to see any areas of abnormality. A biopsy sample may be taken for further investigation.

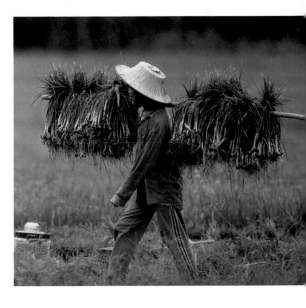

△ In many Asian countries, people live closer to the land and eat high-fibre diets that help protect against colorectal cancer.

TREATMENT OPTIONS

If colorectal cancer occurs, the only chance of a cure is to remove the entire tumour at an early stage. The affected area of the large intestine is removed (a procedure known as a colectomy) and the two free ends joined together. In most cases, surgeons rejoin the two ends of the bowel but sometimes the bowel may be brought up to the abdominal wall to create a temporary opening through which faeces can pass – this is known as a colostomy. Not all colostomies are permanent – some may be done as a temporary measure before the bowel is rejoined in a second operation.

If the cancer is limited to the intestinal wall, more than 90 per cent of people remain free from cancer five years after treatment. If the cancer has spread to the lymph nodes, especially to those within the liver, the survival rate is much lower.

In recent years chemotherapy has prolonged life in advanced cases, but surgery is still the best option. The sooner the operation is carried out, the better the chance of survival. Studies have shown that the biggest time delay in treating colorectal cancer is the time the person spends wondering whether or not to visit the doctor. If you have suspicious symptoms do not delay – see your doctor at once.

Crohn's disease

SEE ALSO
➤ Smoking and your health, p20
➤ Digestive disorders p46
➤ Ankylosing spondylitis, p116

Crohn's disease is a type of inflammatory bowel disease that causes swelling through the whole thickness of the wall of the digestive tract. Over time, this wall becomes thickened and scarred, and a narrowing may form. Crohn's disease can affect any part of the digestive tract from mouth to anus, although it often affects the last part of the small intestine (ileum) and the large intestine (colon). The cause is unknown, although it tends to run in families and smokers are three times more likely than non-smokers to develop the disease.

SIGNS AND SYMPTOMS
➤ Abdominal pain.

➤ Diarrhoea, sometimes with blood.

➤ Fever.

➤ Generally feeling unwell.

➤ Weight loss.

Crohn's disease occurs worldwide but it is more common in the West, where it particularly affects those of Jewish origin. It usually occurs in people between the ages of 15 and 40 and affects both men and women equally. There is no actual cure for the disease, which produces episodic attacks of symptoms with periods of remission in between. However, symptoms can usually be brought under control with drugs.

▽ Contrast X-rays are an effective way of highlighting any abnormalities in the digestive tract, and are helpful in the diagnosis of Crohn's disease.

WHAT MIGHT YOUR DOCTOR DO?
If you visit your doctor with the typical symptoms of Crohn's disease, he or she will check your mouth for ulcers and feel your abdomen, although these may show nothing out of the ordinary. Your doctor may take a sample of blood to do a full blood count, to show the level of inflammation and to check levels of iron, folic acid and vitamin B_{12}. You may also have to supply a stool sample.

You are likely to be referred to hospital for further tests including a colonoscopy, in which a flexible tube is passed through the anus and rectum and used to inspect the length of the colon. Biopsy samples of tissue may be taken. A contrast X-ray may also be performed.

MANAGING CROHN'S DISEASE
If your attacks are relatively mild, you may be treated with standard antidiarrhoeal drugs such as loperamide or codeine. Anti-inflammatory steroid drugs (given as tablets or enemas) and immunosuppressant drugs are the mainstay of treatment. Severe attacks often require hospitalization.

Elemental diets, which contain simple, easily digested nutrients and so serve to rest the digestive tract, may be recommended. Following this type of diet for six weeks can settle an attack of Crohn's; unfortunately, such diets are expensive and unpalatable.

Between 70 and 80 per cent of people with Crohn's disease need surgery, either to

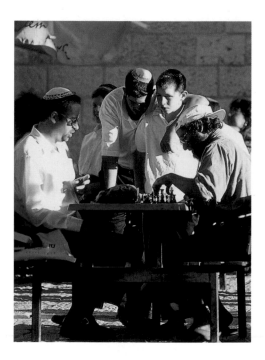

△ Studies show that people of Jewish origin are particularly susceptible to Crohn's disease, but the cause of the condition remains unknown.

remove an affected area not responding to drugs or to remove a narrowing that is causing a blockage. Because many operations may be needed during a person's lifetime, surgery is kept to the absolute minimum to preserve as much of the digestive tract as possible.

Fortunately, attacks of Crohn's disease usually settle down and most people do not need to take any drugs between attacks and can lead normal lives. About ten per cent of people with Crohn's disease will develop other associated disorders. These include a form of arthritis known as ankylosing spondylitis, kidney stones, gallstones, conjunctivitis and skin rashes such as *erythema nodosum*.

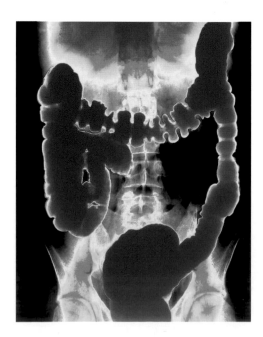

Ulcerative colitis

This type of inflammatory bowel disease affects only the large intestine – that is, the colon and the rectum. The disease often starts in the rectum and then spreads into the colon. The cause is unknown, but ulcerative colitis results in inflammation of the lining of the large intestine, which then breaks down or ulcerates, and bleeds. Ulcerative colitis usually starts between the ages of 20 and 40, and is more likely to affect women than men. As with Crohn's disease, ulcerative colitis tends to occur in distinct attacks with symptom-free periods.

SIGNS AND SYMPTOMS

➤ Diarrhoea with blood and mucus in the stools.

➤ Abdominal pain.

➤ Fatigue.

As in Crohn's disease, severe cases of ulcerative colitis can also affect:

➤ The skin – producing a rash such as *erythema nodosum*.

➤ The eyes – causing conjunctivitis.

➤ The liver – causing fatty deposits.

➤ The kidney – causing kidney stones.

➤ The gallbladder – causing gallstones.

➤ The joints – causing types of arthritis such as ankylosing spondylitis.

Most people with ulcerative colitis take a drug called 5-ASA to minimize the number of attacks and induce remission. Immunosuppressants are sometimes needed. In severe cases, steroids may be given. If drug therapy fails, affected areas of the colon can be removed. In some cases, the whole colon will be removed so that the intestine ends at the ileum (the final part of the small intestine). The surgeon then redirects the ileum into an artificial opening in the abdomen. A bag is attached to this opening, so the bowel contents can be drained.

Surgeons now try to form a new storage pouch from the ileum and connect this to the end of the rectum. This means patients go to the toilet as normal, although motions are looser. However, this does leave a small part of the colon behind, which may be affected by ulcerative colitis in the future.

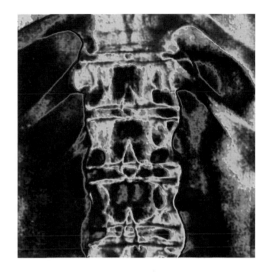

△ This X-ray shows a spine in which the vertebrae have fused together. This is the result of ankylosing spondylitis, which is an inflammatory arthritic condition that can be associated with ulcerative colitis.

COMPLICATIONS

Both Crohn's disease and ulcerative colitis may lead to serious complications.

➤ Perforation – A hole can form in the wall of the digestive tract so the contents of the bowel leak out, causing peritonitis, an inflammation of the abdominal cavity lining.

➤ Toxic dilatation – The large intestine can expand, like a balloon, and then burst. If the ballooning fails to settle, the affected area must be removed. Toxic dilatation is most likely to occur in ulcerative colitis.

➤ Colorectal cancer – Ulcerative colitis increases the risk significantly and so those affected are monitored closely.

HOW A COLECTOMY IS CARRIED OUT

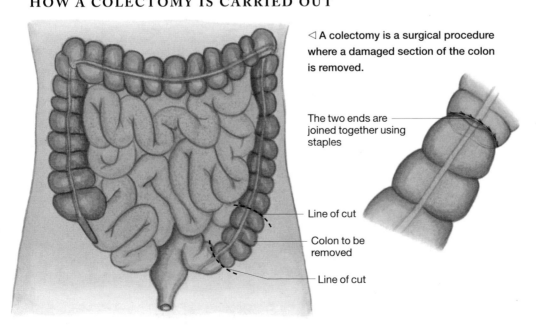

◁ A colectomy is a surgical procedure where a damaged section of the colon is removed.

The two ends are joined together using staples

Line of cut

Colon to be removed

Line of cut

Anorectal disorders

SEE ALSO

➤ Eat healthily, p14
➤ The process of digestion, p44

Many people suffer from an anorectal disorder at some point in their lives. Piles are a particularly common problem – up to 50 per cent of us will suffer from them. Fortunately, disorders that occur around the anus tend not to be serious and are easily treated. Fresh blood in the stool or on the toilet tissue after wiping is almost always due to piles or one of the other conditions below. However, it can be a sign of more serious disorders, so it is extremely important to visit your doctor promptly for a diagnosis if you notice bleeding.

HAEMORRHOIDS

Haemorrhoids or piles are very common. They are due to swollen veins in the anus and rectum, and occasionally these veins can be forced out of the anus. Straining to pass hard stools – often the result of a low-fibre diet – can be the cause. Piles are the most common reason for rectal bleeding.

Piles do not usually hurt, but if a blood clot forms in them they can be extremely painful. Most cases of piles disappear if you eat a high-fibre diet and use soothing anal ointments. Larger more troublesome piles can be destroyed by cutting off their blood supply at the base of the pile with injections and elastic bands.

ANAL ABSCESSES

Mucus-secreting glands around the anus can become infected, and a painful abscess (collection of pus) may form. Anal sex increases the risk of these abscesses.

Antibiotics often fail to cure the infection and many abscesses have to be drained of pus surgically, which is done under a general anaesthetic.

FISTULA

Sometimes an infected anal gland can burst on to the skin and into the anal canal to form an abnormal passage between the inside of the anus and the skin. Unfortunately these passages, known as fistulas, often fail to heal and have to be surgically removed.

ANAL FISSURE

It is quite common for the lining of the anus to tear, such as during the passage of hard faeces. Such tears usually heal. If they are very large, however, they can be pulled apart by the anal sphincter muscle and fail to heal, causing persistent anal bleeding and pain on defecation.

△ Doing pelvic yoga exercises is believed to help protect against anorectal disorders and may be helpful for easing an existing complaint.

A nitrate cream is applied to relax the sphincter muscle and allow the fissure to heal. If this fails an operation is performed to gently weaken the sphincter muscle without affecting control of defecation.

PILONIDAL SINUS

The hair follicles in the cleft between your buttocks can become infected and break down to form an abscess. These abscesses (pilonidal sinuses) do not heal and need to be removed surgically.

REMOVING LARGE HAEMORRHOIDS

▽ The treatment of large haemorrhoids is a straightforward procedure. The doctor passes a short tube (a proctoscope) into the rectum, then grasps the haemorrhoid using forceps. A rubber band is attached to the base of the haemorrhoid, which eventually drops off.

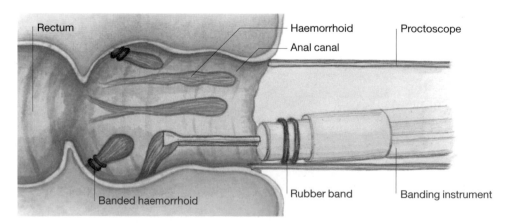

Rectum

Haemorrhoid

Anal canal

Proctoscope

Banded haemorrhoid

Rubber band

Banding instrument

UNEXPLAINED ITCHING

Pruritus ani is anal itching that has no obvious cause but which can be related to poor hygiene, piles or threadworm infestation. The itching makes you want to scratch, which in turn makes the itching worse. Most cases settle if the anus is kept clean and dry, and by avoiding touching the skin. After washing, the anus should be blotted dry (or dried with a hairdryer), not wiped.

4

THE HORMONE SYSTEM

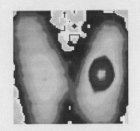

A whole family of hormones is responsible for maintaining constancy within your body's biochemical world. The word "hormone" derives from the Greek term meaning to impel or set in motion. All hormones are essentially chemical messengers that travel in the bloodstream to produce a bodily reaction, either specifically or generally. Occasionally, the glands which manufacture the hormones – known as endocrine glands – are affected by disease or malfunction in some way. Because hormones play such an important role in the functioning of every part of your body there is a wide range of potential endocrinological problems.

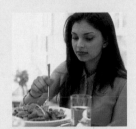

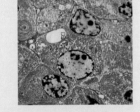

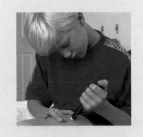

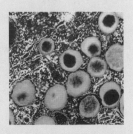

The endocrine glands

SEE ALSO
➤ The cardiovascular system, p28
➤ Diabetes, p66
➤ Diseases of the thyroid gland, p68

Hormones are manufactured by a number of endocrine glands found in different parts of the body. These specialized glands produce and secrete essential hormones which then travel through the bloodstream to their specific site, or sites, of action. For example the adrenal glands produce adrenaline, which affects the heart, brain, blood vessels, muscles, intestines and breathing. The major hormone-producing glands in the body are the pituitary, thyroid, parathyroid and adrenal glands, and the pancreas, ovaries and testes.

Many of the body's hormone-producing glands are controlled by the pituitary – a vital endocrine gland found just beneath the brain. Also called the "master gland", the pituitary produces stimulating factors that prompt other glands to release their hormones into the bloodstream. Disease of the pituitary can have widespread health effects.

A FINE BALANCE

The endocrine system is a complex web of finely tuned mechanisms. The diagram below shows just one aspect of this system – the control of blood sugar by the hormone insulin – in action. In general, things go wrong when these delicate mechanisms are disrupted in some way and the endocrine glands produce either too much (hyper-) or too little (hypo-) of a particular hormone. The most common cause of hormonal disorders is a non-cancerous growth called an adenoma. An adenoma can either block hormone production or it can overstimulate the gland so that it produces far too much.

GLUCAGON AND GLYCOGEN
Any excess glucose in the bloodstream is converted into glycogen so that it can be stored. The hormone glucagon breaks down the stores of glycogen into glucose so that it can be released as needed into the bloodstream.

DIAGNOSING PROBLEMS

Doctors analyse the levels of hormone in a person's bloodstream to compare it with normal values. Such tests also help to monitor hormone or drug therapy. Doctors also use imaging techniques, such as ultrasounds or CT scans, to check endocrine glands for signs of an adenoma.

TREATMENT OPTIONS

The most common endocrine disorders are diabetes mellitus (sugar diabetes) and an underactive thyroid (hypothyroidism). Other disorders are uncommon, and can be treated using one of the following options:
1 Replace or supplement the hormone.
2 Use drugs to block the action of excess amounts of hormone.
3 Remove the offending adenoma surgically or through radiotherapy.

▽ Negative feedback. To maintain correct hormone levels in the blood, the release of most hormones is controlled by a process called the negative feedback loop. This diagram shows how one loop controls our blood glucose levels.

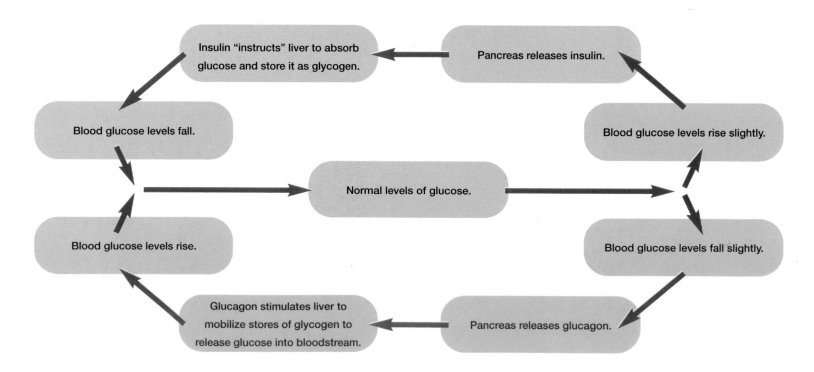

Insulin "instructs" liver to absorb glucose and store it as glycogen.

Pancreas releases insulin.

Blood glucose levels fall.

Blood glucose levels rise slightly.

Normal levels of glucose.

Blood glucose levels rise.

Blood glucose levels fall slightly.

Glucagon stimulates liver to mobilize stores of glycogen to release glucose into bloodstream.

Pancreas releases glucagon.

THE MAJOR ENDOCRINE GLANDS

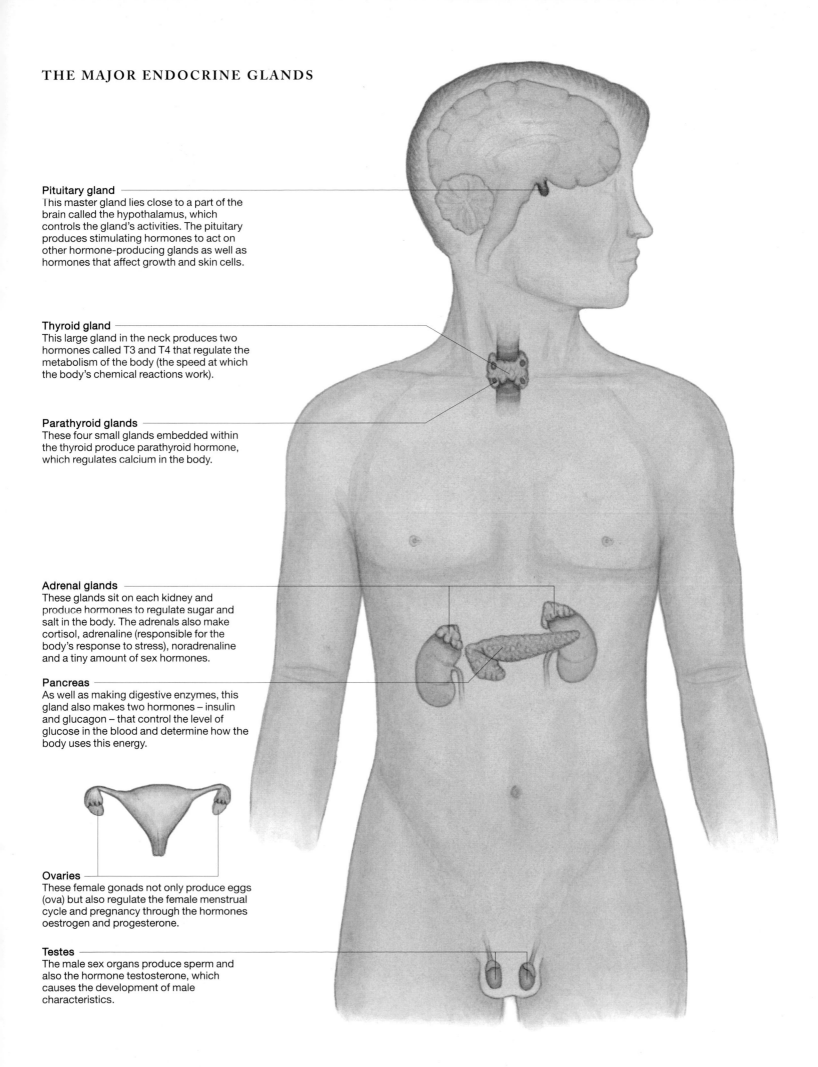

Pituitary gland
This master gland lies close to a part of the brain called the hypothalamus, which controls the gland's activities. The pituitary produces stimulating hormones to act on other hormone-producing glands as well as hormones that affect growth and skin cells.

Thyroid gland
This large gland in the neck produces two hormones called T3 and T4 that regulate the metabolism of the body (the speed at which the body's chemical reactions work).

Parathyroid glands
These four small glands embedded within the thyroid produce parathyroid hormone, which regulates calcium in the body.

Adrenal glands
These glands sit on each kidney and produce hormones to regulate sugar and salt in the body. The adrenals also make cortisol, adrenaline (responsible for the body's response to stress), noradrenaline and a tiny amount of sex hormones.

Pancreas
As well as making digestive enzymes, this gland also makes two hormones – insulin and glucagon – that control the level of glucose in the blood and determine how the body uses this energy.

Ovaries
These female gonads not only produce eggs (ova) but also regulate the female menstrual cycle and pregnancy through the hormones oestrogen and progesterone.

Testes
The male sex organs produce sperm and also the hormone testosterone, which causes the development of male characteristics.

Diabetes

Many people will know diabetes mellitus by its more common name, sugar diabetes. Diabetes results in chronically raised levels of blood sugar because of either a lack of the hormone insulin or of a resistance to it. It is a very common disease affecting 30 million people worldwide and is increasingly widespread in nations of the developed world. In the past, the outlook was fairly bleak for those with diabetes but now, with improved insulin formulations and other drugs to control its complications, people with diabetes have relatively normal and healthy lives.

The hormone insulin is manufactured by specialized cells in a tiny areas of the pancreas called the islets of Langherhans. Insulin makes it possible for every cell in the body to access the sugar glucose from the bloodstream as well as influencing the way in which the liver stores any temporary excesses. All sugars will eventually be converted to glucose, which is one of the body's main fuels.

TYPES OF DIABETES

There are two types of diabetes, known simply as type I and type II.

• Type I – In this form of diabetes the pancreas stops producing insulin or produces only small amounts. This condition usually starts in children and young adults, and mainly affects Europeans and North Americans. Approximately 1 person in 20 has type I diabetes. They will usually be very thin

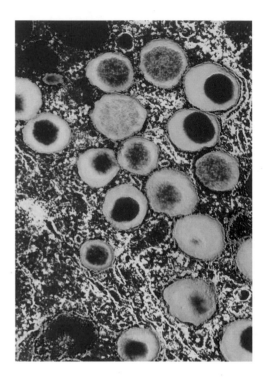

▷ This shows hormone-secreting cells in the islet of Langerhans area of the pancreas. The red circles are hormones (insulin or glucagon) ready to be released into the bloodstream.

SIGNS AND SYMPTOMS

The main symptoms of both type I and type II diabetes are listed below. Type I symptoms tend to develop faster.

➤ Thirst and a dry mouth.

➤ Excessive urination.

➤ Lethargy.

➤ Blurred vision.

➤ Poor-quality sleep because of the need for frequent trips to the toilet.

and will probably first visit their doctor with symptoms of passing a lot of urine (polyuria), thirst and weight loss.

• Type II – This form of diabetes occurs when the pancreas manufactures normal or even increased amounts of insulin but

COMPLICATIONS OF DIABETES

If you have diabetes, you will probably already be aware of its complications. Your doctor will ensure that you have check-ups for signs of these on a regular basis. People who manage their blood sugar levels efficiently will reduce the risk of complications but there are a number of other risk factors:

➤ Vascular disease – Diabetes accelerates the furring up of arteries (atherosclerosis), which makes people with the condition more likely to develop life-threatening complications such as angina, heart

attacks, strokes and gangrene of the foot. It is important to control or minimize any risk factors for atherosclerosis, including high blood pressure, high blood cholesterol levels and smoking.

➤ The nerves – Diabetes damages the small blood vessels supplying nerves. This can lead to a loss of feeling, especially in the feet. The skin of the feet can become damaged without the person knowing it and large ulcers, which do not heal well, can result.

➤ The eyes – Diabetic eye disease (retinopathy) is very common and all people

with diabetes should ensure that they have regular eye checks.

➤ The kidneys – The kidney's small blood vessels can become damaged, reducing the kidneys' ability to function. This damage shows up as protein in the urine, which can be detected with a simple dipstick test.

➤ Infections – People with diabetes, even those who control their blood sugar levels carefully, are prone to infections. The skin, kidneys, bladder and lungs are particularly vulnerable to infection.

the body becomes insensitive or resistant to its actions. Type II is the more common form of diabetes and tends to affect older people of all racial groups. It is sometimes referred to as adult-onset diabetes. (However, doctors are now detecting this type of diabetes in children in developed countries.) In contrast to type I, patients will tend to be overweight but other symptoms are the same in that they will urinate a lot and feel thirsty. Other than that, most patients will complain only of general feelings of tiredness and lethargy.

▽ Many people with type II diabetes can control their blood sugar levels by following a healthy diet and taking regular exercise.

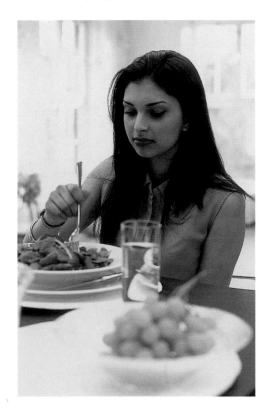

HOW IS IT DIAGNOSED?

First your doctor will want to ask about your symptoms and perhaps perform a physical examination. Usually, you will be asked to supply a urine sample, which can be tested with a simple dipstick while you wait in the doctor's surgery.

After testing a sample of urine for the presence of glucose, your doctor may also take a blood sample. This sample is sent to a laboratory to check its glucose levels. Normally, doctors would want two consecutive measurements to confirm a diagnosis. Such tests are also used to monitor and adjust ongoing treatments.

TREATMENT OPTIONS

All types of treatment aim to maintain glucose levels within a normal range, without too many swings (high or low). Lifelong dietary modification is always essential and may be combined, if necessary, with insulin injections or drug therapy.

• Diet – A good diabetic diet is no different from that considered healthy for everyone. It should be high in fruit and vegetables, low in fat and include complex carbohydrates (such as pasta, rice and bread). Complex carbohydrates release a steady stream of glucose (as do unrefined sugars found in fruit and vegetables) rather than the short-lived surges of glucose from refined sugars (found in sweets and biscuits). Some people with type II diabetes can control their blood glucose levels with diet alone.

• Drug therapy – There are many different types of tablets and they are designed to increase the amount of insulin produced or increase the person's sensitivity to insulin. People with type II diabetes may have to take one or more types of tablets.

• Insulin injections – All people with type I diabetes need regular insulin injections. Some people with type II diabetes also need insulin. Those injecting insulin usually take a long-acting form once or twice a day and a short-acting insulin at meal times. If someone injects too much insulin accidentally, it results in an

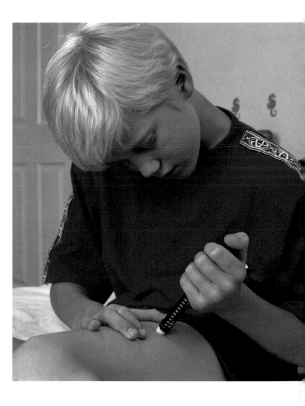

△ Children over a certain age are usually taught to inject insulin themselves. Most diabetics use insulin pens like this one, rather than a syringe.

extremely low blood sugar level, also known as hypoglycaemia. In this state, they become tired, sweaty and confused and may even fall unconscious. To reverse the hypoglycaemia, glucose is given urgently as a sweet, a drink or as an infusion into a vein.

Diseases of the thyroid gland

SEE ALSO

➤ The endocrine
  glands, p64
➤ Pituitary gland
  disorders, p72
➤ Bipolar affective
  disorder, p100

The thyroid gland sits at the front of the neck surrounding the windpipe (trachea). The thyroid hormones regulate the metabolic rate of many tissues. Diseases may cause the thyroid to under- or overproduce the two thyroid hormones called T3 and T4. The thyroid hormones are released into the bloodstream in response to a regulating hormone from the pituitary gland called thyroid-stimulating hormone (TSH). Thyroid disorders are common and often develop gradually. They may lie undetected for months or even years.

HYPOTHYROIDISM

This underactivity of the thyroid gland causes levels of T3 and T4 to be low, while TSH levels remain high.

WHAT CAUSES AN UNDERACTIVE THYROID GLAND?

There are many causes of hypothyroidism.

• Atrophic (autoimmune) hypothyroidism – This is the commonest cause in which the body's own immune system attacks and destroys the thyroid gland. Women are more commonly affected than men.

• Hashimoto's thyroiditis – An auto-immune disease where attacking antibodies cause the thyroid to become enlarged and tender.

• Iodine deficiency – This is common in mountainous areas with little iodine in the water or diet; the thyroid enlarges to form a goitre (see goitres box, opposite).

• Pituitary disease – An underactive pituitary gland will not produce enough

▷ This radionuclide scan of a thyroid shows a non-cancerous adenoma in the right-hand portion of the gland, seen as red and white.

TSH to stimulate the thyroid gland and so in turn causes hypothyroidism.

• Thyroid cancer – Rarely, a cancerous growth destroys the gland.

TREATMENT OPTIONS

Treatment replaces the thyroid hormones T3 and T4 with thyroxine tablets. A low dose is given at first and is then increased until the blood tests show normal levels of thyroid function. Determining the optimal dose is vital for successful treatment. Thyroxine has to be taken for life.

THYROID FUNCTION TESTS

To assess thyroid function, doctors take a sample of your blood and send it to a laboratory for detailed analysis. Such tests measure the levels of:

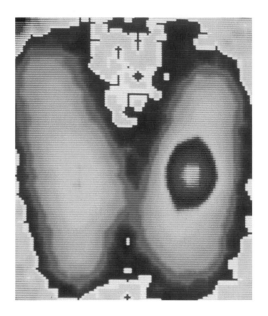

• The thyroid hormones T3 and T4.
• The pituitary hormone TSH.

These test results should enable your doctor to make a diagnosis or if necessary to advise other investigations, such as a radionuclide scan.

THE STRUCTURE OF THE THYROID GLAND

▷ The thyroid gland wraps around the windpipe (trachea) and the four parathyroid glands sit at the back of the thyroid.

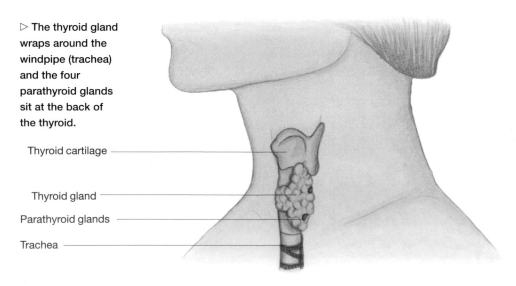

Thyroid cartilage

Thyroid gland

Parathyroid glands

Trachea

SIGNS AND SYMPTOMS OF HYPOTHYROIDISM

Hypothyroidism has various symptoms, many of which are "general". Typical symptoms are tiredness, intolerance of the cold, feeling depressed and gaining weight despite having no appetite.

You may have dry, thin hair, a slow pulse and a swelling in your neck. These are only a few of the features of this disease and doctors often do thyroid function blood tests when they are not sure of the diagnosis.

INVESTIGATING A LUMP IN THE THYROID

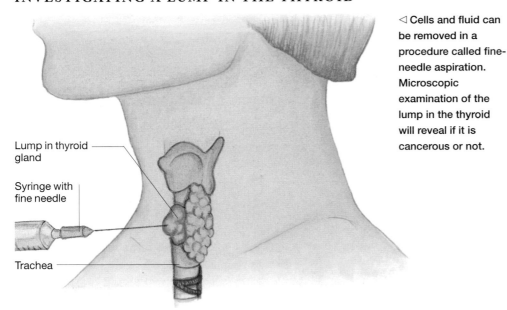

Lump in thyroid gland

Syringe with fine needle

Trachea

◁ Cells and fluid can be removed in a procedure called fine-needle aspiration. Microscopic examination of the lump in the thyroid will reveal if it is cancerous or not.

HYPERTHYROIDISM

An overactive thyroid is quite common and is again more often seen in women. The commonest cause is Grave's disease – an autoimmune disease in which attacking antibodies stimulate the thyroid to release T3 and T4 so their levels in the blood rise.

Rarely, a non-cancerous tumour (adenoma) or thyroid growth produces too much thyroid hormone. Rarer still, a non-cancerous pituitary tumour produces excess TSH, making the thyroid over-secrete.

TREATMENT OPTIONS

Once the cause has been investigated there are three possible options for the treatment of an overactive thyroid gland:

1 Anti-thyroid drugs that block the formation of thyroid hormones.
2 Radioactive iodine to reduce the amount of thyroid hormone produced (this is a sensitive treatment and can easily result in hypothyroidism).
3 Surgery to remove part of the thyroid gland is only an option if drugs fail or produce too many side-effects, or if the patient has a large goitre. It is not always successful and is considered the last resort.

THYROID CANCER

Cancers of the thyroid are rare and thyroid cancer has one of the highest treatment success rates. Treatments vary depending on the growth rate and nature of the cancer.

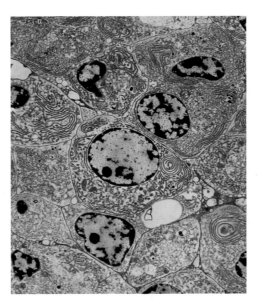

GOITRE (THYROID ENLARGEMENT)

Many diseases can cause goitre and some have already been mentioned, such as Grave's disease, Hashimoto's thyroiditis, iodine deficiency and thyroid cancer. The commonest type is multinodular goitre. This generally harmless condition is caused by the overgrowth of part of the thyroid gland. Goitre can also be a side-effect of lithium, a drug prescribed for people with bipolar affective disorder.

Goitres may produce low, normal or high levels of thyroid hormones, so doctors will often use a standard thyroid function blood test to measure the hormone levels. An ultrasound scan and fine-needle aspiration of the thyroid gland itself will determine the cause of the swelling and whether it is cancerous.

Surgery to remove the goitre is sometimes performed if the goitre is large and unsightly and, in rare cases, when it compresses the windpipe.

▽ The enlarged thyroid gland or goitre in this woman's neck is clearly visible. Most goitres are painless.

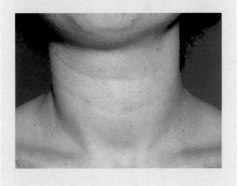

TREATMENT OPTIONS

Usually surgery to remove part or all of the thyroid gland is carried out. This procedure is called a thyroidectomy. If the thyroid gland is removed, and this usually offers the best chance of a cure, a patient will need lifelong thyroxine hormone replacement.

◁ This coloured photomicrograph shows cells taken from a cancerous thyroid. The rapidly-dividing cancer cells have abnormally large nuclei (seen in green).

Adrenal gland disorders

The two adrenal glands sit on fatty pads above the kidneys and consist of two parts – an outer cortex and an inner medulla. The adrenal cortex produces corticosteroid hormones (cortisol and aldosterone) that are involved in regulating sugar, salt and blood pressure; the medulla produces adrenaline and noradrenaline. Diseases occur if there is an insufficient level of a hormone (hypoadrenalism) or if any is present in excess (hyperadrenalism). A non-cancerous adenoma is often the cause of adrenal disorders, which on the whole are rare diseases.

THE STRUCTURE OF AN ADRENAL GLAND

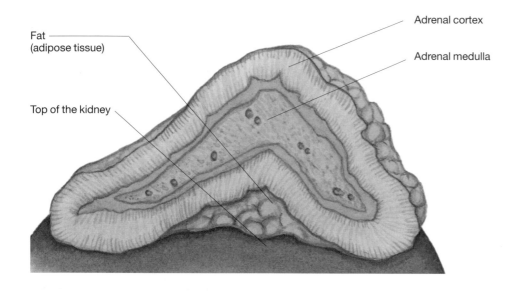

Fat (adipose tissue)

Top of the kidney

Adrenal cortex

Adrenal medulla

△ Located on top of your kidneys, your adrenal glands consist of two parts, each with its own definite functions.

SIGNS AND SYMPTOMS OF ADDISON'S SYNDROME

Symptoms tend to develop slowly and are often just a feeling of ill-health. Other symptoms you may experience include:

➤ Fatigue and weakness.

➤ Loss of appetite.

➤ Fever.

➤ Weight loss.

➤ Skin pigmentation – dark patches of skin on creases of palms, elbows and knees.

Your doctor may also discover you have low blood pressure (hypotension).

ADDISON'S SYNDROME

This is caused by an underactive adrenal gland (hypoadrenalism) and can be due to autoimmune conditions where the body produces antibodies that destroy the adrenal cortex. Rarer causes include HIV and AIDS, tuberculosis and hypopituitarism (underactive pituitary gland). Corticosteroid hormone production can be suppressed in someone taking long-term steroid therapy or who has undergone surgery.

Whatever the cause, the production of corticosteroid hormones in the cortex falls, upsetting the body's chemistry with dangerous consequences. Addison's syndrome is twice as common in women as in men and appears to run in families.

HOW IS IT TREATED?

Synthetic corticosteroids are often prescribed to substitute natural hormones. Occasionally patients have a severe shortage of salt and sugar in their urine and are dehydrated. Their blood pressure is very low and they fall unconscious. This "Addisonian crisis" can be fatal without rapid fluid and steroid replacement. People with Addison's syndrome should always carry a Medic-Alert bracelet, which gives details of their disease if they are found unconscious.

People who have been taking steroid drugs long term for other diseases can also have an Addisonian crisis if they stop their medication suddenly. It is always advisable to step down your dosage of steroids gradually. It is also recommended that you discuss any change in your medication with your doctor first.

▽ Addison's syndrome is twice as common in women as in men and very often the only symptom may be a vague feeling of ill-health.

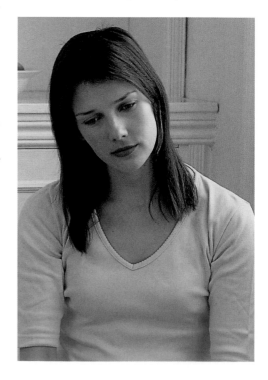

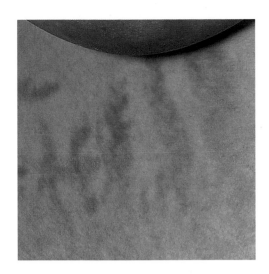

△ Excess levels of corticosteroid hormones in the blood (Cushing's syndrome) can cause streaky marks on the skin, seen here under the breast.

CUSHING'S SYNDROME

In stark contrast to its actions in Addison's syndrome, in Cushing's syndrome the adrenal cortex produces excessive corticosteroid hormones, causing a different upset in the body's chemistry. Cushing's syndrome is more common in women than in men and may be accompanied by depression and other psychological problems.

WHAT CAUSES IT?

It can be caused by an adrenal tumour or by excessive stimulation by adrenocorticotropic hormone (ACTH) from the pituitary gland; ACTH stimulates the adrenals to release their hormones. However, the most common cause is long-term steroid drug therapy. Steroid drugs mimic the action of the body's own adrenal hormones and so, when combined with natural levels, cause dramatically high corticosteroid levels in the body's circulation.

HOW IS CUSHING'S SYNDROME TREATED?

It is vital that Cushing's syndrome is treated as it could be fatal. If the condition is due to steroid drug therapy, your doctor will reassess your dosage or, if possible, discontinue treatment. If a tumour is the cause, your doctor can arrange for the affected gland to be removed surgically.

PHAEOCHROMOCYTOMA

The hormone adrenaline and its counterpart noradrenaline are produced within the adrenal medulla. Adrenaline and noradrenaline increase the heart beat and blood pressure in reaction to times of stress, exertion or fear. Phaeochromocytoma is a rare condition and it is caused by a non cancerous tumour that secretes far too much adrenaline and noradrenaline, and consequently your body behaves as if under constant state of agitation resulting in a variety of distressing symptoms.

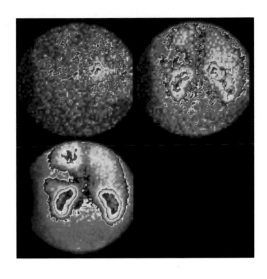

△ This coloured scan shows a tumour of the adrenal gland. The scans are made by injecting the patient with a radioactive "tracer" which shows up any abnormalities.

HYPERALDOSTERONISM (CONN'S SYNDROME)

The adrenal cortex produces the hormone aldosterone, which is involved in the regulation of salt balance and blood pressure. Overproduction of this hormone (known as hyperaldosteronism) results in an accumulation of salt within the body and a loss of the mineral potassium in urine.

Conn's syndrome is often caused by an adenoma in the cortex area of the adrenal gland. Signs and symptoms of hyperaldosteronism include:

➤ Muscle weakness and cramps.

➤ Frequent passage of large volumes of urine.

➤ Thirst.

➤ High blood pressure.

Treatment options include drugs to block the actions of the excessive hormone or removal of a tumour that may be prompting oversecretion.

SIGNS AND SYMPTOMS OF CUSHING'S SYNDROME

People with Cushing's syndrome (or those taking long-term steroids) may develop the following symptoms:

➤ Tiredness.

➤ Excessive facial hair.

➤ The face becomes rounder.

➤ Skin becomes thin and bruises easily.

➤ Tendency to become overweight.

➤ Streaky marks (striae) may develop on the skin.

➤ High blood pressure.

SIGNS AND SYMPTOMS OF PHAEOCHROMOCYTOMA

Physical exercise or heightened emotion can trigger the tumour to release hormones into the bloodstream and also produce typical symptoms such as:

➤ Palpitations.

➤ Nausea and vomiting.

➤ Intense anxiety.

➤ Headache.

➤ Pallid skin.

➤ Profuse sweating.

➤ High blood pressure.

TREATMENT OPTIONS

First, your doctor will treat you to normalize your blood pressure and then look at removing the offending tumour. Surgery is usually successful and people normally make a full recovery.

Pituitary gland disorders

SEE ALSO
➤ The endocrine glands, p64
➤ Cushing's syndrome, p71
➤ Meningitis, p84

The pituitary gland – often referred to as the "master gland" – sits at the base of the brain. It produces many hormones – both releasing factors to stimulate other organs to secrete their hormones and hormones that directly affect the body. Most pituitary disorders are the result of non-cancerous tumours (adenomas) that change the amounts of hormones that the gland produces. Adenomas that secrete growth hormone, adrenocorticotropic hormone (ACTH, for short) and prolactin are the most commonly encountered.

HYPOPITUITARISM

An underactive pituitary gland can affect one or many of the hormones that the pituitary produces. It can be caused by:
• A non-cancerous tumour.
• Infections such as meningitis.
• Trauma, for example a skull fracture.
• Surgery.

The pituitary hormone most likely to be affected by hypopituitarism is the growth hormone, which controls growth rates.

Doctors suspect growth hormone deficiency in a child who fails to grow at the normal rate. A synthetic growth hormone injection can restore normal growth patterns.

PROLACTINOMA

This pituitary tumour causes oversecretion of the hormone prolactin. Prolactin promotes breast development and lactation (milk production in women) and it also helps regulate sexual function. If overproduced, it can cause menstrual disturbance in women and reduced fertility in both sexes.

PITUITARY HORMONES AND FACTORS

➤ Luteinizing hormone (LH) and follicle-stimulating hormone (FSH) – Affect male and female sex organs.

➤ Melanocyte-stimulating factor (MSH) – Affects skin pigmentation.

➤ Adrenocorticotropic hormone (ACTH) – Affects the adrenal glands/body's general metabolism.

➤ Thyroid-stimulating hormone (TSH) – Also affects body's metabolism.

➤ Oxytocin – Affects milk release and uterine contractions.

➤ Antidiuretic hormone (ADH) – Affects kidney function.

➤ Growth hormone – Affects cell division, and bone and cartilage development.

➤ Prolactin – Affects female breast development.

THE STRUCTURE OF THE PITUITARY GLAND

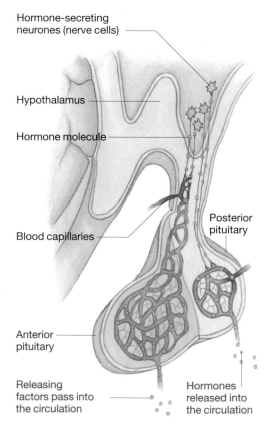

Hormone-secreting neurones (nerve cells)

Hypothalamus

Hormone molecule

Blood capillaries

Posterior pituitary

Anterior pituitary

Releasing factors pass into the circulation

Hormones released into the circulation

TREATMENT OF PITUITARY GLAND PROBLEMS

➤ Replacement of hormone deficiencies.

➤ Reduction of excess hormones, by surgically removing part of the gland or by using drugs to block the formation or effects of the hormone involved.

➤ Removal of the tumour, surgically, with radiotherapy or with drugs that shrink the pituitary gland tumour.

Treatment can lead to hypopituitarism, necessitating lifelong hormone therapy.

ACROMEGALY/GIGANTISM

In children, the overproduction of growth hormone is gigantism, in adults it is called acromegaly. This overproduction from a pituitary tumour causes body parts – usually the tongue, face, hands and feet – to enlarge. The changes happen slowly and may not be obvious. If doctors suspect acromegaly, they may ask for old photographs to compare with your current appearance. People with gigantism can grow more than 2 metres (7 feet) tall.

Other physical changes can include increased growth of coarse body hair, deepening of the voice and excessive sweating. Other symptoms may include headaches and defects of vision as the pituitary tumour presses on the optic nerve.

◁ The pituitary gland has two lobes (anterior and posterior). It hangs from the hypothalamus by a stalk of nerve fibres and a blood vessel network. Releasing factors exit the anterior lobe and the posterior lobe deals with hormones.

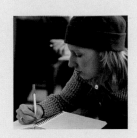

THE NERVOUS SYSTEM

5

The nervous system includes the brain, and the central and peripheral nervous systems. It controls all our body's functions, from vital life support mechanisms, such as breathing, to the ability to sense and react to stimuli. The brain is the control centre that regulates physical functions and makes us conscious and able to feel emotions. Yet, like all our body systems, the nervous system is prey to disorders, from interruption to its blood supply to life-threatening infections. The brain is also prone to subtle chemical change that can cause emotional disturbance and psychological illness.

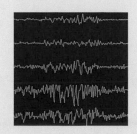

CONTENTS

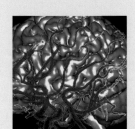

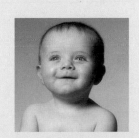

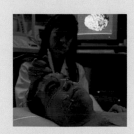

The brain and nerve network

SEE ALSO
➤ Stroke, p80
➤ Multiple sclerosis, p88
➤ Depression, p98
➤ The musculoskeletal system, p106

The brain is the control centre of your body, and other parts of your body play an important role in supporting your brain by feeding it with oxygen and nutrients, for example, and by supplying it with information. The brain functions via billions of interconnected nerve cells and various information-signalling chemicals called neurotransmitters. A fine chemical balance exists in terms of the levels of neurotransmitters in the brain and any shift in balance can cause unusual psychological functions such as mood swings or depression.

Your nervous system can be seen as comprising two parts:
• The central nervous system – The brain and spinal cord.
• The peripheral nervous system – All other nerves throughout the body.

THE BASIC BUILDING BLOCK

The brain is composed of about 100 billion nerve cells, or neurones. Everything you see, feel, think and do depends on their ability to communicate with one another.
Neurones function in different ways:
• Motor neurones – Cause muscles to contract when instructed to by the brain.
• Sensory neurones – Carry sensory information, such as pain or touch, from the body to the brain.
• Interneurones – Connect neurones to each other.

THE STRUCTURE OF THE BRAIN

FAST-TRACKING SIGNALS

Your nerves are made up of bundles of nerve cells, or neurones, which pass information between specific sites in the body and the brain and spinal cord. This information travels as electrical messages along the length of a neurone's axon, and via outgrowths called dendrites. The messages pass from one neurone to another across a gap called a synapse, and are taken across in the form of chemical "neurotransmitters". Doctors are able to measure the electrical activity in the brain by using an electroencephalogram (EEG).

To speed the transmission of nerve impulses, some axons are insulated by a fatty white substance called myelin. In some diseases, such as multiple sclerosis, this myelin insulation is destroyed or damaged, which stops nerve signals getting through.

PROTECTION AND SUPPORT

As your brain and spinal cord perform absolutely vital, finely tuned functions, they have to be well-protected and supported against possible physical injury and infection. The bones of the skull and the vertebrae do a good job of protecting the brain and spinal cord from physical damage. The brain and spinal cord are also enveloped by three protective membranes, called the meninges, and are bathed by a nourishing and lubricating fluid known as cerebrospinal fluid. Both the membranes and fluid act to cushion movements within the head and spine. However, infectious micro-organisms can invade the nervous system. This may lead to inflammation of the membranes – meningitis – and clouding of the cerebrospinal fluid, which can be detected by taking a sample via a procedure called a lumbar puncture.

▽ The brain is divided into two cerebral hemispheres – the left and right hemispheres – which are linked by a network of nerve fibres. This nerve network is called the corpus callosum. Each hemisphere is in turn divided into four areas known as cerebral lobes.

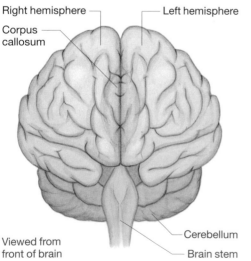

Right hemisphere — — Left hemisphere
Corpus callosum
Viewed from front of brain
Cerebellum
Brain stem

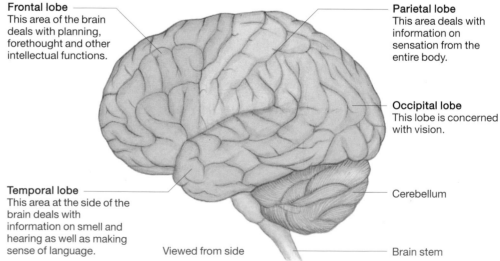

Frontal lobe
This area of the brain deals with planning, forethought and other intellectual functions.

Parietal lobe
This area deals with information on sensation from the entire body.

Occipital lobe
This lobe is concerned with vision.

Temporal lobe
This area at the side of the brain deals with information on smell and hearing as well as making sense of language.

Cerebellum

Viewed from side

Brain stem

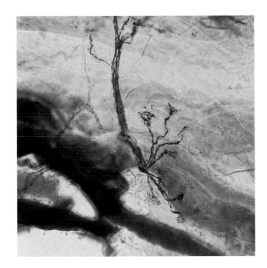

△ This picture shows a nerve–muscle connection – the synapses between a motor neurone axon and the muscle fibres that it controls (the muscle appears as pale bands).

BASIC BRAIN DIVISIONS

The human brain has three divisions:

- Cerebrum – Made up of left- and right-hand cerebral hemispheres.
- Brainstem – Connects the cerebral hemispheres to the spinal cord; it controls the automatic functions of the body, such as heart rate and breathing.
- Cerebellum – This large, flat, tree-shaped area at the back of the brainstem controls and regulates movement.

ANATOMY OF A NEURONE

▽ Neurones of all types consist of a cell body, a long "tail" called an axon and branching projections called dendrites.

Cell body
The nucleus and power-making structures all reside within the cell body.

Axon
Signals from the cell body travel along this to communicate with other neurones, via a synapse and neurotransmitter.

Myelin sheath
A white, fatty substance that helps to speed nervous signals along the axon.

Dendrite
These projections seek out other neurones to make contact and collect information.

Synaptic knob
At the end of each axon branch is a knob that sends signals across a tiny gap (a synapse) to the next neurone.

THE CENTRAL NERVOUS SYSTEM

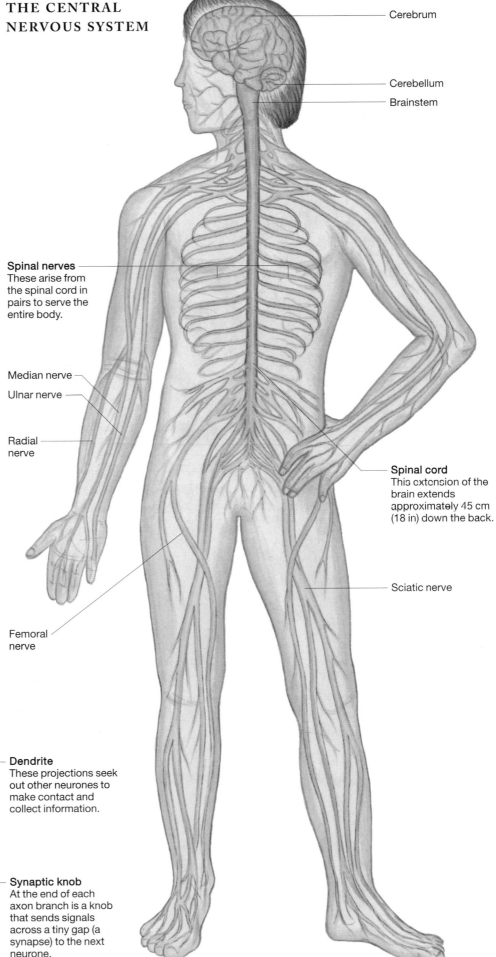

Cerebrum

Cerebellum

Brainstem

Spinal nerves
These arise from the spinal cord in pairs to serve the entire body.

Median nerve

Ulnar nerve

Radial nerve

Spinal cord
This extension of the brain extends approximately 45 cm (18 in) down the back.

Sciatic nerve

Femoral nerve

Headaches and migraine

SEE ALSO

➤ Learn to manage stress, p12
➤ Meningitis, p84
➤ Migraines in children, p230

The majority of people have the occasional headache but this usually disappears spontaneously within a few hours. In some people, though, headaches can persist for longer and cause great distress. The pain itself may focus on the back of the head, the forehead and behind the eyes, and the quality of the pain varies from dull and continuous to sudden and sharp. However, it is rare for a headache to have a life-threatening cause. Most headaches are not serious in nature, although they can be hard to explain and treat.

Doctors tend to talk about four different types of headache:
• Tension headache.
• Analgesic headache.
• Cluster headache.
• Migraine.

A headache may also accompany a feverish illness such as influenza and is an all-too-familiar symptom of the common cold and of sinusitis. Excessive consumption of alcohol can also lead to a headache the following morning.

There are some more serious, but much rarer, causes of headache. These include a brain tumour (benign or malignant), which can be the cause of recurrent headaches, or inflammation of the arteries in the brain, which causes a sudden throbbing pain in one or both temples. Other serious but rare conditions associated with headache include meningitis and subarachnoid haemorrhage.

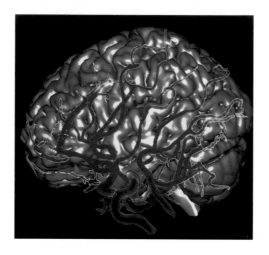

△ Widening and subsequent narrowing of the blood vessels in the brain is a probable cause of the pain of migraine headaches.

It is recommended that you consult your doctor as soon as possible if you experience any of the additional symptoms listed in the box on recognizing serious headaches.

TENSION HEADACHE

This is by far the most common form of headache. Such headaches can be moderately or severely painful. Doctors believe the pain to be due to spasm in the muscles of the scalp and neck. The headache usually feels like tightness across the forehead, often spreading back into the neck. Slight nausea is a common accompanying symptom, although vomiting is not. Usually these headaches last only a few hours but sometimes they can persist. This type of headache generally affects more women than men.

Many factors can trigger tension headaches, including stress, noise, fumes, problems with eyesight and depression. Tension headaches can often result from bad posture and from long periods staring at a computer screen. These headaches respond well to relaxation techniques and over-the-counter painkillers. Tension headaches often improve if you perform some vigorous exercise.

If you suffer from recurrent headaches, your doctor will want to know about the severity and frequency of your symptoms, so it is often useful to keep a note of these. In some cases a CT scan may be carried out in order to discover the underlying cause of recurrent or persistent headaches.

ANALGESIC HEADACHE

It may seem unlikely but painkillers can actually cause a headache. Studies have shown that regular long-term use of painkillers for a headache can in turn lead

▽ Most tension headaches are quickly relieved by over-the-counter painkillers. However, medical advice is needed if headaches recur.

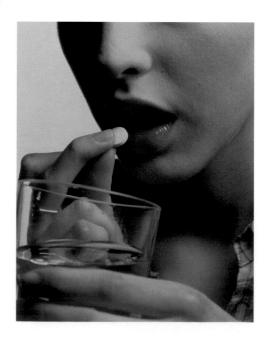

RECOGNIZING A SERIOUS HEADACHE

Seek medical advice without delay if you suffer any of the following symptoms:

➤ A severe headache that develops quickly and suddenly.

➤ A headache that gets worse and worse despite painkillers.

➤ Vomiting after the onset of headache.

➤ Significant numbness and weakness of the limbs.

➤ Blurred vision wiith eye pain.

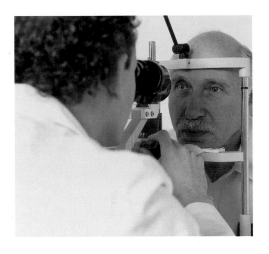

△ Some eye conditions can lead to headaches. An eye examination may be needed in certain cases of persistent or recurrent headaches.

to a pain that is similar to a tension headache. For sufferers there is a temptation to use ever-stronger painkillers, but this will only make the problem worse. This type of headache can be avoided by using painkillers as sparingly as possible. However, if you have a headache that is not relieved by taking simple painkillers, you should always consult your doctor, who will investigate the cause.

CLUSTER HEADACHE

This unusual condition is poorly understood. Sufferers, most commonly men, are often woken in the middle of the night with excruciating pain through one eye. Such attacks generally last 15 to 30 minutes. The headaches tend to follow a pattern and they may occur between one and four times a day.

The pain is exceedingly resistant to painkillers and antimigraine drugs, although lithium, a drug that is also used to treat certain psychiatric disorders, may help prevent attacks and inhaling oxygen may stop an attack. Smoking and drinking alcohol can increase the risk of a cluster headache occurring.

MIGRAINE

This severe form of headache can be extremely debilitating. Millions of people worldwide experience migraines each year. Susceptible individuals usually have their

TYPES OF MIGRAINE

Doctors describe migraine as being either classical or common.

➤ In classical migraine the headache usually affects one side of the head. Many people get a warning – or aura – before the headache starts that usually consists of seeing flashing lights, stars or zigzag lines. About 20 per cent of migraines are classical.

➤ In common migraine, the only symptom may be a one-sided headache.

first migraine before the age of 30 but children as young as three may suffer from this condition. It is rare to experience a first migraine after the age of 40 and the frequency and severity of attacks usually diminishes with age.

Migraine-sufferers usually have other symptoms, such as disturbance to vision, as well as a headache. The cause of the condition is not apparent but it is probably due to the dilation of certain blood vessels in the brain. Just before the symptoms start, small arteries in the brain become narrower, thereby reducing blood flow. For reasons that are not clear, as the headache begins, these small arteries become wider again.

SIGNS AND SYMPTOMS OF A MIGRAINE

As the headache develops there may also be some of the following symptoms:

➤ Vomiting.

➤ Aversion to bright light (photophobia).

➤ Feeling irritable.

Once the migraine has passed, the person will often just want to sleep. It is unusual for a migraine to last for more than 24 hours, although some people suffer recurrent migraines with a day or so gap between them.

POSSIBLE CAUSES

Certain factors seem to trigger a migraine attack in some people, including:

• Stress.
• Foodstuffs such as chocolate, coffee and cheese.
• Red wine.
• Missed meals.
• The contraceptive pill.
• Menstruation.
• Sexual intercourse.

A high percentage of migraine sufferers will have other family members who also suffer from them.

TREATMENT OPTIONS

The priority in the prevention of migraine attacks is to avoid any known precipitating factors. It may help to keep a diary of what you have eaten and other possible factors to help you determine what the cause may be. In many cases, a simple dietary change is all that is needed to prevent a recurrence.

As a migraine begins, painkillers or antimigraine drugs, which act on the brain's blood vessels, can help. Your doctor can recommend antiemetics to quell nausea and/or vomiting, or prescribe drugs that prevent attacks as a long-term treatment.

▽ A variety of relaxation techniques can be effective in cases of tension headaches. Scalp massage is often of benefit.

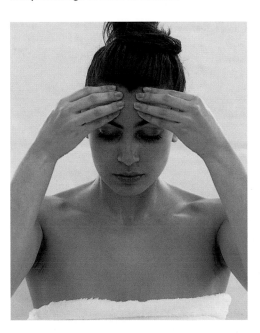

Fatigue

Each day, large numbers of people visit their doctor complaining of tiredness. Yet many come away from consultations feeling that they have had no satisfactory explanation for the way they feel. Fatigue is such a generalized symptom that it is not easy for anyone except the sufferer to assess it, plus it also depends on comparisons with previous energy levels. Fatigue can be caused by a range of conditions, from lack of oxygen in the blood to depression. If there are no other accompanying physical symptoms, then the cause can be very hard to pin down.

COMMON CAUSES OF FATIGUE

➤ Anaemia.

➤ Hypothyroidism.

➤ Diabetes.

➤ Sleep disorders.

➤ Depression.

The first step in a diagnosis is for your doctor to take your medical history in order to find out if there are any other symptoms that may explain your fatigue. If there are symptoms, a physical examination may be carried out to help identify possible causes. Your doctor may then take a sample of blood and send it for laboratory testing. Testing will include:

• A full blood count to check for anaemia.

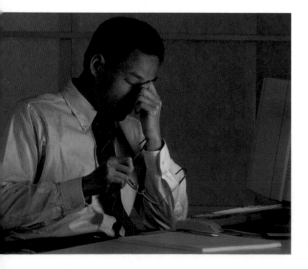

▽ Fatigue may result from long hours in a stressful job or from physical factors such as poor ventilation or glaring computer screens.

• Thyroid function tests to look for an underactive thyroid gland.
• Sugar levels to look for diabetes.

These blood tests are normal in more than 90 per cent of people.

LOOKING FOR CAUSES

Your doctor may not find a physical cause for your lack of energy and may consider whether depression could be to blame. If neither of these seem to be the culprit, then the underlying cause is likely to be stress – probably the main cause of fatigue in the Western world today.

LOOKING AT YOUR LIFESTYLE

Most people live hectic lives, having to cope with demands and strains our bodies were not designed for. Once physical disease and psychological health problems have been excluded, most people feel better if made to recognize that their fatigue may simply arise from the pace of modern life and if they are given some simple, sensible advice to follow. Many of us "burn the candle at both ends" trying to meet the demands of a busy work schedule and home or social life. This may mean you are getting too little sleep, which can lead to a build-up of fatigue. You may be skipping meals or eating too much junk food, thereby missing out on essential nutrients. You should also consider if your alcohol consumption is too high – a major cause of fatigue. Importantly, lack of physical exercise can lead to lethargy and sluggishness. Regular exercise, particularly outdoors, can have a remarkable effect in boosting energy levels.

CHRONIC FATIGUE SYNDROME

Also known medically as myalgic encephalomyelitis (ME), chronic fatigue syndrome is a controversial subject and the symptoms are often vague and non-specific. For this reason the condition is often misdiagnosed. The main symptoms, which may last for about six months, are:

➤ Fatigue and poor quality sleep.

➤ Poor concentration and memory.

➤ Fever.

➤ Aching muscles.

The condition may occur in the aftermath of infection by certain viruses. In other cases it seems to develop in response to severe emotional stress. But in many cases there is no obvious triggering infection or life event. However, many doctors are not convinced that this is a physical illness, preferring a psychiatric or psychological explanation for the symptoms.

Studies have shown that chronic fatigue syndrome occurs most often in women between the ages of 25 and 45, but it is possible for those of either sex or of any age group to be affected.

The treatment for this condition is mainly supportive and psychological, although a programme of graded exercise can be beneficial for many sufferers. Depression is common in people with chronic fatigue syndrome and in such cases antidepressant drugs can be very helpful.

Head injury

SEE ALSO

➤ The brain and nerve network, p74

➤ Epilepsy, p82

➤ The musculoskeletal system, p106

Minor bumps and bangs to the head are extremely common and in most cases leave no long-term ill-effects – the skull is a very resilient structure. As for more serious head injuries, the principal cause of these is road traffic accidents. Many developed countries have made it compulsory for motorcycle riders and drivers to wear helmets and seatbelts respectively. These preventive measures have resulted in significant reductions in the number of road accident-related head injuries. Helmets for cyclists and horse riders also help to minimize injuries.

SIGNS AND SYMPTOMS OF A SERIOUS HEAD INJURY

Look out for any of the following symptoms, which may appear up to 24 hours after the injury:

➤ Vomiting.

➤ Blurred vision.

➤ Loss of memory, especially of events after the injury.

➤ Drowsiness and/or confusion.

➤ Headache that gets progressively worse despite taking painkillers.

If you have injured your head and have any of the symptoms listed in the above box on serious head injury, visit your doctor immediately or go to the nearest accident and emergency department.

TYPES OF INJURY

The brain can be injured by:

• Shearing and rotation, which means that the brain's nerve cells are battered and bruised inside the skull. This is the commonest form of brain injury.

• Direct nerve damage caused by penetrating injuries.

• Swelling of the brain as a result of inflammation.

• Lack of oxygen to the brain while the patient is unconscious.

• Raised intracranial pressure, which can occur if the pressure within the skull rises. This may be caused by an expanding blood clot from a torn blood vessel, for example. As a result the brain is forced out of the bottom of the skull, causing severe damage.

INVESTIGATING HEAD INJURIES

Doctors may examine you physically and ask about the incident and any symptoms. They may X-ray your skull to look for fractures, although this will reveal little about any underlying brain damage.

Most minor head injury patients are allowed home if someone can keep an eye on them. Serious problems can develop in the first 24 hours and so monitoring is vital.

TREATMENT OPTIONS

If the head injury is severe, the patient may be kept in hospital for observation. In such cases, a brain scan may be done to look for brain damage.

In severe head injuries, the patient may remain unconscious for a long time. In a

▽ When taking part in any activity with a risk of head injury it is advisable to wear a helmet to prevent serious damage if an accident occurs.

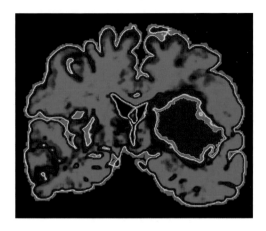

△ A computer-enhanced scan of the brain shows bleeding within the brain (red area). This may be caused by a serious head injury.

few cases the problem lies with an expanding blood clot or haematoma, which needs to be removed by a neurosurgeon.

The key treatment is to assist a person's breathing so that the brain gets plenty of oxygen and nutrients. Drugs may be given to prevent the brain swelling. Recovery from a severe brain injury may take weeks or months and the degree of recovery is variable and not easy to predict early on.

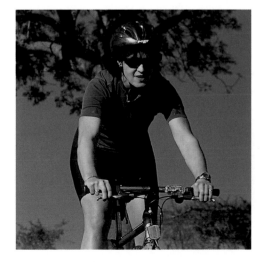

POSSIBLE COMPLICATIONS AFTER A HEAD INJURY

The commonest complication is post-head injury syndrome – consisting of headache, nausea and tiredness – which can occur even after very minor head injuries. In most cases this settles with a few weeks' rest. More serious possible long-term consequences can include epilepsy, loss of higher brain function, personality changes and hydrocephalus (water on the brain).

Stroke

Brain damage caused by an interruption in the brain's blood supply – and therefore its oxygen supply – is a common cause of death in many developed countries and a major cause of long-term disability. Stroke is more common in those over 70 and the risk of stroke increases with age.

It can occur with little or no warning and have devastating effects, depending on which part of the brain is affected. With the help of staff in specialized rehabilitation units, stroke victims often make a full recovery, although about a third may be left with some form of disability.

Strokes, also known as cerebrovascular accidents (CVAs), can be caused by several different types of disruption to the blood supply to the brain. The main types of stroke are:

• Cerebral infarction – This is the commonest form of stroke and occurs when a blood vessel in the brain becomes blocked – either by a clot formed within the blood vessel (thrombus) or by a clot that has formed elsewhere in the body and has travelled to the brain (embolus). The area of the brain supplied by that blood vessel dies and the functions that were provided by that area are affected. The main underlying cause of this type

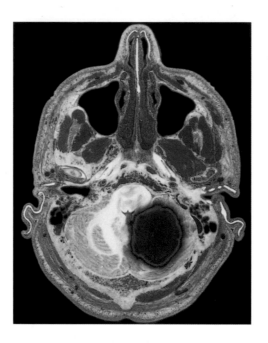

△ The red colouring in this scan of the brain indicates the area affected by a cerebral haemorrhage in the cerebellum.

of stroke is atherosclerosis – where fatty plaques (atheroma) form on the lining of blood vessels, which encourages the formation of blood clots in the brain and elsewhere. Less common causes of cerebral infarction include disorders such as sickle-cell disease, in which the blood tends to form clots too easily, and disorders of heart rhythm or heart valves.

• Cerebral haemorrhage – In this form of stroke a blood vessel in the brain bursts and as a result blood leaks out and causes damage to the surrounding brain tissue. This can occur as a result of an underlying weakness of the blood vessels in the brain, and is perhaps exacerbated by high blood pressure, or if the blood-clotting process is impaired – for example by drug treatment.

SIGNS AND SYMPTOMS

➤ Loss of consciousness.

➤ Weakness or inability to move on one side of the body.

➤ Blurred or fuzzy vision or loss of vision in one eye.

➤ Numbness on one side of the body.

➤ Loss of control of fine movements and tremor.

➤ Speech difficulties.

➤ Difficulties maintaining balance and vertigo.

RISK FACTORS FOR STROKE

There are several adjustments that you can make to your lifestyle in order to reduce your risk of atherosclerosis and stroke. These are some of the risk factors that can be controlled by you:

• High blood pressure – This increases the risk of atherosclerosis by putting strain on the blood vessels in the brain.

• Smoking – As well as the many other risks associated with it, smoking leads to narrowing of the blood vessels and encourages the formation of blood clots.

• High blood cholesterol levels – This condition, which may be the result of an inherited tendency or a high fat diet, can lead to atherosclerosis.

• High alcohol intake – Although drinking small amounts of alcohol may be beneficial for the circulation, studies have shown that regular high alcohol consumption increases the risk of stroke.

MINI-STROKES

Also known by doctors as transient ischaemic attacks (TIAs), mini-strokes are short-lived versions of a stroke that may last from a few seconds to an hour. Symptoms are often similar to those of a stroke but they disappear over 24 hours. They are caused by lack of oxygen to the brain due to temporary blockage of a blood vessel. Sudden visual loss in one eye and bouts of confusion, that usually pass in a few hours, are characteristic of such mini-strokes.

After a series of mini-strokes, doctors often perform a Doppler ultrasound scan of the carotid arteries in the neck to see if they are furred up with atheroma. Treatment options include aspirin, surgical removal of the plaques or balloon angioplasty to widen the arteries narrowed by atheroma.

- Inactive lifestyle – Taking regular exercise reduces the formation of atherosclerosis and helps to maintain healthy blood pressure.
- Diabetes – This condition carries an increased risk of atherosclerosis. So it is important that a diabetic's blood pressure is monitored very carefully.
- Obesity – There is a strong correlation between being severely overweight and circulatory problems of all kinds.

AREAS OFTEN AFFECTED BY STROKE

In theory, any brain function could be affected by a stroke but certain areas of the brain are more at risk. These areas include:

- Motor strip – This region is concerned with muscle control and damage to this area on one side of the brain results in weakness and/or paralysis on the opposite side of the body.
- Broca's and Wernicke's areas – These areas of the left side of the brain are principally concerned with speech. People affected by strokes in these areas have difficulty understanding speech or find it difficult to find the right words.
- Brainstem – In this area, which controls vital functions such as breathing, the nerve fibres are tightly packed as they pass into the spinal cord and even very small strokes can cause life-threatening damage. Victims of strokes in this part of the brain rarely survive in the long term.

▽ Fast foods and convenience dishes are often very high in fat. Controlling your fat intake is an important way of reducing your risk of stroke.

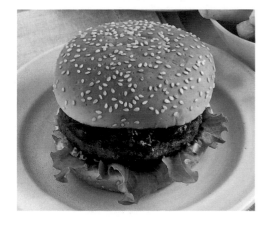

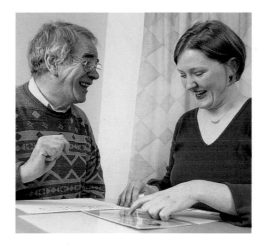

△ Special therapists can help those recovering from the effects of a stroke. Activities and games are used to rebuild speech, cooordination and thought processes.

DIAGNOSING A STROKE

There are rarely any warning signs of a stroke, although someone who has experienced repeated transient ischaemic attacks or mini-strokes is at increased risk. Anyone displaying symptoms of a stroke requires immediate medical attention. A doctor may be able to diagnose the condition from the obvious physical symptoms or after making a detailed physical examination to find out whether any functions are not working as normal and by taking a medical history. The precise site of the stroke can be confirmed by a CT or MRI brain scan.

TREATMENT OPTIONS

If a cerebral infarction is picked up early the main aim of treatment will be to try to minimize damage and reduce the long-term ill effects. Specific treatment to reverse the stroke may not always be possible, although drugs to reduce blood pressure or to combat inflammation may be administered.

Long-term treatment following a cerebral infarction may include regular low doses of aspirin to prevent further clots forming. Once the victim's condition has stabilized following a stroke, the focus of treatment is likely to be rehabilitation and returning the patient to as near normal life as possible.

STROKE REHABILITATION

The brain has an amazing capacity to "rewire" itself and bypass damaged areas so that most people who have had strokes recover some of the lost function, although to what extent is variable and unpredictable.

Rehabilitation following a stroke starts soon afterwards with physiotherapy to get your body moving again. It is important to regain mobility as quickly as possible because there is a greater the chance that surviving nerve cells can remodel themselves to acquire lost functions. Specialist interventions may also include hydrotherapy and speech therapy.

Once an individual is ready to leave hospital, an occupational therapist will help to implement any adaptations that may be needed in the home, such as grab rails or a stair lift, in order that as much independence can be retained as possible. If necessary, speech therapists and physiotherapists continue to visit the patient after discharge from hospital to pursue their programme of treatment.

THE LONG-TERM OUTLOOK

Improvements to functions damaged by stroke can continue to happen for as long as six months after the stroke. However, any remaining disability after this time is more likely to last. Some people are severely disabled by stroke and require long-term, full-time nursing care. One person in five dies within a month of a stroke.

▽ Taking regular exercise throughout adult life, and particularly later in life, can make a vital contribution to the health of your blood vessels.

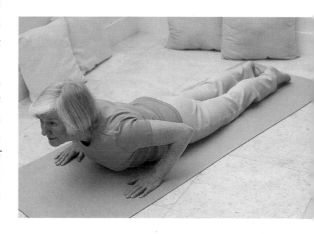

Epilepsy

SEE ALSO
➤ Dementia, p90
➤ Stroke, p80
➤ Febrile convulsions, p231

An epileptic fit or seizure occurs when part or all of the brain's nerve cells create electrical signals in an uncontrolled manner. If you have an isolated seizure this does not necessarily mean that you have epilepsy. Doctors need evidence of recurrences of such seizures on two or more occasions to carry out a proper diagnosis. Epilepsy is a very common condition, affecting 2 per cent of the population in developed countries. Many people with epilepsy lead normal lives, although some activities, such as driving, are prohibited.

Epileptic seizures can be categorized into two types – these are generalized seizures or partial seizures:

- Generalized seizures are the most common and there are two sub-categories – tonic-clonic and absence. A tonic-clonic (or grand mal) generalized seizure may start with a vague sense of foreboding (an "aura"), after which the

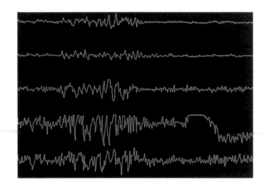

△ Traces produced by an EEG (electroencephalography) show increased electrical activity during an epileptic seizure.

▽ During an EEG electrodes are placed on the scalp. The electrodes monitor and record electrical activity in the brain.

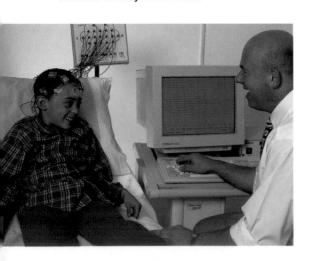

person suddenly becomes rigid and falls to the ground, often uttering a cry. They may bite their tongue, lose control of their bowel or bladder and start to shake all over. Finally, as the fitting subsides and ends, the person becomes very drowsy. Fits usually occur one at a time; fits that follow on from one another are a dangerous sign and the person needs to go to hospital as soon as possible.

- Absence (or petit mal) generalized seizures are more common in childhood and adolescence. In such cases the child "goes blank", often with the eyes open and staring, for up to 30 seconds.

- Partial seizures are less common. In this case the fit is limited to just one part of the brain. The person may simply look blank or vacant for a few minutes, may experience odd sights or smells, or may have uncontrolled movement of one part of their body.

CAUSES OF EPILEPSY

In most people no obvious cause for epilepsy is found, although the condition does tend to run in families. Most epileptics experience their first seizure as children and many outgrow the condition during adolescence. A person who has a first fit in adulthood is unusual and this should be investigated further.

Other causes of seizures include:

- Brain trauma or surgery.
- Brain tumour.
- Drugs and alcohol.
- Alzheimer's disease.
- Stroke.

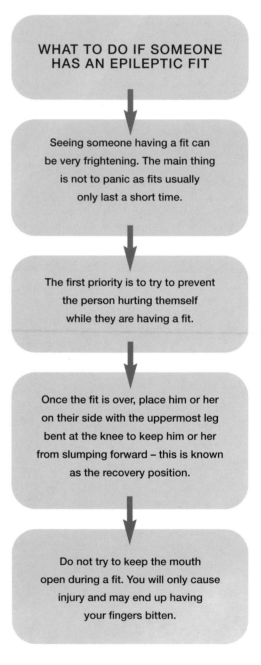

WHAT TO DO IF SOMEONE HAS AN EPILEPTIC FIT

↓

Seeing someone having a fit can be very frightening. The main thing is not to panic as fits usually only last a short time.

↓

The first priority is to try to prevent the person hurting themself while they are having a fit.

↓

Once the fit is over, place him or her on their side with the uppermost leg bent at the knee to keep him or her from slumping forward – this is known as the recovery position.

↓

Do not try to keep the mouth open during a fit. You will only cause injury and may end up having your fingers bitten.

- High fever – Young children with a fever can have a fit, which is known as a febrile convulsion, but this is a fairly normal response and there is little risk of this developing into epilepsy as an adult.

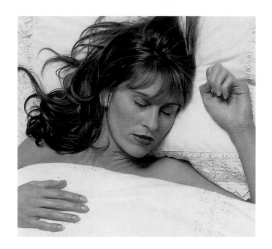

△ Lack of sleep can trigger seizures. Most epileptics benefit from an ordered lifestyle with regular meals and low stress levels.

Some things can trigger a seizure or make it more likely, and these include strobe lighting, excessive stress and lack of sleep.

DIAGNOSIS AND TREATMENT OPTIONS FOR EPILEPSY

Epilepsy can be confirmed with a tracing of the electrical activity of the brain, called an electroencephalogram or EEG. Brain scanning may also be performed to shed light on any physical defects that could be causing the epilepsy, such as a brain tumour.

In the long term there are a wide range of anticonvulsant drugs to control the fits. The correct dosage varies greatly between individuals and it may take a little while for the doctor to find the optimum dose to control fits in each case. Most people with epilepsy have no or very few fits once they are stabilized on medication.

The danger to other road-users means that in many countries people with epilepsy must have had three fit-free year before they can drive again. Commercial drivers, such as lorry drivers and bus drivers, may be prohibited from driving altogether. Anyone who has suffered from epilepsy should seek medical advice before undertaking potentially dangerous sports such as rock climbing or scuba diving.

Brain tumours

SEE ALSO

➤ Lung cancer, p136

Brain tumours can either originate in the brain or spread from a cancer elsewhere, such as the lungs or breast. Tumours can be cancerous or non-cancerous, but because of the restrictions of the skull any such growth may affect brain function. Fortunately, such tumours are rare.

If your doctor suspects a brain tumour from your symptoms and a thorough physical examination, then you will be referred to a neurologist and for brain scanning. In certain cases, additional tests such as

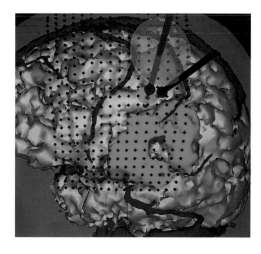

△ The green area in this MRI (magnetic resonance imaging) scan shows a tumour in the motor cortex (blue dotted area) of the brain.

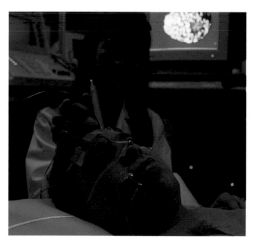

△ A technician prepares a patient for brain surgery by creating a computerized map of the brain, which is then used to guide the surgeon.

SIGNS AND SYMPTOMS
Symptoms often appear due to compression of part of the brain by the growing tumour; they include:

➤ Headache, usually worse in the morning.

➤ Nausea and vomiting.

➤ Blurred vision.

Symptoms are often specific to the part of the brain affected, including:

➤ Difficulty reading or writing.

➤ Slurred speech.

➤ A change of personality.

cerebral angiography or a brain biopsy (in which a sample of tissue is removed for analysis) are carried out.

Some benign brain tumours may be removed surgically and recovery chances tend to be good. Removing benign tumours may pose operative risks, such as brain damage, as they lie close to vital structures, such as the brain stem. Radiotherapy to shrink the brain tumour, may be advised. Depending on its location and spread, a cancerous tumour may be removed surgically. If surgery is not possible, the tumour may respond to radiotherapy, but the outlook in cases of brain tumours that have spread from other organs is poor.

Meningitis

Meningitis is the inflammation of the membranes surrounding the brain (the meninges). It is usually caused by an infection. Viral meningitis is the most common, and less dangerous, form and generally affects young adults. Bacterial meningitis is a more serious condition that mainly affects children. This life-threatening condition often begins with symptoms similar to those of a common cold or flu. However, the child's condition rapidly worsens and the classic symptoms of the disease, described below, develop.

Meningitis is the result of an infection by one of a number of different viruses or bacteria. In rare cases, usually among those with reduced immunity, it may also be caused by a fungal infection. Although treatment depends on the type of infection, all forms of the disease are serious and any suspected case of meningitis warrants immediate medical assessment and possible admission to hospital.

MAKING THE DIAGNOSIS

A doctor will usually make a provisional diagnosis based on observation of the symptoms and an examination of the

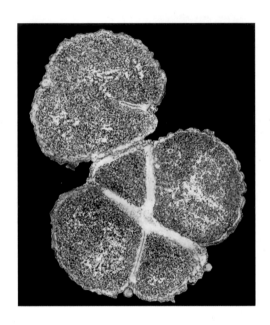

△ *Neisseria meningitidis*, seen here in the process of dividing, is the bacterium that causes meningococcal meningitis.

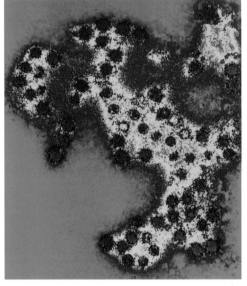

△ The coxsackie virus shown here is a common cause of colds as well as being a frequent cause of viral meningitis.

SIGNS AND SYMPTOMS

If the infection is due to a virus, the symptoms tend to develop gradually. In bacterial meningitis, however, symptoms appear rapidly. Symptoms of meningitis include the following:

➤ Fever.

➤ Headache.

➤ Neck stiffness.

➤ Dislike of bright lights (photophobia).

➤ Sometimes a rash will develop.

In addition, children and babies may be:

➤ Very drowsy and unrousable.

➤ Floppy.

➤ Have a high-pitched cry.

Fitting may occur if treatment is not given as soon as possible.

patient. Further investigations, which may be carried out after treatment has already started, are likely to include a lumbar puncture, in which a sample of cerebrospinal fluid is removed from around the spinal cord in the lower back and examined under the microscope for signs of infection. In some cases a brain scan may be carried out.

TREATMENT OPTIONS

Viral meningitis generally requires no specific treatment beyond analgesics to provide pain relief and reduce fever. Full recovery from the condition takes one to two weeks.

In cases of suspected bacterial meningitis, prompt administration of intravenous antibiotics is essential. Time is vital and minutes can save lives. In some cases, corticosteroids may be given to reduce inflammation. Recovery from the bacterial form of the disease is much slower than from viral meningitis, but recovery times vary from case to case. Even with the best treatment, approximately 15 per cent of patients die from the condition.

WHAT ARE THE LONG-TERM EFFECTS?

Although most people make a full recovery from viral and bacterial meningitis, some people are left with long-term problems following bacterial meningitis. These include hearing loss and impaired memory.

PREVENTING MENINGITIS

Many people are concerned, when there is a case of meningitis locally, that they or their children may be at risk. However, bacterial meningitis is actually quite difficult to catch from another person. You would need to be breathing the same air as the affected person for a number of hours to be even slightly at risk. The spread of infection among such close contacts is usually effectively prevented by the administration of a two-day course of antibiotics.

Children in many developed countries now receive immunization against *Haemophilus influenza* type B (HIB) bacterium, which is a common cause of meningitis. The meningococcal bacterium has two main strains that cause meningitis in Europe. There is now a vaccine to the C strain and it is part of the standard childhood vaccination programme. A vaccine for the more common B strain is likely to be available shortly.

HOW TO RECOGNIZE A MENINGOCOCCAL RASH

It is possible that meningitis resulting from infection with meningococcal bacteria may also result in an infection in the blood stream. This sometimes leads to a characteristic purpuric rash which looks like a bruise, appears suddenly and spreads quickly. The rash consists of small, blotchy dark-red-purple spots. One of the factors that may help you recognize this rash is that it does not "blanch" (seem to disappear) when it is pressed – typically using the side of a glass tumbler. However, if you have any doubts at all about the nature of a rash, particularly if it is accompanied by any of the other symptoms, consult a doctor, or take your child to hospital, as soon as possible.

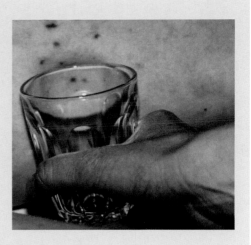

△ The tumbler test is the best way to find out if it is a meningococcal rash. Press the side of a glass over the affected area. If the rash does not disappear when pressed, then you must seek medical advice immediately.

Viral encephalitis

SEE ALSO
➤ Viral infections, p218

This viral infection of the brain tissue itself results in inflammation and raised intracranial (inside the skull) pressure. It is a rare condition that is usually fairly mild in nature and settles rapidly. Viral encephalitis most commonly affects babies and the elderly.

This condition may develop as a complication of another viral illness and is often caused by the same viruses that cause mumps and measles. It may also be caused by the herpes simplex virus. This form of the disease can be life-threatening. In some parts of the world there are more severe forms, such as Japanese encephalitis in South-east Asia, California encephalitis in the US and Ross River fever in Australia.

If your doctor suspects viral encephalitis, immediate hospital admission is necessary. A lumbar puncture to take a sample of cerebrospinal fluid may be necessary. A CT or MRI brain scan may also be carried out. In some cases, an electroencephalogram (EEG) is done.

There is no specific treatment for some forms of viral encephalitis and most patients recover spontaneously. However, acyclovir may be given intravenously in cases of herpes simplex infection. A vaccine exists for preventing Japanese encephalitis.

SIGNS AND SYMPTOMS

Typical symptoms of viral encephalitis include the following:

➤ Fever.

➤ Headache.

➤ Drowsiness.

These symptoms are similar to those of meningitis and a doctor's main concern will be to discount this possibility as quickly as possible.

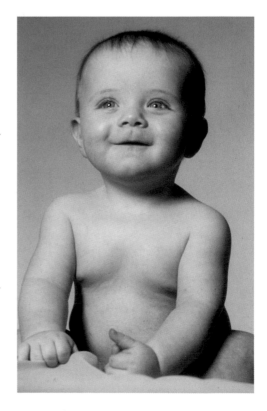

▷ Babies are among those most susceptible to viral encephalitis. Fever and drowsiness are the most common symptoms.

Prolapsed disc and sciatica

SEE ALSO

➤ Exercise for life, p18
➤ The brain and nerve network, p74
➤ Backache, p117

The intervertebral discs sit between the bones of the back (vertebrae). These discs consist of a tough, fibrous ring that holds the bones together and a spongy centre that acts as a shock-absorber. A prolapsed disc, which is also known as a slipped or herniated disc, occurs when the fibrous ring splits and some of the spongy centre is forced out; this in turn presses on the nerves leaving the spine, thereby causing pain. A slipped disc very often leads to a common condition called sciatica – severe nerve pain felt in the buttocks and legs.

SIGNS AND SYMPTOMS OF A PROLAPSED DISC

➤ Pain in the back that radiates down one leg.

➤ Weakness and numbness in a leg.

PROLAPSED DISC

The symptoms of a slipped disc may appear to develop suddenly but this condition arises from long-term changes in the discs caused largely by poor posture and exercise habits. The normally plump and resilient discs can dry out and become brittle as a result of poor circulation in the spine and strain from long periods spent sitting. The affected discs then become vulnerable to

▽ Doing regular toning and stretching exercises, and working on maintaining good posture, will dramatically decrease the risk of developing sciatica.

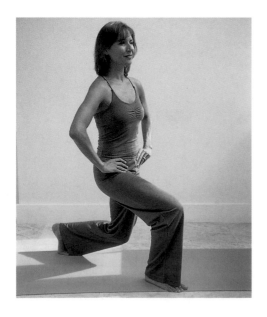

damage, often from relatively minor strains such as bending to pick something up.

To check for a slipped disc, your doctor will consider your medical history and make a thorough examination. A classic sign is that you experience pain when you are lying down and try to lift one leg straight up in the air. A CT or MRI scan of your back can identify the location of the slipped disc.

TREATMENT OPTIONS FOR A PROLAPSED DISC

Most slipped or prolapsed discs will settle after a few weeks of rest and some gentle activity. It is important to keep comfortable and to have adequate pain relief. Many people find that treatment by a physiotherapist is helpful.

If the pain fails to settle or if there is any weakness or numbness, an MRI scan of the back can show how big the prolapse is. It may be necessary to have an operation (microdiscectomy) to remove the affected disc and release the pressure on the nerves.

SCIATICA

This form of pain can be felt anywhere along the course of one of the sciatic nerves that run from the lower back, through the buttocks and down the back of each leg. The pain may be brought on by twisting the back and is made worse when coughing or sneezing. Rarely, there may be weakness and numbness of the leg.

CAUSES OF SCIATICA

In the majority of cases, sciatica is caused by a slipped vertebral disc but other causes can include severe degenerative bone

THE SCIATIC NERVE

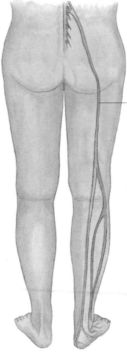

Sciatic nerve

◁ The sciatic nerves extend the length of each leg and end in branching nerve pathways in the foot. The nerves originate from the branching nerve roots in the lower part of the spinal cord. (Note: although occurring in each leg, the nerves are shown in one leg only for simplicity.)

changes to the spine. In rare cases, secondary bone tumours press on spinal nerves and this may affect both legs and the nerves to the bladder and bowel.

TREATMENT OPTIONS

Persistent sciatica should always be assessed by a doctor. If you suffer from sciatica and have difficulty passing urine or opening your bowels, see your doctor immediately or go straight to the hospital. You may need an operation to remove a disc from your spine to prevent paralysis of the legs.

In less severe cases, once a serious underlying condition has been excluded, rest and painkillers are usually the only treatments required.

Spinal injuries

SEE ALSO
➤ The brain and nerve
  network, p74
➤ Backache, p117

Injuries to the spinal cord are often the result of a major trauma such as a fall or a road traffic accident. If the impact was severe, the spinal cord may be damaged beyond repair. The spine is most likely to be damaged at its most mobile parts, which are the neck and lower back. The consequences of a severe spinal cord injury are profound because all muscle and sensory function is usually lost from the point of the injury downwards. A more common and less severe form of spinal injury is whiplash – also caused mainly by road traffic accidents.

Injuries to the neck vertebrae at the top of the spine are immediately fatal because the nerves supplying the breathing muscles are paralyzed. In damage below the fourth neck vertebra, breathing can continue as the nerves to the diaphragm are unaffected. Injuries to the spinal cord in the neck produce quadriplegia (paralysis of all four limbs) whereas lower back injuries can cause paraplegia (paralysis of the legs).

People with spinal cord injuries are also prone to bladder and chest infections and can develop pressure sores on the heels and buttocks due to immobility and the lack of pain sensation.

WHIPLASH INJURY

This common spinal injury occurs when the neck is quickly and violently bent forwards and/or backwards. It usually occurs after a road traffic accident, particularly one in which there is impact from behind. The effects can be long-lasting and debilitating.

THE SPINAL NERVES

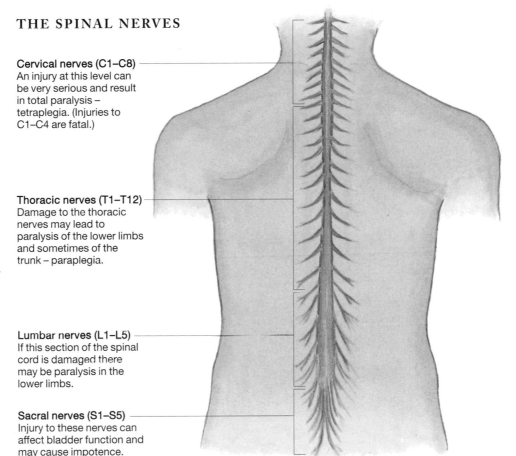

Cervical nerves (C1–C8)
An injury at this level can be very serious and result in total paralysis – tetraplegia. (Injuries to C1–C4 are fatal.)

Thoracic nerves (T1–T12)
Damage to the thoracic nerves may lead to paralysis of the lower limbs and sometimes of the trunk – paraplegia.

Lumbar nerves (L1–L5)
If this section of the spinal cord is damaged there may be paralysis in the lower limbs.

Sacral nerves (S1–S5)
Injury to these nerves can affect bladder function and may cause impotence.

△ The vital spinal nerves enable your body to move and function, so any damage to them can have serious consequences.

SIGNS AND SYMPTOMS OF WHIPLASH INJURY

There may be no pain initially, but neck pain and stiffness start to develop after a few hours. Other symptoms may include:

➤ Headache.

➤ Swelling of affected area.

➤ Shoulder pain.

Seek urgent medical advice if you develop numbness or weakness in your arm or if pain persists or suddenly gets more severe.

It is very often the case that the pain in the neck may not develop until a day or two after the accident.

It is important to seek medical advice if you have been involved in a traffic accident that has affected your neck. Your doctor may refer you to a specialist for an X-ray to assess the extent of any damage.

TREATMENT OPTIONS

Most people with a whiplash injury simply require bed rest, and painkillers to relieve the pain and discomfort. Non steroidal anti-inflammatory drugs such as ibuprofen are most effective. It is advisable that anyone who has had a previous neck problem, or someone whose symptoms do not show any sign of settling after two weeks, should return to their doctor, who may refer them for physiotherapy.

For a long time it was usual practice to issue soft neck collars to whiplash victims however, doctors now know that these tend to stiffen the neck which slows down the healing process, so that it takes much longer for the pain to subside.

Multiple sclerosis

SEE ALSO

➤ The brain and nerve network, p74
➤ The roles of blood and lymph, p200
➤ Autoimmune diseases, p211

Many of the nerve cells in the brain and spinal cord are insulated by sheaths of a fatty substance called myelin, which speeds signals along the nerves. In multiple sclerosis, damage is caused to these myelin sheaths. This is due to abnormal activity of the immune system and the trigger may be infection, but genetic factors may also play a role. This means that the nerve cells cannot function properly. In some cases steroids and the drug beta-interferon can reduce the severity and length of a relapse, but there is no long-term cure for the condition.

SIGNS AND SYMPTOMS

➤ Weakness and/or numbness of limbs.

➤ Loss of coordination.

➤ Urinary frequency, and sometimes incontinence.

➤ Blurred vision.

The symptoms of multiple sclerosis tend to develop in young people over the age of 20. There are two main forms of this disease. The most common is the relapsing-remitting form, in which there are frequent attacks of disabling symptoms with periods of recovery between. Over time, recovery between attacks becomes less complete and there is increasing disability. In the chronic-progressive form, the disabling symptoms advance more slowly and there are no periods of recovery in between.

Doctors may not make a diagnosis until two or more episodes of symptoms have occurred. An MRI brain scan will probably show areas of damage within the brain. If this is unhelpful, taking a sample of the fluid from the spinal cord can aid diagnosis.

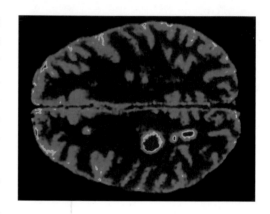

△ This brain scan shows damage, coloured red and yellow, caused by multiple sclerosis. The symptoms vary depending on which nerves have been damaged.

Motor neurone disease

SEE ALSO

➤ The brain and nerve network, p74

This rare progressive disease affects the nerves in the brain and spinal cord that control movement – the motor neurones. Also known as amylotrophic lateral sclerosis, this debilitating disease usually develops after the age of 40. It is more common in men.

SIGNS AND SYMPTOMS

Initially, someone affected by motor neurone disease may not realize anything is wrong. Symptoms develop slowly and insidiously. Over time, a person may start to stumble or notice a weaker grip or increasingly stiff muscles. As the condition progresses, muscles that are involved in swallowing and speech control may be affected. The condition results in severe physical disability but despite this a person's senses and intelligence remain intact.

It may take some time and several visits before your doctor can diagnose motor neurone disease, as the symptoms tend to be general and so could point to a number of different diseases.

You may undergo several investigations before a firm diagnosis is made. These include an MRI scan of the spine and a lumbar puncture (taking a sample of cerebrospinal fluid to check for inflammation). Electromyelography – a test that monitors electrical activity in the muscles – may be performed to show if nerves supplying muscles are damaged.

TREATMENT OPTIONS

As there is no cure for this condition, treatment focuses on relieving any symptoms. Antidepressants may be prescribed and antibiotics may be needed to treat chest infections, to which motor neurone disease sufferers are particularly prone. Physiotherapy to maintain mobility for as long as possible is likely to be offered as well as practical support in dealing with the patient's increasing disability. People with this condition have been known to survive for as long ten years, but a higher proportion die within three years.

Other neurological problems

SEE ALSO

➤ Diabetes, p66
➤ Diseases of the thyroid, p68
➤ Rheumatoid arthritis, p114
➤ Acupuncture, p245

Many neurological problems are localized and affect only the very limited area of the body served by a particular nerve or nerves. They may be painful and distressing and, in some cases, difficult to treat. Symptoms may result from inflammation of nerves as a result of infection or other factors. In other cases the nerve problem is caused by compression from surrounding tissues. Although none of these conditions is a threat to general health, medical advice is needed to obtain effective treatment, possibly including surgery.

TRIGEMINAL NEURALGIA

The trigeminal nerve transmits sensations from parts of your face to the brain as well as controlling muscles that move your jaw. If this nerve is compressed, inflamed or damaged, sharp shooting pains may be felt in the cheeks, lips or one side of the face.

This condition is common among elderly people and its cause is unknown. Pain occurs in short bursts which then subside. Attacks may be triggered by activities such as washing, being out in a cold wind or eating. If painkillers do not help, your doctor may prescribe an anticonvulsant drug called carbamazepine. In a few cases surgery is required.

BELL'S PALSY

The facial nerve carries taste sensations from the front of the tongue and controls muscles of expression in the face. If this nerve is compressed, inflamed or damaged, it causes paralysis of muscles on one side of the face and loss of taste on the front part of the tongue. Often the eyelid and the corner of the mouth will droop. In some cases, the symptoms appear over the course of 24 hours. It may be caused by a virus and usually settles in a couple of weeks, with no after-effects. A course of steroid drugs may help to resolve the paralysis problem. The front of the eye (cornea) needs to be protected if the eyelids cannot be closed and you may have to use artificial tears.

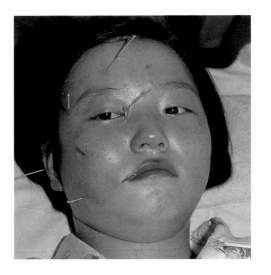

△ Acupuncture, a traditional Chinese therapy, is being used here to treat Bell's palsy, but the symptoms of this condition often disappear without any treatment at all.

THE BRANCHES OF THE TRIGEMINAL NERVE

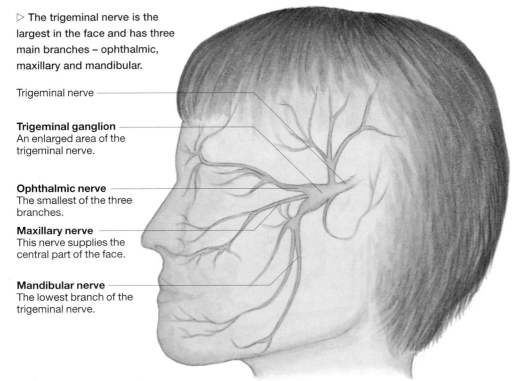

▷ The trigeminal nerve is the largest in the face and has three main branches – ophthalmic, maxillary and mandibular.

Trigeminal nerve

Trigeminal ganglion
An enlarged area of the trigeminal nerve.

Ophthalmic nerve
The smallest of the three branches.

Maxillary nerve
This nerve supplies the central part of the face.

Mandibular nerve
The lowest branch of the trigeminal nerve.

CARPAL TUNNEL SYNDROME

The carpal tunnel is a narrow space in the bones of the wrist and the median nerve runs through it on its way to the hand. If the median nerve becomes trapped and/or constricted it can cause pain and tingling in the hand and forearm. Carpal tunnel syndrome is a common condition. Typically it causes weakness of the thumb and pins and needles in the index, middle and ring fingers, which may be worse first thing in the morning. In most cases there is no obvious cause, although carpal tunnel syndrome is sometimes related to hypothyroidism, diabetes, pregnancy, obesity and rheumatoid arthritis.

Splints and steroid injections can be helpful, but an operation to relieve the pressure on the nerve may be required in some cases.

Dementia

Dementia is a deterioration in mental ability due to a disorder of the brain. It has a combination of symptoms – memory loss, confusion and intellectual decline. It is common and becoming more so as a larger section of the general population is living longer. In severe cases, it is very disabling and distressing for both patients and their friends and families. Dementia usually affects those over 70, but can occur in younger people. Some disorders, such as depression, behave like dementia but once identified and treated, the dementia symptoms soon disappear.

SIGNS AND SYMPTOMS OF DEMENTIA

The following are typical symptoms of dementia and are all related to the loss of higher brain functions:

➤ Impaired memory, particularly of recent events.

➤ Loss of the ability to think.

➤ Noticeably reduced verbal and conversational skills.

➤ Inability to learn new skills or facts.

➤ Loss of emotional control.

➤ Increasing restlessness and a tendency to wander.

➤ Behavioural difficulties.

➤ Depression and/or anxiety.

There is no single test to identify dementia or its specific cause. If your doctor suspects an underlying condition is causing symptoms of dementia, then he or she will arrange for tests to confirm or exclude the suspected diagnosis.

Your doctor may take a sample of blood to send for laboratory analysis, in order to determine the possibility of a vitamin deficiency. Brain scanning may provide revealing information and rule out the more uncommon causes of dementia. Your doctor may also carry out a detailed questioning session aimed at assessing mental ability.

The commonest causes of dementia are Alzheimer's disease and multi-infarct dementia. Rarely, dementia is caused by Creutzfeldt-Jakob disease, known as CJD. Conditions that can cause symptoms similar to those of dementia include vitamin deficiency or anaemia, and adverse reactions to certain drugs.

TREATMENT OPTIONS

There is no specific treatment for any of the forms of dementia and the symptoms get progressively worse with time. Recently, new drugs have become available that improve the symptoms for a short time, but unfortunately in the long term there is nothing that can be done to halt the progress of the disease.

Treatment is based on caring for the increasingly dependent sufferer and most patients end up requiring full-time supervision and nursing care for the remainder of their life.

It is also vital to care for the needs of those looking after a person with dementia.

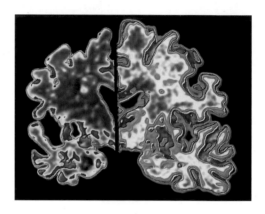

△ A brain affected by Alzheimer's disease (left) is considerably shrunken compared with a normal brain (right).

The impact on carers can be profound, especially if a loved one becomes violent or is unable to remember the carer. No matter how devoted someone is, all carers need plenty of support from medical advisers and social services, and the opportunity to take a break from their responsibilities by taking advantage of respite care.

ALZHEIMER'S DISEASE

This is the most common cause of dementia. This is a progressive degenerative brain condition that causes 70 per cent of the cases of dementia. It results from the loss of nerve cells in the brain, a reduction in neurotransmitter levels and the development of "protein tangles" around the nerve cells. These abnormalities can be detected by a brain scan, which can distinguish Alzheimer's disease from other possible causes of dementia. The underlying cause of the condition is not known, but studies have shown that the tendency to develop Alzheimer's disease may be genetic because it appears to run in families.

▽ Alzheimer's disease is the most common cause of dementia and it is most likely to develop later in life, specifically in those over 70 years of age.

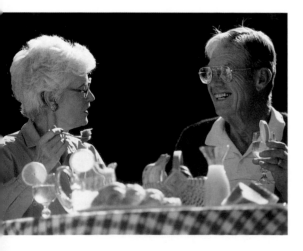

SIGNS AND SYMPTOMS OF ALZHEIMER'S DISEASE

➤ Limited memory. Short-term memory of a few minutes may be intact, but long-term memory is lost with the most recent events being affected first. Many people with dementia can recall their early lives in great detail, but are unable to remember anything that happened to them on the previous day.

➤ Inability to learn new information or use previously learned information.

➤ Loss of language skills.

➤ Inability to perform complex muscular activity, even though muscle function remains normal.

➤ Inability to recognize objects.

➤ Rapid mood swings.

➤ Personality changes.

➤ Wandering off and getting lost, even in familiar surroundings.

➤ Neglect of personal hygiene.

occurs as the result of small ischaemic episodes, which mean there is an inadequate supply of blood reaching a part of the body. These episodes result in oxygen deprivation in the surrounding areas of the brain, causing the gradual death of nerve cells and loss of the functions that they control. Like other forms of stroke, the underlying cause is usually atherosclerosis (the furring up and narrowing of arteries), which is usually the result of lifestyle factors such as a high-fat diet, heavy smoking and lack of exercise. High blood pressure is also a very important risk factor.

The precise nature of the symptoms of this dementia depends on the area of the brain that has been affected, but the process of the condition is gradual and there are not usually any neurological symptoms such as weakness or slurred speech.

MAKING THE DIAGNOSIS

This form of dementia can often be diagnosed from the pattern of symptoms, but in most cases a CT or MRI brain scan is usually carried out to confirm the diagnosis and rule out other possible causes of the symptoms of dementia.

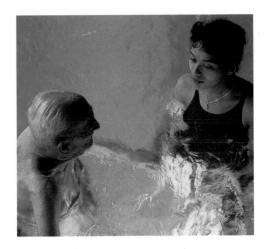

△ Regular gentle exercise such as swimming is particularly important for sufferers from multi-infarct dementia as it can help to reduce the risk of future attacks.

TREATMENT OPTIONS

Brain damage caused by multiple infarcts cannot be repaired. Treatment is therefore focused on the prevention of future episodes and most importantly the risk of a potentially fatal major stroke. Drugs are usually prescribed to reduce blood pressure and regular doses of aspirin may also be taken to reduce the chance of the formation of blood clots.

HOW THE CONDITION PROGRESSES

The symptoms of the disease develop very gradually, and the person will start to become increasingly forgetful and absent-minded. As the disease progresses, among the most distressing symptoms are personality changes and the failure to recognize family and close friends.

Although modern drug treatment can help some symptoms and slow the progress of the disease in certain cases, most Alzheimer's disease sufferers do not survive for longer than ten years following the initial diagnosis.

MULTI-INFARCT DEMENTIA

This condition is also known as vascular dementia. Multi-infarct dementia is the second most common cause of dementia. It

CREUTZFELDT-JAKOB DISEASE (CJD)

An unusual infectious agent called a prion causes this rare disease. It causes spongy areas to develop in the brain, leading to dementia and ultimately death in around six months. Other symptoms include:

➤ Depression.

➤ Unsteadiness and poor coordination.

➤ Seizures.

➤ Impaired vision.

This disease has a very long incubation period and may occur anything up to 20 years after the initial infection. A new variant of CJD (vCJD) has also developed that tends to affect younger people. Scientists have linked vCJD with eating meat from animals infected with "mad cow disease" – bovine spongiform encephalopathy (BSE).

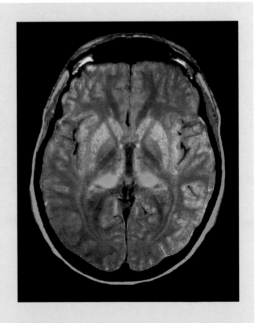

△ This MRI scan shows a section through a CJD-affected brain. The diseased parts of the thalamus (areas of grey matter in the front of the brain) are indicated in green.

Parkinson's disease

SEE ALSO

➤ The brain and nerve network, p74
➤ Dementia, p90
➤ Depression, p98

The symptoms of this common neurological condition, which mainly affects the elderly, are the result of degeneration of nerve cells in a part of the brain that controls movement. The degeneration means that the affected area of the brain no longer produces sufficient dopamine, a chemical neurotransmitter that normally works in balance with another neurotransmitter called acetylcholine, to fine-tune your muscle control. The resulting chemical imbalance in the brain is the cause of the typical symptoms of Parkinson's disease.

SIGNS AND SYMPTOMS OF PARKINSON'S DISEASE

Typical symptoms are:

➤ Tremor of a hand, arm or leg on one side of the body, which may stop as the person attempts a task. Over time both sides may be affected.

➤ Rigidity of the muscles.

➤ Difficulty in initiating movement.

➤ A stooped, shuffling walk.

➤ Expressionless or mask-like face.

➤ Slurred speech.

➤ Depression.

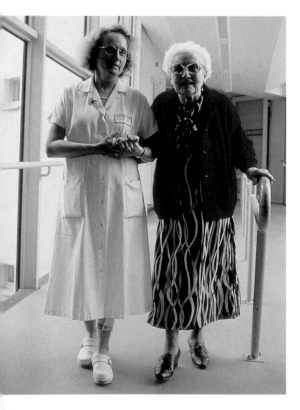

◁ Mobility problems are among the chief symptoms of Parkinson's disease. Plenty of support is needed to maintain an active life.

The underlying cause of the spontaneous degeneration of the nerve cells in the basal ganglia, the part of the brain affected by Parkinson's disease, is unknown. What is known is that susceptibility to the disease appears to run in families and that men are more commonly affected than women. Parkinsonism – which has symptoms similar to those of Parkinson's disease but is due to identifiable factors – can be caused by certain drugs or by head injuries.

HOW THE DISEASE PROGRESSES

In 1817, James Parkinson described this disease as the "shaking palsy", which quite accurately conveys the classic symptoms of this disease – tremor and stiffness. These symptoms develop very gradually. As these movement difficulties grow progressively worse, it can become almost impossible for individuals to perform even the most simple everyday tasks. Many people with Parkinson's disease develop depression and some also develop dementia.

HOW IS IT DIAGNOSED?

Because Parkinson's disease often develops gradually it may take some time for your doctor to diagnose the condition, based on a medical history and physical examination. Long-term observation of muscle activity may be needed to make a definite diagnosis. Blood tests can be carried out to eliminate other conditions. Further tests may include brain scans to establish if the symptoms are caused by a stroke or a brain tumour.

WHERE DAMAGE OCCURS

▽ The area of the brain affected by Parkinson's disease is the basal ganglia. It is this part of the brain that controls smoothness of movement.

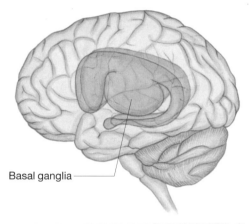

Basal ganglia

Questions will be asked about various factors including exposure to drugs or viruses to establish if it is Parkinsonism.

TREATMENT OPTIONS

Parkinson's disease is usually treated primarily by drugs. The drug most commonly prescribed is levodopa, which is converted to dopamine in the brain and

FUTURE THERAPIES

Some patients undergo brain surgery but this procedure is still experimental. Scientists are currently experimenting with the use of stem cell implants in the treatment of Parkinson's disease. Another possibility for treatment in the future is a pacemaker-type implant that dramatically reduces tremor by stimulating the brain directly. However, none of these therapies are currently used routinely.

restores levels of this neurotransmitter. In excess, this drug can cause unpleasant side effects and the dose is carefully tailored to each patient. In some cases the dose needed to control symptoms is so high that the side effects are unacceptable. In such cases, an alternative drug is prescribed.

Another group of drugs that are sometimes used are anti-cholinergic drugs. These block the effects of acetylcholine, thereby bringing it back into balance with the reduced levels of dopamine. It may take some time to find the right dose of drug for each person and side effects such as dry mouth and impaired vision can create difficulties for some people.

In some cases, most commonly when the disease affects a younger person, surgery

▽ A computer image of a dopamine molecule. Lack of this chemical in the brain is responsible for the symptoms of Parkinson's disease.

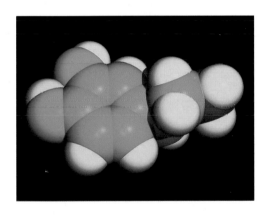

CAUSES OF PARKINSONISM

The symptoms of this condition are very similar to those of Parkinson's disease and can be produced by:

➤ Certain drugs, such as some antipsychotics.

➤ Rare viral infections, such as the strain of flu virus that caused an epidemic in the 1920s.

➤ Abuse of the drug known as MPTP.

➤ Head injury, particularly repeated head injuries such as those sustained by boxers.

BENIGN ESSENTIAL TREMOR

This is a common inherited condition where the tremor usually affects the upper limbs of elderly people. The condition displays symptoms similar to Parkinson's disease but the two are actually not related.

In most cases, treatment may not be needed, although small doses of alcohol or beta-blocker drugs can help reduce the severity of symptoms.

may be considered. The aim of such treatment is to destroy tissue in the area of the brain that governs the tremor. Other more experimental treatments include brain cell transplantation and electrical stimulation of the brain.

SUPPORTIVE MEASURES

Maintenance of mobility is of utmost importance to people with this condition. Parkinson's disease sufferers should try to take as much gentle exercise as possible, including stretching exercises such as yoga, taught by a qualified practitioner. Many people benefit from physiotherapy to help with mobility problems. Rest is also important, as excessive tiredness can make symptoms worse.

As the disease progresses, an individual with Parkinson's disease may also need various physical aids to make everyday tasks achievable. It is important to make clothing, cutlery, chairs, shoes and floors as easy as possible to use. An occupational therapist can advise on adaptations to equipment and to the home that will help to maintain independence. Speech therapy may also be useful. Increasing depression is a common feature of the disease, and in such cases plenty of support from health professionals, as well as family and friends, is very important.

Although Parkinson's disease is debilitating and reduces quality of life, people with the condition can survive for many years following the diagnosis.

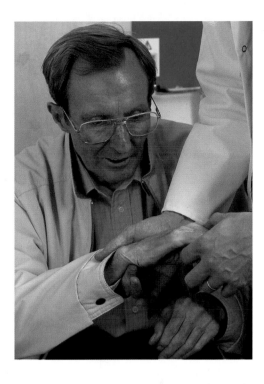

△ A doctor examines the hand of a Parkinson's disease patient. A tremor is one of the classic symptoms of this condition.

HUNTINGTON'S DISEASE

Also known as Huntington's chorea, this rare inherited brain disorder causes jerky, uncontrolled muscle movements and increasing dementia. The disease is caused by the presence of an abnormal gene. The Huntington's disease gene is "dominant", which means that, to be affected, a person has to inherit the defective gene from only one parent. A genetic test, which can be done at any age, can tell you whether you have the abnormal gene.

In those who carry the gene for Huntington's disease, symptoms commonly develop between the ages of 30 and 50. The diagnosis can be confirmed by a CT or MRI scan of the brain, which can detect the type of degeneration that is characteristic of the condition. Drug treatment can ease the spasms and jerks, but the disease gets progressively worse over time, with most patients requiring high levels of care in the later stages. Most sufferers do not survive for more than 10–20 years following the onset of symptoms.

Anxiety

We all experience feelings of nervousness or apprehension in different situations at different times in our lives and this is a completely normal response – whether it is butterflies in the stomach before a big test or exam or worrying about a job interview. Such feelings often lead us to perform better but if anxiety persists or becomes a common response to everyday situations, it can start to have a detrimental effect on normal life. In such cases, particularly when feelings of anxiety occur without apparent cause, professional advice is needed.

SIGNS AND SYMPTOMS
Common symptoms of anxiety are:

➤ Feelings of general unease and agitation.

➤ Inability to relax.

➤ Disturbed sleep.

➤ Episodes of panic.

➤ Feelings of being unable to cope.

A number of factors can contribute to persistent feelings of anxiety but often no underlying cause can be clearly identified. A susceptibility to this condition may be inherited or be brought about by events and experiences in early childhood.

The inherent ability to cope with everyday stress in your life is also influenced by a number of other factors:
• The levels of support available from family and friends.
• Socioeconomic circumstances.
• The number of factors provoking anxiety.
• The intensity of those provoking factors.

Symptoms of anxiety may be felt intermittently when the immediate cause is present (for example when exposed to the object of a phobia) or when the cause is uppermost in a person's mind (reading a bank statement when you have financial problems, say). In other cases there may be almost constant feelings of agitation and fear with no readily discernible cause. In extreme circumstances, when a person cannot cope with overwhelming feelings of anxiety, they may suffer from acute episodes of anxiety known as panic attacks.

Anxiety can result in hyperventilation or overbreathing. This occurs when the stress of a situation causes you to take conscious control of your breathing and you overdo it. The levels of carbon dioxide in the blood fall and your automatic breathing mechanism switches off. The sensation of not being able to breathe is extremely distressing and makes you take deeper breaths. Breathing in and out of your mouth into a paper bag breaks the cycle and normalizes oxygen and carbon dioxide levels in the blood. Hyperventilation is a common feature of panic attacks.

THE CAUSES OF ANXIETY
Common causes of anxiety are:

➤ Relationship problems.

➤ Loss and bereavement.

➤ Health problems.

➤ Financial worries.

➤ Work-related problems.

➤ Unresolved conflicts.

➤ Phobias or obsessive-compulsive disorder.

➤ Physical causes, such as hyperthyroidism.

Anxiety may also accompany or alternate with depression, or may be part of a more serious psychiatric disorder such as schizophrenia. Often, however, no particular cause can be found.

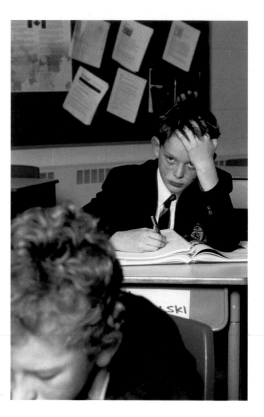

△ The stress of exams and of school life in general can easily lead to anxiety in children and teenagers. It is never too early to learn how to recognize the symptoms and how to deal with what is causing the anxiety effectively.

TREATMENT OPTIONS
The first step in treatment is to consider whether your anxiety may have a root cause in a set of complex physical and/or mental health problems. In the first instance, discussing your situation with your doctor or with a counsellor could help shed some light on the factors that may be important in your case. It is also possible that your doctor may decide to arrange blood tests to rule out the possibility of a physical cause for your symptoms, such as excess production of thyroid hormone.

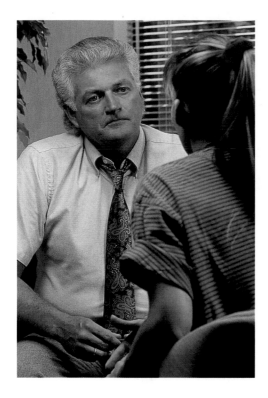

△ Professional counsellors are skilled at helping to discover the root of a problem. Tackling the cause of anxiety is an important part of the treatment for sufferers.

Some patients are reassured when their doctor tells them their symptoms are anxiety-related, as they may have thought that they had developed a serious heart condition, for example. Shortly afterwards, their symptoms may settle and the anxiety is likely to abate.

There are two courses of recognized treatment for anxiety – drug therapy and supportive therapies:

• Drug therapy – The most commonly used anti-anxiety drugs belong to the benzodiazepine family. These drugs can be beneficial in the short term for anxiety and disturbed sleep but the danger is that they are highly addictive and can have counter-productive side effects, so long-term use is not an option. In cases where a patient's anxiety is associated with a depressive illness, antidepressant drugs may be prescribed.

• Supportive therapies – Counselling may allow an affected person to focus on the root causes of his or her anxiety. A psychological approach (cognitive-behavioural therapy) tries to alter the individual's reactions to anxiety-provoking situations. If a phobia or obsessive-compulsive disorder is at the root of the anxiety, specialist therapy to overcome the underlying psychological problem may be recommended.

LONG-TERM OUTLOOK

In most cases, the earlier a person suffering from anxiety receives treatment, the faster they recover from the condition. Without appropriate treatment the anxiety could become ingrained and develop into a lifelong condition.

SELF-HELP

In addition to specific medical treatment and professional counselling, anxiety-sufferers often find that they benefit from making a variety of lifestyle changes. Scientific studies have shown that increasing the amount of regular physical activity taken helps to burn off excess adrenaline, and also provides a healthy outlet for feelings of restlessness. Studies have also shown that exercise helps to

▽ Studies have shown that it is often beneficial for people who suffer from anxiety to own a pet. Caring for and petting an animal has been shown to have a calming influence.

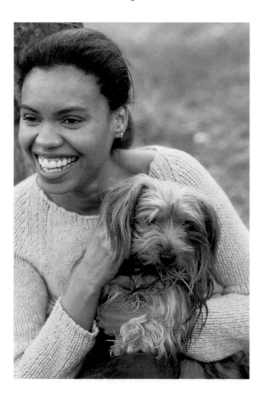

lighten mood and encourage a more positive outlook. Forms of exercise that incorporate relaxation techniques, such as yoga, are particularly effective for dealing with anxiety. In addition, cutting down consumption of stimulants such as caffeine can often dramatically reduce the physical symptoms of anxiety.

PANIC ATTACKS

Someone with an anxiety disorder may suffer from episodes of severe physical symptoms that result from high levels of adrenaline being released into the bloodstream in response to a fear-provoking situation. (Under normal circumstances, this neurotransmitter is released in order to prepare the body for "fight or flight" when confronted by a threatening situation, by increasing the heart rate and breathing rate and causing blood to be diverted to the muscles from other parts of the body.) Typical symptoms of a panic attack are:

➤ Palpitations.

➤ Tightness and pains in the chest.

➤ Difficult or rapid breathing.

➤ Light-headedness and faintness.

➤ Sweating, trembling and nausea.

➤ Heaviness in the arms.

➤ Tingling in the fingers.

➤ Sense of impending death.

Panic attacks may result from exposure to the object of a phobia or they may be a recurring feature of a generalized anxiety disorder.

A panic attack can be alarming to witness and may be hard to distinguish from a heart attack. Although a panic attack usually passes without any harm to the sufferer, if you are present when someone has such an attack and are unsure whether it is a panic attack or something more serious, it is best to summon medical help without delay.

Phobias

SEE ALSO
➤ Anxiety, p94
➤ Panic attacks, p95

A phobia is an irrational and intense fear that is focused on one specific object, activity or situation. There are many common phobias, such as fear of spiders, flying, or heights. Some people become fearful of leaving their home. Certain phobias are minor and, because they do not have a significant impact on daily life, they require no treatment. In other cases the phobia presents a major obstacle to everyday life, preventing the sufferer from pursuing normal activities, and this is where treatment is essential in order to restore quality of life.

When a phobia develops, an affected person will often go to considerable lengths to avoid a specific object or animal, or a fear-provoking situation such as flying or going to the doctor. Exposure to the provoking factor tends to result in hysteria or a panic attack.

WHAT CAUSES PHOBIAS?

It is often not easy to identify the cause of a phobia. A bad experience in early life may result in phobic symptoms. People who are already anxious are more likely to develop phobias, which may be an expression of an underlying generalized anxiety disorder.

TREATING PHOBIAS

Phobias often respond very well to a gradual process of treatment called desensitization. While being given support by your doctor or therapist, you are exposed in stages of increasing intensity to the provoking object or situation. At first, you will experience anxiety but as the treatment progresses you will gradually learn to overcome these feelings. Simple phobias usually respond very well to such treatment, but more complex phobias may be more difficult to treat in this way and therefore require a range of psychological and/or psychiatric interventions.

EXAMPLES OF DIFFERENT PHOBIAS

- Acrophobia – Heights.
- Agoraphobia – Open spaces.
- Arachnophobia – Spiders.
- Aviophobia – Flying.
- Claustrophobia – Enclosed spaces.
- Hydrophobia – Water.
- Latrophobia – Doctors.
- Nosophobia – Becoming ill.

Post-traumatic stress disorder (PTSD)

SEE ALSO
➤ Anxiety, p94

This condition may occur after a person has been exposed to a particularly stressful and upsetting event. Common trigger events include an assault, and witnessing or being involved in a serious accident or disaster. This disorder is more likely to develop in anxiety-prone people.

SIGNS AND SYMPTOMS

These symptoms can develop at any time after the trigger event and tend to persist for months or years afterwards:

➤ Preoccupation with the event and/or flashbacks.

➤ Anxiety and panic attacks.

➤ Depression and poor concentration, often with signs of withdrawal and detachment.

This condition has been more widely recognized in recent years. Effective support and/or counselling following involvement in a traumatic event can help to prevent it from occurring or at least minimize its severity. People with this disorder often respond well to a few months of counselling in conjunction with antidepressant medication. The support of family and close friends is an invaluable aid to recovery.

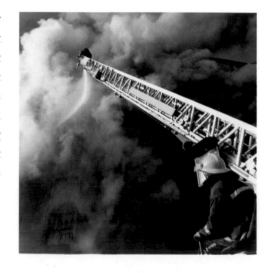

▷ Emergency workers such as firefighters are at risk from post-traumatic stress disorder because of the nature of their work.

Obsessive-compulsive disorder

SEE ALSO
➤ Learn to manage stress, p12
➤ Anxiety, p94
➤ Addictive behaviours, p102

This psychiatric disorder, or neurosis, is one in which a person experiences anxiety in connection with a persistently recurring thought, feeling or impulse. As a result of this there is often an irresistible urge (compulsion) to carry out rituals, such as the repeated washing of hands, excessive cleaning and constant checking of keys, gas controls or water taps. The affected person will very often understand that their behaviour is irrational but simply cannot control it. The rituals usually have an anxiety-reducing and containing function.

Obsessive-compulsive disorder is relatively common. Doctors believe it affects about 1 in 100 people in developed countries. However, the exact numbers affected are difficult to estimate because many people who suffer from this form of psychiatric disorder do not seek medical help.

WHAT TRIGGERS OBSESSIVE-COMPULSIVE BEHAVIOUR?

Many of us enact harmless rituals that often started in childhood – for example, always avoiding treading on the lines of paving stones or always taking precisely the same route home. This kind of ritualized behaviour is not a problem if it is not accompanied by extreme anxiety or fear of the consequences if the ritual is not carried out. It is only when the need to perform the ritual dominates a person's life and takes priority over other needs such as work that a person can be said to have this condition.

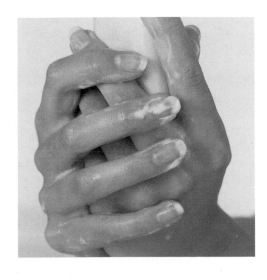

▽ The ritual of obsessive handwashing may be the result of an excessive fear of germs or a feeling of being unclean.

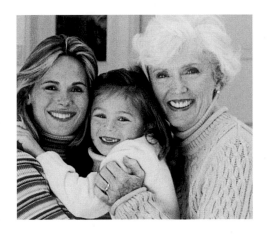

△ Some families are prone to obsessive-compulsive disorder, but it is unclear whether it is an inherited tendency or learned behaviour.

Obsessive-compulsive disorders often first appear in adolescence and many cases can be linked to stress or stressful events in a person's life. It sometimes runs in families. Some people are said to have an obsessive-compulsive personality, meaning that these people continually strive for perfection and disregard other people's feelings. People with such personality types are more likely to suffer from this problem.

WHEN TO SEE YOUR DOCTOR

In severe cases of obsessive-compulsive disorder, a person may perform rituals such as handwashing hundreds of times a day, which may interfere with everyday life such as going out to work or doing household chores. The anxiety that often accompanies the behaviour can be very distressing for the affected person. If you are worried about the fact that you are experiencing uncontrollable thoughts and are carrying out compulsive rituals, then it is a good idea to talk things through with your doctor.

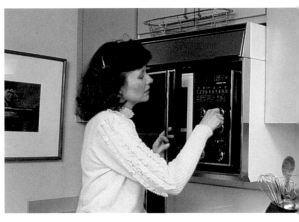

△ The excessive checking of switches or dials is a classic manifestation of an obsessive-compulsive disorder.

WHAT MIGHT YOUR DOCTOR DO?

Your doctor may suspect obsessive-compulsive disorder from a description of your feelings and behaviour. A range of psychotherapeutic approaches may be helpful – cognitive and behavioural therapies can be highly successful. Such therapy is designed to help you confront and control your compulsions to carry out rituals. You may find that things get worse for a short time before you start to experience an improvement in your condition. Your therapist or doctor may also prescribe a course of antidepressants.

WHAT IS THE OUTLOOK?

The majority of people with obsessive-compulsive disorder start to show substantial improvement once they are receiving appropriate therapy. Some people, such as those with an obsessive-compulsive personality, are prone to persistent or recurring episodes of such behaviour over many years.

Depression

SEE ALSO
➤ Learn to manage stress, p12
➤ Eat healthily, p14
➤ Exercise for life, p18
➤ Sensible drinking, p22

Feelings of sadness are normal emotions that are experienced by all of us to some degree during our lives. Depression is a psychological state in which these feelings become intense and start to interfere with everyday activities. It is one of the most common mental health problems and affects twice as many women as men. Depression often clears spontaneously after a few days or weeks, but in other cases it requires professional help and support. Severely depressed people may need to be admitted to hospital to protect them from self-harm.

SIGNS AND SYMPTOMS
➤ General loss of interest and apathy.

➤ Low levels of energy.

➤ An inability to cope.

➤ Persistent low mood.

➤ Early morning waking.

➤ Loss of libido.

➤ Loss of appetite.

➤ Low self-esteem.

➤ Guilt.

➤ Anxiety.

➤ Morbid preoccupations.

➤ Thoughts of self-harm.

such as low levels of thyroid hormone (hypothyroidism) or the hormonal disruption that can occur after childbirth or around the menopause. In other cases lifestyle factors such as excessive alcohol consumption or drug abuse are the cause of the problem. However, depression may also develop suddenly in a person who has no clearly identifiable risk factors or who has not experienced any triggering life events. This is known as endogenous depression.

NON-DRUG TREATMENT
It is important to seek your doctor's advice if you are feeling persistently depressed. It is also vital that someone who has contemplated suicide obtains medical help as a matter of urgency.

You may find it helps to clarify things in your own mind by discussing your

△ Feelings of despair, futility and worthlessness are the hallmark of depression. Such feelings are more severe than just being "down".

situation with your doctor or, perhaps, a member of your church where this is appropriate. It is often therapeutic if a neutral person listens to your problems without being judgemental or critical.

Causes of depression are many and varied. There is evidence that some people inherit a genetic predisposition towards developing depression that may then be triggered by any or a combination of provoking events. Common triggers include:
• Loss and bereavement.
• Relationship problems and breakdown.
• Poor health.
• Acting as a carer for long periods.
• Financial worries.
• Work-related problems.
• Unresolved conflicts.

Sometimes depression develops when the accumulated load of problems becomes too much for a person to bear. In some cases depression is caused by physiological factors

JUST A BAD MOOD?
Depression is part of the full spectrum of different moods that people experience – we all have our ups and downs in life and this is often reflected in how we feel. It is quite normal to feel sad every now and then, but if this becomes a persistent feeling, then that is depression, and there is something wrong with the balance of neurotransmitters in your brain that needs to be addressed. Likewise, everyone has periods of elation but if this became a permanent state of euphoria and excessive activity, known as mania, your mental function would suffer and you would need medical help to normalize brain function and behaviour. Below is a simplified medical interpretation of the full range of states of mind.

▬▬ Normal range of mood
▬▬ Abnormal range of mood

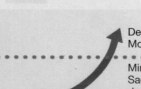

Mania

Mild euphoria
Cheery, hopeful, happy

Depressive psychosis
Moderate depression

Minor depression
Sad, gloomy, despondent

Your doctor may also suggest an assessment with a counsellor or a psychologist. A fair amount of overlap exists between these two disciplines. A counsellor tends to focus on your feelings and helps you to understand them, while a psychologist attempts to change negative patterns of thinking and channel them in a more positive direction.

Support from a range of sources is helpful. Immediate family and friends may be a ready source of day-to-day support, encouragement and help. However, not everyone is fortunate enough to have a supportive circle of people available to help them at such a time.

ANTIDEPRESSANT DRUG THERAPY

Your doctor may prescribe a course of antidepressants and you may take them in conjunction with psychological therapy. Antidepressants alter the balance of the chemicals in the brain and there are several different types. Your doctor will choose a drug suitable for your situation and needs. Although certain benefits, such as improved sleep, may be noticed immediately, it takes at least two weeks for most antidepressant drugs to start to lift mood. However, minor side effects may be noticed straight away. If

▽ Certain life-stages, such as leaving home to cope with the pressures of student life, often lead to stresses that in turn trigger depression.

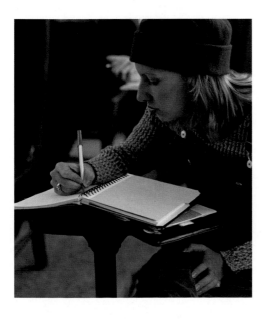

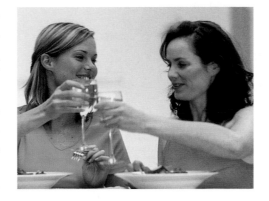

△ Talking to, and being around, friends can help to stave off depressive feelings, though medical help may also be necessary.

such side effects are troublesome you should contact your doctor, who may be able to find an alternative drug that is more suitable for you.

Once an antidepressant is working, initial improvements are often sustained and a person gradually becomes more able to cope with everyday life. Most doctors recommend that antidepressants are taken for at least four to six months. The decision to stop taking medication depends on how well you respond, along with a number of other factors. If the factors that caused the depression in the first place have not been resolved, or if a period of counselling is proving to be quite stressful, it is usually better to wait until things have settled down before discontinuing medication.

Antidepressants do not take away the ability to feel the natural spectrum of human emotions, and they are not addictive. People often confuse them with tranquillizers, which are addictive and are of no help in managing depression.

SELF-HELP

The effectiveness of any treatment for depression can be increased in many cases by attention to lifestyle and daily routine. It is important to establish that day to day you take plenty of exercise, preferably outdoors, and that your diet is healthy. Filling each day with interesting and enjoyable activities is important, although care should be taken not to take on too much too quickly.

SEASONAL AFFECTIVE DISORDER

Many people with recurrent depression tend to develop marked feelings of unhappiness and low mood during winter. This is known as seasonal affective disorder (SAD), and it is thought to be linked to low levels of light during the winter months.

Most people notice a lowering of mood in winter and this usually improves markedly with the brighter conditions of spring. Animals and plants are much less active during the cold months of winter and it may be that your body has a natural urge to slow down but modern lifestyles make no allowance for such reduced activity in winter.

Light therapy, which involves treatment with ultraviolet light, can improve the mood of people with SAD. If this fails, a course of antidepressant drugs may be prescribed.

▽ People who are affected by SAD often benefit from specialized treatment that involves being exposed to high-intensity light panels for several hours each day.

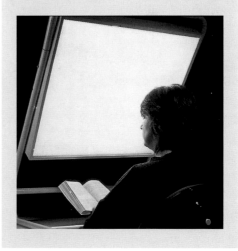

THE LONG-TERM OUTLOOK

In the majority of cases, depression either passes without any need for treatment or it is resolved with supportive therapy, counselling and/or medication. Some people, however, will continue to suffer from episodes of depression throughout their lives and often require long-term specialist treatment.

Bipolar affective disorder

Many people experience considerable swings of mood – episodes of low mood alternating with periods of elation and enthusiasm. Previously known as manic-depression, bipolar affective disorder is the condition in which this tendency to mood fluctuation becomes extreme. An affected person switches from periods of profound depression to episodes of extremely energetic activity (mania), often with very bizarre behaviour that may include excessive expenditure on unnecessary goods, personal neglect, and/or outbreaks of violence.

Bipolar affective disorder often becomes apparent during a person's early 20s. Researchers believe that some individuals may have a genetic predisposition toward developing this condition and that it may be triggered or unmasked by one or a number of adverse life events.

GETTING HELP

While in the depressed phase of this condition, the person may feel so despairing and demotivated that they can see no

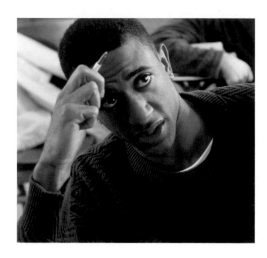

△ Inability to concentrate is a common symptom during the manic phase of bipolar affective disorder.

purpose in seeking help. They may feel so worthless that they do not believe that they deserve to be helped. At such times it is important for family and friends to make every effort to persuade the person to see their doctor.

During the manic phase, the person may feel completely well and have no insight into the abnormal nature of their behaviour or mood. They are likely to blame others for any difficulties that they are experiencing. In cases where the manic behaviour leads to aggression or violence, compulsory admission to hospital for treatment may be required.

TREATMENT OPTIONS

During the depressive phase, antidepressant drugs are usually prescribed. However, doctors must maintain a balance so that they control the depression without elevating the mood so much that a person becomes manic.

Treatment of the manic phase of this condition is more difficult because the person often does not accept the need for treatment. Severe mania is usually effectively controlled by treatment with antipsychotic drugs.

Individuals who are particularly prone to recurrent episodes of bipolar depression may respond well to lithium, a drug that tends to stabilize mood swings and prevent relapses. Certain anticonvulsant drugs also have mood-stabilizing properties and doctors sometimes prescribe these as an alternative treatment.

People with bipolar affective disorder need regular check-ups to monitor mood changes and fine-tune drug treatment.

▽ Periods of depression alternate with mania. As with other forms of depression, low mood is not helped by excessive alcohol consumption.

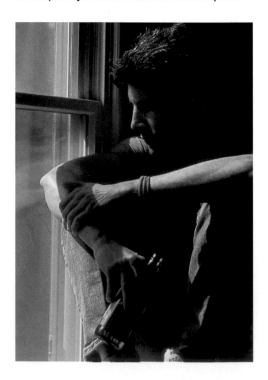

SIGNS AND SYMPTOMS

Bipolar affective disorder is characterized by alternating episodes of depression and mania. These episodes will last for varying lengths of time and are usually interspersed with periods of complete normality.

During the depressive episode, symptoms are the same as those experienced during depression and the severity of these symptoms will vary.

Episodes of mania are characterized by the following symptoms:

➤ High levels of energy and activity.

➤ Elation.

➤ Delusions of grandeur.

➤ Inability to concentrate.

➤ Lack of insight into the situation.

➤ Spending sprees.

➤ Lack of sexual restraint.

➤ Lack of self-care.

Schizophrenia

SEE ALSO
➤ Anxiety, p94
➤ Addictive behaviours, p102

This serious mental disorder affects about 1 in every 100 people and affects both men and women. Sufferers have a skewed view of reality and are unable to function socially. The causes of schizophrenia are uncertain but researchers believe that genetic factors may play a significant part in the condition's development. Adverse life events, such as a bereavement, may unmask a schizophrenic illness in someone with a genetic predisposition. Taking mood-altering drugs, such as Ecstasy, can also trigger schizophrenia in predisposed individuals.

SIGNS AND SYMPTOMS

The most common time for men to be diagnosed with schizophrenia is during the late teenage years and early 20s. Women tend to develop the condition later in life, during their 30s and 40s. The symptoms may become apparent gradually over many months but it is possible for them to appear suddenly in someone with no previous history.

Common symptoms include:

➤ Hearing imaginary voices.

➤ Paranoia.

➤ Having irrational beliefs.

➤ Becoming withdrawn.

➤ Agitation.

➤ Having rambling thoughts and ideas.

➤ Lack of insight.

Some of these symptoms, such as hearing voices, will often relate to a patient's personal belief system.

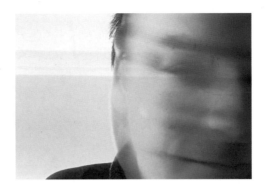

△ Disconnection from reality, isolation and inappropriate emotional responses are typical symptoms of schizophrenia.

Schizophrenia is a serious form of psychological illness. Its name, meaning split personality, does not, in fact, describe this condition accurately. The characteristic features of this disorder are a loss of connection with reality, which leads to irrational beliefs, bizarre behaviour and emotional disturbance. Hallucinations, particularly hearing voices, are common in cases of schizophrenia. In many cases the person believes that their thoughts are being controlled by someone or something outside themselves. He or she may ascribe unwarranted significance to minor events or things. The symptoms described above may occur in distinct episodes or be present continuously.

TREATMENT OPTIONS

A person with suspected schizophrenia needs medical help. Someone displaying signs of schizophrenia may be admitted to hospital for initial assessment and treatment. Investigations may include brain scans to eliminate other possible causes of the disturbed behaviour.

Once the condition is diagnosed, treatment with antipsychotic drugs is usually given, which in most cases helps to control symptoms and effectively prevent relapses. However, long-term treatment with such drugs can produce a variety of adverse effects such as tremors and other involuntary movements. These problems can sometimes be alleviated by an adjustment in dosage or the administration of other drugs to counter these effects. A range of newer drugs seem to have far fewer side effects than those associated with the older antipsychotic medications.

People living with schizophrenia usually require regular long-term follow-up care to ensure their wellbeing and to try to detect episodes of relapse before they become problematic. Family and friends prove invaluable in such situations. Supportive therapies such as counselling may help to reduce the levels of stress and anxiety triggered by this condition.

WHAT IS THE OUTLOOK?

About 20 per cent of affected people have one isolated episode of schizophrenic illness with no further episodes of the condition. For the remaining 80 per cent, however, the condition is a life long problem in which periods of apparent normality are interspersed with periods of schizophrenic illness of varying severity, which often require long periods of hospitalization.

▽ Schizophrenia requires doctors and other healthcare professionals to cooperate in working out the best long-term care strategy for the patient.

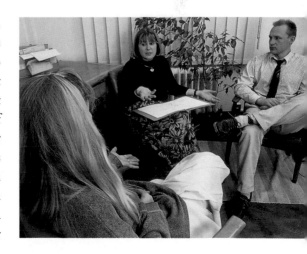

Addictive behaviours

Addiction is dependence on a particular substance or behaviour to the extent that fulfilling that dependence becomes a dominant preoccupation in a person's life. Substance misuse, most commonly involving alcohol and drugs, is an increasing problem worldwide. It causes a range of health problems as well as a variety of social problems, including the breakdown of families and increased levels of crime. Addictive behaviours, such as compulsive shopping or gambling, are likely to cause social rather than physiological problems.

For many people, obtaining and consuming an addictive substance or pursuing an addictive behaviour takes precedence over family relationships and breaks through social restraints, often leading to criminal behaviour. The addiction may be physical, in that withdrawal of the substance produces symptoms such as diarrhoea and vomiting, or the dependence may be psychological, producing craving and agitation if the consumption of the substance or behaviour is prevented. Most addictions to substances such as drugs and alcohol are a combination of both.

DRUG ADDICTION

Children and young people are influenced by parents, peers and role models. People who have difficulty dealing with anxiety and other emotions may find that drugs help control their symptoms and allow more effective social functioning. Children growing up in such an environment are vulnerable, and studies have shown that they are more at risk of succumbing to addictive patterns of behaviour.

DRUGS OF ABUSE

There is a wide range of illicit substances available. Commonly used stimulants are amphetamines, Ecstasy, crack and cocaine. These drugs stimulate the nervous system and induce a sense of power and energy. They allow the user to keep going for long periods without sleep but may also induce a sense of anxiety and paranoia. Exhaustion results from continuous use and there may be long-term psychological damage.

Many people believe that cocaine is a social drug with no potential for addiction, but crack and cocaine are extremely addictive. Cravings for crack are almost impossible to control and usually result in destructive behaviour designed to perpetuate the addiction.

Some drugs have a relaxant effect. The most commonly used is marijuana (cannabis) but heroin and the anaesthetic ketamine are widely used, too. Tranquillizers that are legally prescribed for the short-term treatment of anxiety may also be abused and have addictive potential. The long-term health risks of smoking cannabis are not fully known, but regular consumption may impair judgement and can induce long-term psychological

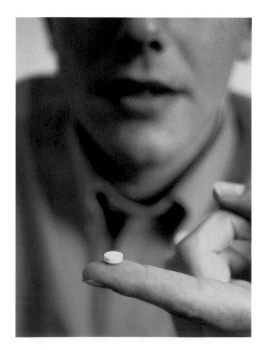

◁ The exact constituents of illicit drugs is usually unknown, which increases the risk of dangerous and unpredictable side effects.

SIGNS AND SYMPTOMS OF DRUG ABUSE

Tranquillizers such as benzodiazepine cause drowsiness, shallow breathing and a weak pulse. Stimulants such as cocaine and amphetamines cause extremely excitable behaviour and the shakes. Narcotics such as heroin cause confusion, tiny pupils and shallow breathing. Hallucinogens such as LSD cause sweating and hallucinations. Alchohol causes flushed skin, a weak pulse and, at worst, coma.

Withdrawal from any drug can cause a variety of symptoms including muscle aches and pains, diarrhoea and vomiting.

problems such as demotivation and depression, and it may also cause COPD (chronic obstructive pulmonary disease).

SOCIAL CONSEQUENCES

Users of drugs such as crack and heroin often develop physical dependence and become involved in crime to pay for their habit. Addiction has a destructive effect on relationships and employment. An addict may lose everything of value and face legal proceedings, often ending up in prison.

DRUG ABUSE HEALTH RISKS

People who inject drugs such as heroin risk contracting a range of infections. Where needles and syringes have been shared there is a high risk of catching:
• Hepatitis B.
• Hepatitis C.
• HIV.

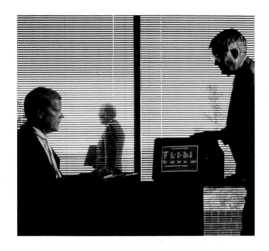

△ In much of the world today, work is a central part of many people's lives and long hours are the norm. In this climate, it is easy for work to dominate and turn into a kind of addiction.

Other common infections among injecting drug-users are:
• Septicaemia (blood poisoning).
• Endocarditis (infection of the valves inside the heart).
• Cellulitis (infection of the skin and subcutaneous tissues).
• Abscesses, especially at injection sites.

ALCOHOLISM

Alcohol is a central nervous system depressant that is an accepted part of everyday life in most societies around the world. Taken in moderation it can induce relaxation and ease inhibitions. In excess, it can severely impair judgement and coordination, and sometimes leads to violent behaviour. Regular heavy alcohol consumption may produce physical and psychological dependence, often preventing the person from working effectively and leading in some cases to loss of employment and severe disruption of family relationships The many health problems associated with heavy drinking include:
• Liver damage.
• Vitamin deficiencies.
• Peptic ulcers.

SIGNS OF ALCOHOLISM

It is not always easy to distinguish between regular social drinking and the excessive drinking that indicates alcoholism. The amount of alcohol consumed is only a rough indicator, although a person who drinks enough to be noticeably intoxicated several times a week is likely to have become dependent. Other indicators of a potential drinking problem include:
• Gradually increasing alcohol intake.
• A compulsion to drink and anxiety or physical symptoms if this is not possible.

TREATMENT OPTIONS FOR ADDICTION

It is very rare for any addictive behaviour, and particularly drug addictions and alcoholism, to improve spontaneously and addicts cannot begin their recovery programme until they admit that they have a problem and seek help. The addict may often need to be admitted to a special clinic where there is no access to the addictive substance or opportunity to pursue addictive behaviour. Supportive counselling and other specialized therapies such as cognitive and behaviour therapy also play an important part in the treatment process. The first step in the treatment of any addiction is to try to establish the root cause of the behaviour. Many specialists believe that there is such a thing as an "addictive personality", which might be partly genetic. However, there is also much evidence to support addiction as a learned behaviour.

If you know someone who has an addiction, you can go to your doctor to discuss how you should handle the problem

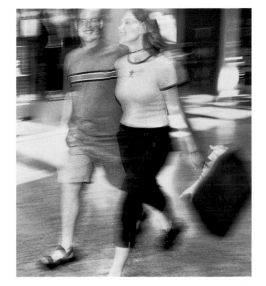

COMPULSIVE GAMBLING
Some people have an intense and compulsive desire to gamble and this urge dominates their lives. It more commonly affects men and often appears before the age of 25. Compulsive gamblers, also known as pathological gamblers, continuously increase the amounts of money they bet in order to experience the desired level of excitement. This kind of behaviour can destroy a person's life, affecting personal relationships, work, family and friends. In certain cases, gamblers lie, cheat or steal money for more gambling, regardless of the effects it may have on anyone close to them. Therapy via self-help groups, with encouragement from close friends and family members, can be successful.

▽ The motivation for compulsive gambling may be the "high" from the expectation rather than the win itself.

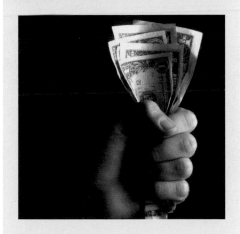

and how the addict can get help. Your doctor will be able to give you information and direct you to the many appropriate specialized services that have been developed to support and treat people with addictions.

However, the fact remains that any treatment can only be effective in the long term if the addict wants to stop and acknowledges their need for therapy.

◁ One form of addictive behaviour is obsessive "retail therapy", where shoppers feel highs and lows much like a drug addict. This can create all kinds of problems, including vast debt.

Eating disorders

SEE ALSO
➤ Eat healthily, p14
➤ Weight control, p16
➤ Depression, p98

Eating disorders are most common in Western cultures, which place great emphasis on being slim. Such problems are especially prevalent among the middle or upper social classes and are a particular occupational hazard for models, dancers, actors and certain athletes, who are required to maintain a slim body. There are two main types of eating disorder: anorexia nervosa and bulimia. About 1 per cent of teenage girls develop anorexia. Once considered a largely female problem, eating disorders are now seen increasingly in teenage boys and young men.

ANOREXIA NERVOSA

Anorexia usually affects teenage girls or young women. It is potentially life-threatening and 5 per cent of sufferers die from complications linked to severe weight loss. Women with anorexia even stop menstruating, as the condition affects their hormone balance. There may be muscle-wasting and loss of bone density. Depression is common. The affected person has a false body image, which makes them feel overweight and desperate to lose weight even when they are, in fact, very thin. Anorexics often hide their condition by wearing baggy clothes. They may show interest in food and cooking, while at the same time not eating.

BULIMIA

Bulimia is a less dangerous condition as it rarely leads to extreme weight loss. It tends to develop in young women who worry about their weight but, rather than diet

▽ Most sufferers of eating disorders are young women. This woman is being encouraged to look in a mirror in order to help her correct any distorted ideas she has about her body shape.

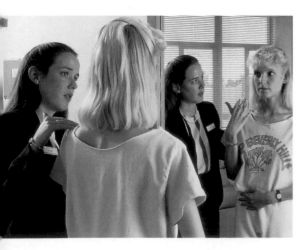

SIGNS AND SYMPTOMS OF EATING DISORDERS

Symptoms of anorexia nervosa include:

➤ Dieting and exercising excessively.

➤ Using laxatives and inducing vomiting.

➤ Using weight-reducing drugs, such as amphetamines.

Symptoms of bulimia include:

➤ Food cravings and binge eating.

➤ Eating induced by guilt and/or anxiety.

➤ Inducing vomiting.

➤ Excessive use of laxatives.

Other physical symptoms of eating disorders may include:

➤ Swollen ankles.

➤ Erosion of tooth enamel, on front teeth especially.

➤ Scars or bruises on the fingers from bouts of self-induced vomiting.

moderately, they follow an extreme regime of bingeing and starving themselves. There may be phases of anorexia and bulimia in the same person.

TREATMENT OPTIONS

Treating people with eating disorders can be difficult, especially when they refuse to acknowledge that they have a problem. Such treatment is highly specialized and is usually managed by a team of people with specific experience in dealing with eating disorders. Approaches that they use include:
• Counselling.
• Psychotherapy such as cognitive and behaviour therapies.
• Psychiatric support.
• Family therapy.

RECOVERY RATES

About 20 per cent of people with anorexia recover completely. But in two-thirds of patients, the condition persists or recurs.

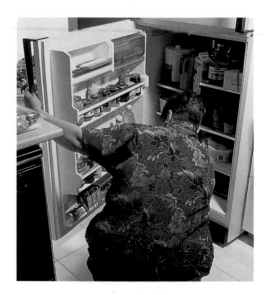

△ Secret binge eating is one of the key features of bulimia. A person with this condition is not usually underweight.

Symptoms often become especially apparent during times of stress and conflict. Bulimia can often be controlled – in four out of five cases the frequency of bingeing is reduced by therapy.

THE MUSCLES AND SKELETON

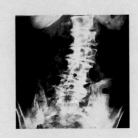

The bones of the skeleton provide the body with structural support, protection for the major internal organs and, combined with the muscles, enable our bodies to move. Each joint where bones meet allows flexibility and movement, and muscles are joined to bones at the joints by tough fibres called ligaments. Your muscles operate by contracting and relaxing to pull on the bones and so move the body around. Even a minor injury can cause major disruption to this complex structure, and regular exercise and a healthy diet will do much to keep the system functioning well.

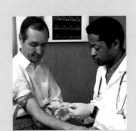

CONTENTS

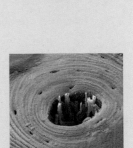

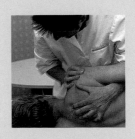

The musculoskeletal system

SEE ALSO

➤ Exercise for life, p18
➤ Osteoporosis, p108
➤ The function of the ears, nose and throat, p166

The musculoskeletal system is made up of the bones of the skeleton, joints that link the bones together and the muscles that enable the body to move. At birth, a baby has around 350 bones, some of which fuse together as it grows. Adults usually have 206 bones, though some have extra ribs and others have fewer. The body's largest bone is the femur in the thigh and its smallest is the tiny stapes in the ear. The muscles and ligaments act with the bones to produce a range of movements, from precision threading of a needle to the most vigorous exercise.

BONE STRUCTURE

There are two types of bone structure. Compact bone is smooth and hard. Spongy or cancellous bone has a honeycomb structure that makes it much lighter. A long bone has an outer layer of compact bone around a layer of spongy bone. Blood vessels run through cavities in the bone carrying oxygen and nutrients. Red bone marrow lies in the centre of flat and irregular shaped bones such as the ribs, vertebrae and skull.

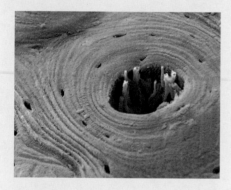

△ Blood vessels and nerves run through a cavity in a section of compact bone.

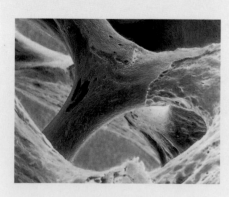

▽ Cancellous (spongy) bone from the femur. The cavities in the bone are filled with bone marrow.

Bone is a living part of the body that is constantly growing and changing. It has an immense and intricate blood supply, which is why major fractures can cause considerable blood loss. Bone consists of a mesh-like network of collagen, a protein that is the main building block of the body. Into this mesh, bone-making cells called osteoblasts deposit calcium and these give bone its hardness and strength. After death the collagen decays, and only the calcium element of the bones remains.

Most bone develops from cartilage (cartilage is the tough, gristly material found at the ends of ribs, in the outer ears and the tip of the nose). When a baby is still in the womb, cartilage starts to harden into bone in a process called ossification. As a child grows, the process continues. Bone growth occurs at the ends of the long bones as new cartilage is continually laid down before it goes through the hardening process. The skeleton is not fully formed until around 30 years of age.

THE FUNCTION OF BONES

The bones of the skeleton provide structural support for the body and work with the muscles to move it. Bones also have other functions:

• Some bones protect the vital organs. The skull acts as armour for the brain, and the pelvic bones keep abdominal organs from being damaged. The movement of the ribs aids the process of breathing and they also protect the organs of the chest, such as the heart and lungs.

• The bones of the ear help with hearing. They act as amplifiers when sound passes from the outside world through the ear on its way to the brain.

• The bone marrow inside flat bones, such as the shoulder blades and breastbone, produces a range of blood cells.

PHYSIOTHERAPY

Treatment for many diseases affecting the musculoskeletal system involves physiotherapy. During physiotherapy the muscles, bones and joints are encouraged to recover through regular and systematic exercises, performed either by the patient or with manipulation by the physiotherapist. The trained physiotherapist also has access to ultrasound and heat treatments, as well as a range of supports and splints. The aim is to return the affected area of the body to health and get it working normally again as fast as possible.

THE JOINTS

A joint is the junction between two or more bones. Some joints are fixed, such as those of the skull, while others, such as the cartilaginous joints between the vertebrae of the spine, have hardly any movement. However, most joints in the body move freely and are known as synovial joints. The ends of the bones meeting at synovial joints are covered with a thin layer of cartilage to stop them grinding against each other. They are lubricated, to allow smooth movements, by a thin layer of fluid called synovial fluid. The ligaments are strong fibrous strips that hold bones together at the joint and stop them from moving too far apart.

TYPES OF JOINTS

There are six types of joint and each joint has a different range of movement.

Type of joint	Where in the body
Ball and socket	Shoulders and hips.
Ellipsoidal	Links the radius to the wrist.
Hinge	Knees, elbows and fingers.
Plane or sliding	Links the carpal bones in the wrists and the tarsal bones in the feet.
Saddle	Base of the thumb.
Pivot	Links the first two vertebrae in the neck.

MUSCLE POWER

There are about 640 skeletal muscles in the body, forming up to half of the body's weight. Muscles cover the framework of the skeleton to give the body its shape. Skeletal muscles link two bones and pass across the joint between them. Each muscle is made up of muscle fibres that can be up to 30 cm (12 in) long but are thinner than a hair. There are three different types of muscle:

- Skeletal muscles – The bulk of the body's muscles are skeletal muscles, which move the body. Skeletal muscles are voluntary muscles – they do not contract on their own. In response to a nerve impulse from the brain, the muscle contracts, pulling on the bone and moving it. Muscles can only pull and never push so they work in pairs. When the biceps contracts it pulls the forearm towards the upper arm, bending the arm at the elbow. The triceps on the opposite side of the upper arm relaxes, allowing this to happen. When the triceps contracts, the biceps relaxes and the movement is reversed.
- Smooth muscles – Situated in the walls of the body's hollow organs, such as the digestive tract, they perform automatic tasks such as propelling food along.
- Cardiac muscle – This forms the non-stop pump that is the heart.

THE MUSCLES AND SKELETON

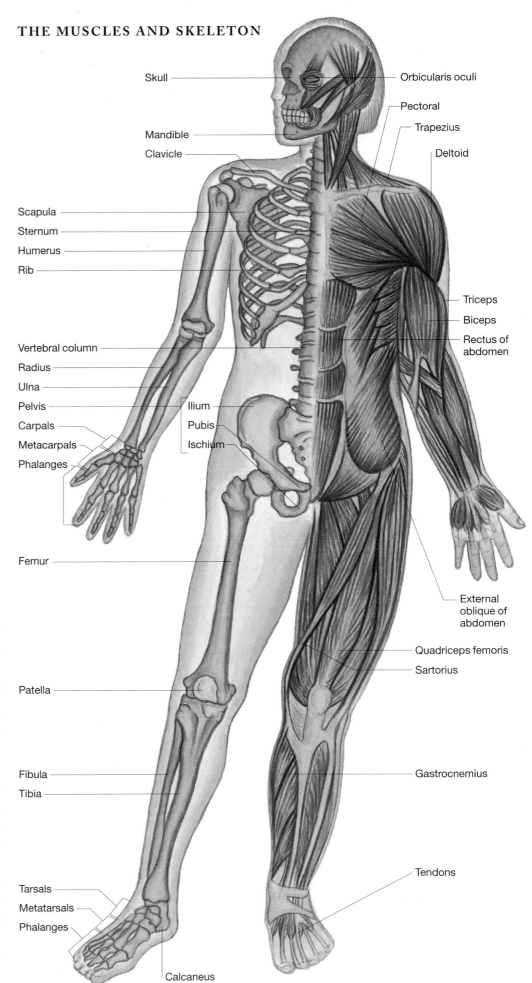

Skull

Mandible

Clavicle

Scapula

Sternum

Humerus

Rib

Vertebral column

Radius

Ulna

Pelvis

Carpals

Metacarpals

Phalanges

Femur

Patella

Fibula

Tibia

Tarsals

Metatarsals

Phalanges

Calcaneus

Orbicularis oculi

Pectoral

Trapezius

Deltoid

Triceps

Biceps

Rectus of abdomen

Ilium

Pubis

Ischium

External oblique of abdomen

Quadriceps femoris

Sartorius

Gastrocnemius

Tendons

Osteoporosis

Osteoporosis is a common condition in which the bone tissue loses calcium. This means the bones are brittle and more liable to fracture. Throughout life the body breaks down the bone and then builds it up again and this process promotes growth and repair. In young people the rate at which new bone is formed is faster than the breaking down process. This begins to change in early adulthood and from middle age onwards the breaking down process is accelerated and rebuilding slows down, so that bones become less strong and much lighter.

Osteoporosis affects one in twenty people, and it is four times more likely to affect women than men. This is probably because oestrogen levels fall in women after the menopause, often resulting in severe osteoporosis. Many people do not realize that they have osteoporosis until they have a minor fall that results in a fracture, most commonly of the wrist or hip. Other osteoporotic fractures are crush or compression fractures of the spine and fractures of the femur (thigh bone), which are a major cause of disability in elderly women and can be life-threatening.

BUILDING STRONG BONES

There are many strategies to keep your bones strong and healthy and prevent osteoporosis before a fracture happens.

➤ Avoid alcohol and stop smoking.

➤ A diet rich in milk, cheese and dark, leafy vegetables provides calcium which is vital for bone formation and can improve bone density.

➤ Depending on your BMD (bone mineral density), your doctor may advise low-impact activities, such as walking or yoga, rather than high-impact ones like jogging or aerobics. Weight training to tone and build muscle helps prevent osteoporosis by improving support to the joints.

➤ Hormone replacement therapy (HRT). If this is taken for five to ten years after the menopause, HRT can reduce the risk of fractures. It can slow down or halt osteoporosis and may help to prevent fractures.

WHO IS MOST AT RISK?

Age-related osteoporosis affects people with differing degrees of severity and the condition usually develops gradually over a period of 15 to 20 years. Postmenopausal osteoporosis takes only ten years to develop and is more common in women who have an early menopause.

▽ A fractured femur from an osteoporosis patient. The dark areas show where the bone lacks minerals and fractures are likely.

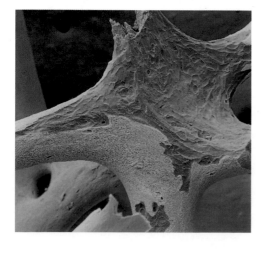

Other risk factors include:
• Low body weight.
• Smoking.
• Excess alcohol consumption.
• Long-term corticosteroid drug therapy.
• Lack of exercise.
• Overactive thyroid.
• Family history of osteoporosis.
• Rheumatoid arthritis.
• Chronic kidney failure.

DIAGNOSING OSTEOPOROSIS

Your doctor may only detect signs of osteoporosis when examining an X-ray of a fracture. The patient will be sent for a scan to test bone mineral density (BMD) – the level of bone density is measured in the femur and wrist to confirm the diagnosis.

TREATMENT OPTIONS

You may be referred to a physiotherapist, who will advise on bone-building exercises. If you've had a fracture due to osteoporosis, you may receive the following treatments:

• HRT (hormone replacement therapy). This may halt the condition in women.
• Calcium tablets combined with a special drug, to encourage the bone to take up extra calcium.
• Vitamin D supplements can be effective, but their use must be monitored with blood tests.

▽ Many osteoporosis sufferers develop a "hunchback" appearance. Their excessively curved spines are the result of crush fractures.

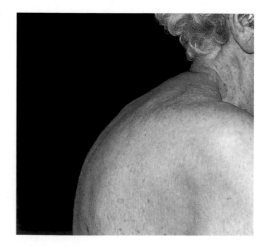

CALCIUM AND BONE HEALTH

An inadequate supply of calcium over a lifetime is believed to play a significant role in the development of osteoporosis. Studies show that low calcium intakes appear to be associated with low bone mass, rapid bone loss and high fracture rates. National nutrition surveys have shown that many people consume less than half the amount of calcium recommended to build and maintain healthy bones. Good sources of calcium include:

• Dairy products, such as low-fat yogurt, milk and cheese.
• Dark green, leafy vegetables, such as broccoli, watercress and spinach.
• Tinned fish with soft, edible bones.
• Tofu.
• Almonds and sesame seeds.

• Fresh parsley and thyme.
• Foods fortified with calcium, such as orange juice, cereals and breads.

Depending on how much calcium you get each day from food, you may need to take a calcium supplement, but most people do not need supplements so always check with your doctor or pharmacist first.

Your body's need for calcium changes as you get older. The need is at its greatest during childhood and adolescence, when the skeleton is growing rapidly, and during pregnancy and breastfeeding, when a mother passes calcium to her baby. With age, the body becomes less efficient at absorbing calcium. Older men and postmenopausal women need extra calcium because they lack adequate vitamin D, which is required for calcium absorption. Older adults with chronic medical problems may be taking drugs that impair calcium absorption.

THE EFFECT OF GRAVITY ON BONES

Having to support your own body weight against the effects of gravity stimulates bone growth. If you have a period of immobility due to illness your bones become temporarily weaker. Astronauts have great problems with loss of bone mass during space flights, although NASA has now developed a series of resistance exercises to counteract this effect. The exercises simulate gravity's bone-stimulating effects.

Osteomalacia and rickets

SEE ALSO
➤ Osteoporosis, p108

Osteomalacia is a weakening and softening of the bones that can lead to severe deformity. It is due to a vitamin D deficiency which causes a lack of calcium and phosphorus – minerals essential for bone growth. In children, the disease is known as rickets.

The commonest cause of osteomalacia is a shortage of vitamin D. Essential to enable the body to deal with calcium and phosphorus, vitamin D is found in green vegetables, fortified margarines, milk and fish. It is also made in the skin by exposure to sunlight.

A lack of vitamin D may occasionally occur in people on a vegetarian diet who do not eat dairy products or in people who are lactose intolerant (have trouble digesting milk products). Symptoms of osteomalacia are bone or muscle pain and tenderness.

Rickets is fairly rare. It is most likely to occur in young children around 6 to 24 months old, where the body demands high levels of calcium and phosphorus. Symptoms include forward projection of the breastbone (pigeon chest) and bow legs.

Both conditions can be confirmed by blood tests and X-rays. Treatment aims to increase intake of vitamin D and encourage increased exposure to sunlight.

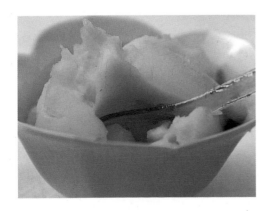

◁ Most margarines are fortified with vitamin D. This vitamin is essential in allowing the body to absorb calcium and phosphorus.

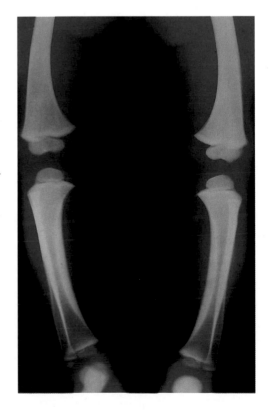

▷ Bow-leggedness caused by weakening of the bones in a child with rickets. Walking may be painful and the bones are prone to fracture.

Bone cancer

SEE ALSO
➤ The musculskeletal system, p106
➤ Lung cancer, p136

Cancers that originate in the bone, called primary bone cancers, are very rare. They most often occur in children and adolescents. Cancerous tumours in the bone "eat" their way through surrounding structures and spread quickly around the body, so early diagnosis is essential. If detected early, surgery can be carried out to remove the tumour, and most patients have only a slight chance of the disease recurring within five years, and after that recurrence is not likely. However, most cases are not diagnosed early and the prognosis is not good.

The causes of primary bone cancer are not yet known, but there may be a genetic link because it often seems to run in families. This form of cancer most often occurs in the leg, with a painful swelling just above or below the knee. The pain may be worse while standing or while in bed at night.

HOW IS IT DIAGNOSED?
Patients will be referred to a specialist to have X-rays taken and further tests such as a computerized tomography (CT) scan or magnetic resonance imaging (MRI) will be carried out so that the diagnosis can be confirmed. The most common primary bone cancer is called osteosarcoma.

Tumours are highly malignant and the disease will often spread to the lungs, so patients may also be sent for a chest X-ray.

TREATING BONE CANCER
In most cases the tumour is surgically removed and any bone that is taken away is replaced either by artificial bone or by a section of bone from elsewhere in the body or from a compatible donor. Radiotherapy or chemotherapy is normally given after surgery to get rid of any remaining cancer.

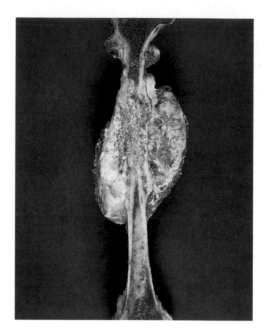

▷ This specimen of a femur – thigh bone – shows a cancerous growth. Bone tumours are highly malignant and the cancer often spreads quickly to the lungs.

Bone metastases

SEE ALSO
➤ Bone cancer, above

Bone metastases or secondary bone cancer are terms for tumours that have spread from other parts of the body. Cancers prone to metastasize to bones include breast, lung, thyroid, prostate and kidney cancers. Bone metastases are more common than primary bone cancers.

Bone metastases tend to occur in elderly people and most often affect the ribs, pelvis, skull and spine. There is a tender swelling of the area and severe bone pain, which is usually worse at night. The affected bones are weakened and may easily fracture.

Patients who have already been diagnosed with cancer elsewhere in the body may have an X-ray or radionuclide scanning to discover if the cancer has spread to the bones. If this is the first sign of cancer, further such tests may be necessary to locate the site of the primary cancer from which the metastases developed.

Treatment focuses on the primary site. A bone fracture may be fixed with metal plates or screws. Once cancer has spread to the bone any treatment is palliative not curative – chemotherapy, radiotherapy or hormone therapy may relieve pain only.

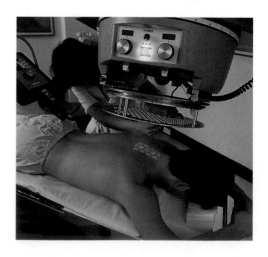

▷ A patient with secondary bone cancer has radiotherapy. The machine can be positioned very precisely so that the area to be treated is targeted accurately.

Arthritis

Arthritis refers to a group of conditions characterized by inflammation that causes pain and stiffness in one or more of the body's joints. The condition may be acute – typically sharp, severe and short-lived pain – or chronic – a constant dull ache. Arthritis may be linked to other complaints such as Crohn's disease or psoriasis. Treatment will largely depend on the severity and type of arthritis. Most treatments rely predominantly on painkillers to relieve the discomfort but as yet nothing can be done to cure the condition.

There are several different types of arthritis, and each type has its own characteristics:

- Osteoarthritis – The cartilage at the ends of bones is worn away and replaced by bony growths. It affects weight-bearing joints such as knees and hips and also the hands. It tends to occur in people over 60 and is twice as common in women.

- Rheumatoid arthritis – This causes the synovial membranes to become inflamed. The joints become swollen and stiff and ultimately deformed. It is most common between the ages of 40 and 60 and is four times as likely to affect women than men.

- Gout – This arthritis is due to deposition of uric acid crystals in the joints. The base of the big toe is most commonly affected. Gout is 20 times more common in men.

- Pseudogout – This is similar to gout in that crystals are deposited in the joints, but in pseudogout the crystals are formed from a chemical called pyrophosphate. This is more common in women.

- Psoriatic arthritis – The skin disease psoriasis can cause a form of arthritis similar to rheumatoid arthritis.

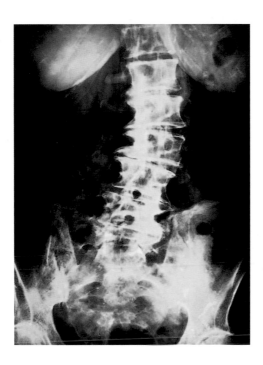

△ The spine of an 80-year-old woman with osteoarthritis shows a prominent curve and the growth of osteophytes – bony projections – between the vertebrae (upper left of picture).

- Ankylosing spondylitis – This arthritic condition can affect joints and may be associated with inflammatory bowel diseases such as Crohn's disease and ulcerative colitis. Ankylosing spondylitis is four times more likely to occur in men than in women.

- Septic arthritis – This type of arthritis results from infection in a joint, caused by a wide variety of bacteria. The joint involved is hot, swollen and painful to move. Young children and older people are most likely to develop this condition.

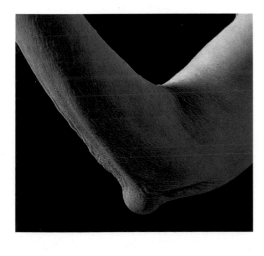

◁ A rheumatoid nodule on the arm of an elderly patient with rheumatoid arthritis. The soft nodule has been formed as a result of physical stress on the elbow joint.

- Irritable hip – In young children, a viral infection such as a cold can sometimes cause hip discomfort, difficulty walking and a limp which resolves spontaneously over a few days. However, a doctor should be consulted as there may be a problem with the hip joint called Perthes' disease where the blood supply to the joint can be affected, and a different treatment is required.

SELF-HELP FOR ARTHRITIS

A doctor will often prescribe strong drug treatments to relieve the pain but there are other treatments and self-help therapies that you may wish to consider:

- Consult a complementary practitioner in osteopathy, chiropractic or acupuncture, especially electro-acupuncture.

- Low-impact exercises such as yoga, t'ai chi and qi gong have all been shown to benefit arthritis sufferers.

▽ A finger-diameter gauge being used to measure arthritic knuckle joints. This helps to assess if a particular course of drug treatment is successfully reducing the painful swelling.

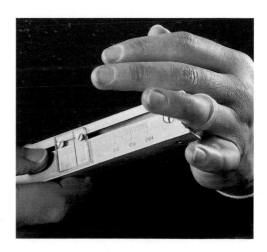

Osteoarthritis

SEE ALSO

➤ Weight control, p16
➤ Exercise for life, p18
➤ Complementary therapies and their uses, p244

Osteoarthritis is the commonest form of arthritis. It is due to the thinning and wearing away of the smooth cartilage at the ends of the bones at joints. It tends to affect the major weight-bearing joints such as the hips and knees, but very mobile joints, such as the shoulder and neck, can also be affected. Doctors once thought that osteoarthritis was simply wear and tear. However, the current theory is that it is a disease of the cartilage itself, and so new drug treatments to prevent a loss of cartilage are now in development.

If a joint has been damaged by infection or fracture, or an injury has caused damage to the cartilage pads, it is much more likely that osteoarthritis will develop in that joint later in life.

DIAGNOSING OSTEOARTHRITIS

It is possible that your doctor might suspect osteoarthritis straight away simply by taking note of your symptoms. However, in the over-55 age group, eight in ten people will probably have osteoarthritis but will not have any symptoms. No single test can confirm the diagnosis, so your doctor will want to know about pain, stiffness, and joint function, and how this has changed over time. It is also important for the doctor to know how the condition is affecting the patient's work and daily life. The patient may then be sent for an X-ray of the affected joint. X-rays can show such things as cartilage loss, bone damage and bone spurs. An X-ray will not necessarily give an accurate idea of the level of pain and disability being experienced by the patient. Your doctor may recommend a blood test to rule out other types of arthritis, such as rheumatoid arthritis.

SIMPLE SELF-HELP MEASURES

Your doctor may suggest a few simple measures to help ease osteoarthritis:
• Carrying extra body weight puts added pressure on the joints, so a healthy diet to lose weight is often recommended.
• Low-impact exercises, for example swimming, yoga and walking can be beneficial. Studies have shown that exercise improves mood and outlook. It also increases supplenesss and flexibility, as well as easing pain, and improving heart function and blood flow. It helps maintain a healthy weight and boost general physical fitness. If done correctly, it should have no negative side effects. The amount and type of exercise will depend on which joints are involved, how stable those joints are, and whether a joint replacement has already been carried out. Some doctors recommend t'ai chi, a Chinese form of exercise that is gaining popularity in the West. It is easy to learn and easy to practise at home, and it involves slow, rhythmic movements that improve balance and concentration, which will help to reduce the risk of falls in the elderly. The weight-bearing aspects of this exercise have the potential to stimulate bone growth and strengthen connective tissue. Studies have shown that it also lowers blood pressure and reduces pain and inflammation.
• Wearing well-fitting, supportive shoes gives increased comfort when walking.
• Regular massage sessions bring relief.
• Warm baths, ice packs or heat pads can soothe joint pain.

HOW THE HIP JOINT IS AFFECTED

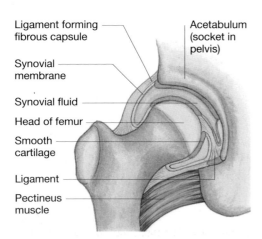

Ligament forming fibrous capsule
Synovial membrane
Synovial fluid
Head of femur
Smooth cartilage
Ligament
Pectineus muscle
Acetabulum (socket in pelvis)

△ In normal hip joints the ligaments, membrane and fluids work together to keep the joint moving smoothly.

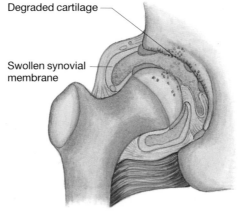

Degraded cartilage
Swollen synovial membrane

△ In an osteoarthritic hip joint, the swollen synovial membrane bulges outwards and smooth cartilage is degraded and worn away.

CERVICAL SPONDYLOSIS

This form of osteoarthritis affects the upper spine. As the cartilage between the backbones degenerates, bony growths develop on the neck vertebrae, which may press on spinal nerves in the neck. This causes pain in the neck and sometimes down the arms. Inflamed joints may restrict neck movement. It mainly affects people over the age of 45 and appears to be more common in men.

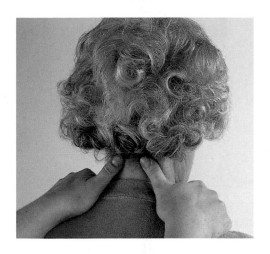

△ A neck massage provides relief. However, it is important to seek professional advice about this because massaging arthritic areas can cause damage if it is not properly done.

HOW IS IT TREATED?

Most successful programmes involve a combination of treatments tailored to the patient's individual needs, lifestyle and health. There is no cure for osteoarthritis and so treatment has four main goals:

• To control pain through drugs and other measures.
• To improve joint care through resting and gentle exercise.
• To maintain an acceptable body weight.
• To achieve a more healthy lifestyle.

There are a number of treatment options and these include:
• Taking simple painkillers.
• Taking anti-inflammatory painkillers. These drugs can cause stomach ulcers if used long term, so are combined with other drugs that protect the stomach.
• Glucosamine and chondroitin sulphate dietary supplements are among the latest treatments for osteoarthritis. These nutrients are found in small quantities in food and are components of normal cartilage. Studies have not yet shown that they affect the disease, though they may relieve symptoms in some patients.
• Physiotherapy.
• Walking aids, including walking frames.
• Steroid injections into the joint.
• Surgery to replace the joint.
• Many people find that osteopathy or

JOINT REPLACEMENT

Surgery may be required in cases where the damage to the joints is severe. A range of operations is available and they include fusing the joint, removing and replacing the affected joint and correcting any deformity. Joint replacement is the most advanced treatment. Hip and knee joints are routinely and successfully replaced. Elbow and shoulder joints can be replaced but are generally less successful.

In a hip replacement, a metal ball and stem is cemented into the top of the femur to recreate the "ball" of this ball-and-socket joint, while a plastic "socket" is cemented into the pelvis. This operation is very successful and replacement hips last approximately 15 years.

Knee replacements tend to be slightly less successful than hip replacements. A new metal end is attached to the lower end of the femur (thigh bone) and a plastic top to the tibia (shin bone). Knee replacements can last up to ten years.

Further operations to insert new replacements when the originals have worn out are much more difficult. For this reason surgeons operate as late as possible in a patient's life to minimize further operations.

▽ This is a prosthetic (artificial) hip joint. Hip-replacement operations can transform the lives of osteoarthritis sufferers, although the artificial joint may loosen with time.

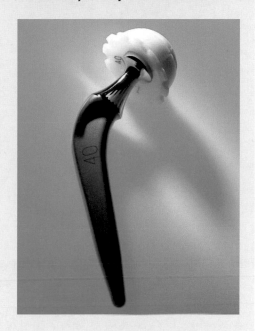

chiropractic manipulation helps ease pain and keep them mobile.
• Research shows that acupuncture is effective in some osteoarthritis patients, reducing pain and improving mobility. Licensed acupuncture therapists insert very fine needles into the skin at various points on the body. The needles are believed to stimulate the brain to produce natural painkilling chemicals.

THE IMPORTANCE OF REST

Regularly scheduled rest is important for good joint care. Patients must learn to listen to their body's signals, and know when to slow down or stop to prevent pain caused by over-use. Some patients benefit from using splints or braces to provide extra support for weakened joints during sleep or while active. Splints are used for limited periods only because joints and muscles must be exercised to prevent stiffness.

SIGNS AND SYMPTOMS

The symptoms are generally mild at first and slowly worsen over the years. The number of joints affected dictates the level of pain, discomfort and restricted mobility. Often only one or two joints are affected but it can be more widespread. The main symptoms are:

➤ Pain and tenderness, which worsens during periods of activity.

➤ Swelling around the joint.

➤ Joint stiffness.

➤ Restricted movement.

➤ Crackling noise on moving the joint, which is known as crepitus.

➤ The joints become increasingly immobile and deformed.

Rheumatoid arthritis

SEE ALSO

➤ Joint replacement, p113

➤ Anaemia, p202

➤ Autoimmune diseases, p211

Rheumatoid arthritis is a chronic inflammation of the synovial membrane that lines the joints. It is an autoimmune disease, a condition in which the body produces antibodies that attack its own tissues. This joint-destroying disease develops slowly and damages the ends of the bones and the cartilage that covers them within a joint. Continued inflammation results in damaged tendons and ligaments, which make the joint unstable and, ultimately, deform the joint. This condition can run in families and more commonly affects elderly women.

Rheumatoid arthritis is a serious disorder where symptoms may be set off by illness, stress or injury. Symptoms vary in severity and often worsen gradually.

Any joint in the body can be affected by rheumatoid arthritis, but the fingers, wrists, knees and ankles are most susceptible. There may be rheumatoid nodules (lumps of tissue under the skin), but the main indicators are pain and stiffness in the joints. Most people find that the pain and stiffness is worse in the morning but gradually improves during the day. Eventually, the damage may be so great that the joints develop characteristic swelling and deformities.

Other tissues of the body, including the eyes, skin, lungs, nerves and brain, kidneys,

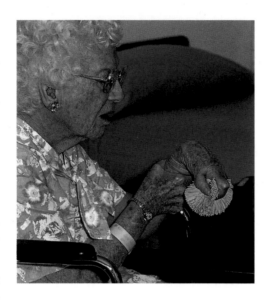

△ An elderly lady exercises her arthritic hand during a physiotherapy session. Gentle exercise can help ease pain and prolong mobility.

heart and spleen, can also be affected by rheumatoid arthritic inflammation.

TREATMENT OPTIONS

There is as yet no cure for rheumatoid arthritis, but doctors can prescribe a range of highly effective drug therapies. Disease-modifying drugs, that act on the auto-immune disease, are usually the first line of treatment. Nonsteroidal anti-inflammatory drugs may be given to relieve pain and reduce swelling. These treatments decrease the inflammation and the deformity, and slow down the progress of the disease. Regular check-ups are advisable to monitor the drug's action and any possible side effects, which may include slight ulceration of the stomach.

In addition to drug therapy, your doctor may recommend wearing a brace or splint to support a troublesome joint and to slow

DIAGNOSIS

It is important to diagnose rheumatoid arthritis early in the disease in order to be able to treat it most effectively with disease-controlling drugs. The usual methods of diagnosis are to perform a physical examination and check X-ray images. A blood sample will be taken to test for the presence of certain antibodies known as rheumatoid factor. Rheumatoid factor is present in about 80 per cent of rheumatoid arthritis sufferers, but it can also be found in other conditions such as gout.

down the development of deformities. Patients may also be referred to a physiotherapist for guidance on regular gentle exercises to help keep symptoms at bay and joints mobile during periods of disease remission.

In the case of an acutely painful joint, the doctor may ease the pain using a corticosteroid drug, which is injected into the joint. Where joints are severely damaged, surgery may be necessary to release contracted tendons, allowing greater movement, or the inflamed synovial membrane is removed in a process called synovectomy. Sometimes joint replacement surgery is carried out on severely deformed, immobile and painful joints.

THE OUTLOOK

Many people with rheumatoid arthritis learn how to cope with the disease and lead normal lives but about 10 per cent of sufferers become severely disabled.

SIGNS AND SYMPTOMS

The main symptoms are pain, swelling and stiffness of the joints. Other symptoms may include:

➤ Fever.

➤ Pallor.

➤ Anaemia.

➤ Loss of appetite and energy.

The joints of the hands and feet are often affected first. Rheumatoid arthritis commonly affects the wrist and many of the hand joints, but usually not the joints closest to the fingernails, except the thumb. It can also affect the elbows, shoulders, neck, knees, hips and ankles. Both sides of the body are usually affected to the same extent.

Gout

Also known as crystal-induced arthritis, gout is an extremely common condition, particularly in the developed world, affecting men more than women. Gout is an inflammation of the joints caused by high levels of a waste product called uric acid. Formerly a leading cause of painful and disabling chronic arthritis, gout has been all but conquered by advances in research. Unfortunately, many people with gout continue to suffer because knowledge of effective treatments has been slow to spread to patients and their doctors.

SIGNS AND SYMPTOMS

Gout can cause a very painful arthritis of any joint, but for reasons that are not yet fully understood, it tends to affect the base joint of the big toe. The joint becomes hot, red, swollen and extremely tender to touch. In some cases gout can affect the earlobes and the skin around a joint, especially the finger joints or the back of the heel.

Gout is the result of an excess of uric acid in the body. This excess can be caused by a failure of the kidneys to eliminate uric acid or by increased intake of foods containing substances called purines, which are metabolized to uric acid in the body. Purines are found in certain meats, seafood, dried peas and beans. Drinking alcohol may also significantly increase uric acid levels and trigger gout attacks.

In most people there is no immediately obvious cause for a sudden attack of gout, although it does tend to run in families. It is more prevalent in cases of obesity, where people eat a high-fat diet or drink large amounts of alcohol. It is also common in people with heart disease or high blood pressure. The incidence of gout tends to increase with age but is most common between the ages of 30 and 50.

Other conditions, including kidney disease and hypothyroidism, as well as diuretic drugs, may also lead to gout.

With time, as levels of uric acid in the blood rise, deposits collect around joints. Eventually, the uric acid forms needle-like crystals in the joints, leading to acute gout attacks. Uric acid may also collect under the skin in pockets called tophi, or in the urinary tract as kidney stones.

HOW IS IT DIAGNOSED?

The diagnosis of your condition may be obvious from your symptoms, but it is not always easy to distinguish gout from other types of arthritis. The definitive diagnosis depends on a blood test to confirm the presence of uric acid crystals in the joint

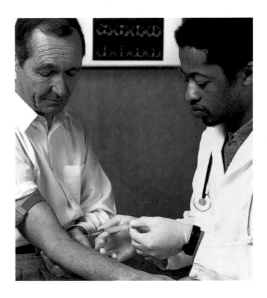

△ A blood sample is taken to confirm diagnosis of gout. The test will confirm if there are high levels of uric acid in the blood.

fluid during an acute attack. However, uric acid levels in gout sufferers are not always significantly high, and the diagnosis is made more complicated by the fact that a blood test for a non-gout sufferer may also show high uric acid readings.

TREATMENT FOR GOUT

Fortunately, an attack of gout will usually settle rapidly following a course of treatment with nonsteroidal anti-inflammatory drugs (NSAIDs), and this is the only treatment that most people require.

In patients who have suffered from multiple gout attacks, or who have developed tophi, the doctor may prescribe a drug to help the kidneys eliminate uric acid or to block its production in the body. This treatment must be started with care as it can cause an acute attack of gout when it is first used.

▽ This patient's left knee is affected by an attack of gout, causing pain and swelling. Gout is sometimes associated with other complaints, such as kidney stones and diabetes.

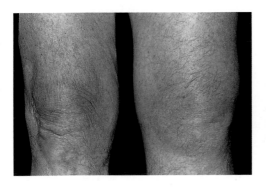

▽ This light micrograph shows uric acid crystals in a gouty joint, where they are causing an intensely painful attack of arthritis. Gout usually occurs in a single joint in the body.

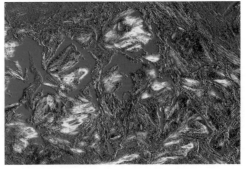

Ankylosing spondylitis

SEE ALSO

➤ Exercise for life, p18
➤ Crohn's disease, p60
➤ Ulcerative colitis, p61
➤ Urinary tract infections, p142

Ankylosing spondylitis primarily affects the pelvis and lower spine. It causes chronic, progressive inflammation of the joints and ligaments that normally permit the spine to move. The vertebrae may fuse and grow together, causing the spine to become rigid and inflexible. Other joints, such as the shoulders, knees or ankles, may also be involved. Men and women are affected equally, mainly in young adulthood, but the disease is usually more severe in men. There may be an inherited factor as ankylosing spondylitis can run in families.

SIGNS AND SYMPTOMS

Symptoms appear most commonly in men between the ages of 16 and 35. In women, the disease is often milder and is therefore more difficult to diagnose. The first symptoms are usually pain in the pelvis, knees, heels and big toes, followed by back pain and stiffness. Fatigue, mild fever and weight loss are also common.

Ankylosing spondylitis may take the form of intermittent back pain throughout life, or it may be a severe chronic disease that attacks the spine, peripheral joints and other body organs. It can eventually result in severe joint and back stiffness, loss of mobility and deformity.

▽ An X-ray of the pelvis and lower spine of a person with ankylosing spondylitis shows the joints in the pelvis are fused. Inflammation begins here and moves up the spine.

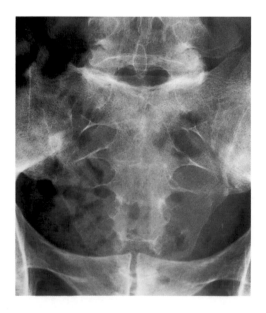

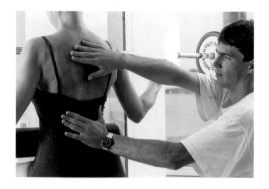

△ A physiotherapist adjusts the posture of a woman learning back exercises. Good posture while walking and standing minimizes pain.

The cause of ankylosing spondylitis is not yet known, but 90 per cent of people with the disease share a common genetic marker, called HLA-B27. In some cases, the disease is believed to be triggered in these predisposed people after exposure to infections of the bowel or urinary tract.

Symptoms usually first appear in late adolescence and early adulthood and then gradually develop over the course of months or years. In severe cases, bone starts to grow between the bones of the spine so that the vertebrae fuse together. In the long term, this leads to loss of mobility and a hunched-over appearance.

HOW IS IT DIAGNOSED?

Diagnosis of the disease is often delayed because symptoms may be attributed to more common back problems. A sudden and severe loss of flexibility in the lumbar region of the spine is an early symptom of ankylosing spondylitis.

Back problems may be followed by the development of inflammatory bowel disease, and sometimes by fever, exhaustion, weight loss, anaemia and inflammation of the eye. Malfunction of the heart valve is involved in some severe cases.

A diagnosis may be confirmed by an X-ray examination of the pelvis and spine. Blood tests can help determine the severity of the inflammation and detect the presence of genetic factor HLA-B27.

TREATMENT OPTIONS

The severity of the disease varies widely from one patient to another. Early, accurate diagnosis and treatment may spare years of suffering and disability.

Treatment is usually with nonsteroidal anti-inflammatory painkillers. These help control the symptoms, while physiotherapy sessions strengthen back muscles and help prevent stiffness and deformity of the spine.

Even with the best care and treatment, some patients will develop a permanently stiff or ankylosed spine. However, they can still retain mobility if the fusion keeps the spine upright. Ankylosing spondylitis is a lifelong problem and continuing care is essential if permanent posture and mobility losses are to be avoided.

SELF-HELP

Those with ankylosing spondylitis need to take proper rest and exercise. A physiotherapist will help with correcting a patient's posture and walking position as well as providing abdominal and back exercises to maximize joint flexibility. Deep-breathing exercises improve lung capacity and general health, and swimming offers gentle aerobic exercise.

Backache

SEE ALSO
- ➤ Weight control p16
- ➤ Exercise for life, p18
- ➤ Prolapsed disc and sciatica, p86
- ➤ Osteopathy and chiropractic, p246

Human beings are particularly prone to back pain, especially pain of the lower back because this is the part of the spine that supports most of the body's weight. This tendency may be explained by the fact that human beings walk upright when their spines are designed for moving around on all fours. After the common cold, backache is the cause of the most lost work days in adults under 45. Four out of five adults experience low back pain at some point, and it is one of the most frequent problems treated by orthopaedic surgeons.

The lower or lumbar spine is an important structure because it provides both mobility – allowing turning, twisting or bending movements – and the strength to stand, walk and lift. Smooth functioning of the lower back is vital for practically all the activities of daily life. Pain or stiffness in this area can severely restrict normal functioning, reduce work capacity and degrade quality of life.

DIAGNOSING BACK PAIN

Most types of back pain can be diagnosed by questioning and physical examination in the doctor's surgery. If the pain is severe and unresponsive to treatment, or if there is serious leg pain, imaging tests may be needed. For conditions that involve soft tissues such as the lumbar disks or nerves, a CT (computerized tomography) scan or MRI (magnetic resonance imaging) may be needed to make a diagnosis. A bone scan can assess bone activity and EMG (electromyography) tests can detect nerve or muscle damage.

HOW IS IT TREATED?

In most people lower back pain settles in a few days. Contrary to popular belief, bed rest or lying on a hard surface are not recommended. Rest simply stiffens the back and prolongs the healing process. It is better to continue with gentle activity combined with painkillers to relieve the symptoms.

In cases of recurrent backache the best treatment is physiotherapy, though many people consult alternative practitioners such as chiropractors, osteopaths or cranial osteopaths. In some cases combined local anaesthetic and corticosteroid injections to affected joints may be necessary. Surgery on the lower back can remove the pressure from a prolapsed disc when it causes severe nerve and leg pain.

PREVENTING BACK PAIN

Back pain is a major cause of disability and the options for treatment are limited, so prevention is crucial.

- ➤ Never bend or stoop forward to pick up something. Bend your knees and lift by using your thigh muscles while keeping your back straight.
- ➤ Sit for short periods only. Sitting puts great strain on the back and can be compounded by bad posture. Keep your back straight and if you have to sit for a long time, while driving for example, support the lower back with a pillow.

Special "Mackenzie D rolls", available from physiotherapists, provide excellent lumbar support.

- ➤ Lose excess weight. Your lower back supports most of the weight of your upper body, so less weight equals less stress on your back.
- ➤ Sleep on a firm, supportive mattress. Sleeping on a soft, sagging mattress will often lead to back problems.
- ➤ Practise regular stretching and bending exercises, such as yoga.

SIGNS AND SYMPTOMS

Pain in the lower back can be sharp and sudden or it can be persistent and dull. Backache is sometimes called lumbago, while a pain in the back that also sends stabbing pains down the leg is referred to as sciatica. Backache can be caused by damaging the back muscles when lifting something heavy incorrectly but it is more commonly due to long-term wear and tear of the ligaments, joints and discs and the softer bone tissue between the vertebrae.

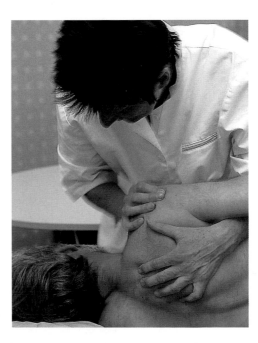

▽ An osteopath manipulates the back and shoulder of a patient. Osteopathy also involves stretching and applying pressure to affected parts of the body.

Frozen shoulder

SEE ALSO
➤ The musculoskeletal system, p106
➤ Diabetes, p66

A frozen shoulder is a chronic inflammation of the tendons and synovial capsule around the shoulder joint. In many cases the condition develops for no obvious reason, but it may be the result of an injury. The joint can also freeze up if the shoulder has been kept immobilized for a period of time, such as after a stroke. The pain is long-standing and gets worse on moving the shoulder. Movement is severely restricted. The condition occurs more often in people over 40 and affects more women than men. People with diabetes are particularly susceptible.

The ball-and-socket joint at the shoulder is prone to injury because of its huge range of movement. Any injury or damage to this joint can cause a frozen shoulder.

In a frozen shoulder, the capsule around the joint contracts and reduces movement at the joint. Movement becomes more and more restricted, and there is severe pain whether the joint is moved or not.

SIGNS AND SYMPTOMS

Pain is slight to start with and gradually worsens. Movement is difficult and it may be impossible to lie on the affected shoulder. In time, the pain may subside but the joint becomes increasingly stiff.

HOW IS IT TREATED?

Treatments that may help to ease stiffness and improve mobility of a frozen shoulder include a course of physiotherapy or manipulative treatment carried out by an osteopath or chiropractor. Nonsteroidal anti-inflammatory drugs may be prescribed to relieve pain and reduce inflammation. Your doctor may inject the shoulder with corticosteroids and this can act quickly, and may sort out the problem completely. However, in severe cases an injection may only give temporary relief and further manipulative treatments may be necessary.

Many cases of frozen shoulder eventually settle within three months, although it is possible for residual stiffness to last for much longer.

INJECTING A FROZEN SHOULDER

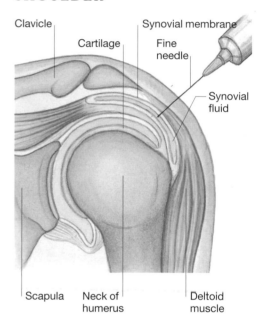

Clavicle · Cartilage · Synovial membrane · Fine needle · Synovial fluid · Scapula · Neck of humerus · Deltoid muscle

Bunions

SEE ALSO
➤ Osteoarthritis p112

A bunion is a thickened lump of soft tissue and bony overgrowth at the base of the big toe. This deformity is also known as hallux valgus. Bunions are painful and can affect either sex. They are more common in women and may be a result of wearing pointed, high-heeled shoes.

Bunions can often become inflamed and painful, making shoes uncomfortable and walking difficult. Underlying the bunion is a deformity of the bone that forces the big toe to point inwards towards the other toes. The cause of bunions is not yet known. They sometimes run in families and may be due to wearing tight shoes. Well-fitting shoes, and walking barefoot as often as possible, may ease the discomfort.

TREATMENT OPTIONS

For painful bunions the only solution is surgery in which the joint is straightened and fused. People normally make a full recovery within six weeks. Untreated bunions increase the risk of developing osteoarthritis in that joint in later years.

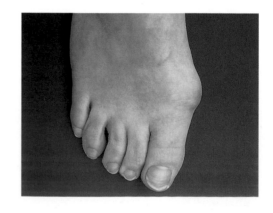

▷ A bunion can cause the big toe to point inwards and crush its neighbour. A cotton wool pad between the toes can help to correct this.

Repetitive strain injury

SEE ALSO
➤ Exercise for life, p18
➤ Rheumatoid arthritis, p114

Repetitive strain injury (RSI) is a common condition among people who do repetitive work, or play regular sport, that places strain on a particular part of the body. This painful condition is especially common in the muscles and tendons of the arms and hands and is caused by repeating the same movement over and over again, especially if that movement is rapid and forceful. RSI affects people in a range of occupations that place stress on joints and muscles – from keyboard operators and assembly line workers to musicians and athletes.

SIGNS AND SYMPTOMS
The symptoms of RSI develop gradually and include pain, aching and tingling in the affected limb during the key activity. In the early stages the pain often disappears during rest periods, though in the later stages, it is constant and severe.

Repetitive strain injury is much easier to treat in the early stages of the disease, so it is vital to act on symptoms as soon as they appear. If untreated, RSI may worsen, leaving the patient with permanent damage and unable to use the affected limb to work or play sport. This may mean an enforced change of lifestyle and, if symptoms are related to occupation, a change of jobs.

HOW IS IT DIAGNOSED?
Diagnosis is by questioning the patient and examination of the tender muscles or joints. There may be a blood test to rule out other diseases, such as rheumatoid arthritis.

TREATMENT FOR RSI
In many places of work, advice is given on posture and most will organize special equipment to reduce the likelihood of repeated symptoms. In all cases, there are steps to take to minimize the effects of RSI, or to prevent it in those at risk. Simple exercises such as swimming, walking, yoga and stretching routines can improve suppleness and mobility. Massage therapy is a relaxing way to reduce strain and prevent current discomfort from turning into chronic disabling pain.

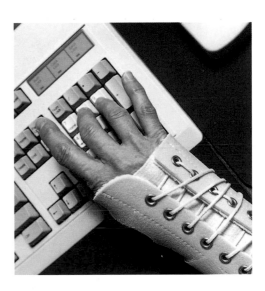

▽ Anyone working with computers is at risk from RSI because of the strain placed on the wrist by typing. If the disease has developed, wearing a wrist support may be recommended as well as exercises to avoid repetitive strain.

Fibromyalgia

SEE ALSO
➤ Learn to manage stress, p12

Fibromyalgia is a muscle disorder that causes sharp pains and aching all over the body. It has no obvious cause, but may be brought on by intense stress. Patients may also suffer from conditions such as chronic fatigue syndrome, irritable bowel syndrome and depression.

Fibromyalgia affects women more commonly than men, but is rarely diagnosed because it causes no visible abnormality in the muscle tissue. It is often misdiagnosed as chronic fatigue syndrome. No doctor would dispute that fibromyalgia can cause suffering, but medical opinion is divided as to the basis of physical and psychological factors.

WHAT MIGHT YOUR DOCTOR DO?
After a physical examination, a blood test may be taken to rule out other disorders, such as rheumatoid arthritis.

TREATING FIBROMYALGIA
Pain may be treated with therapies such as deep tissue massage and locally applied heat, or an injection with a local anaesthetic.

Painkillers must be used sparingly. Low-intensity exercise is recommended, such as walking, yoga or t'ai chi. Any related conditions, such as depression and irritable bowel syndrome, are treated accordingly. Psychological treatments, such as cognitive therapy, are often very helpful and many patients are able to make a complete recovery.

Fractures

SEE ALSO
➤ The musculoskeletal
   system, p106
➤ Osteoporosis, p108

Any bone can be fractured (break or crack) if enough force is applied to it, but fractures tend to occur at weaker spots in certain bones. Fractures are more likely to occur in children and the elderly. Children's bones are softer and tend to crumple on one side – a greenstick fracture – rather than snap. In the elderly, especially elderly women, bones can become brittle (osteoporotic) and even a minor injury can smash the bone into fragments. Spontaneous fractures in bones affected by cancer tumours are called pathological fractures.

There are two main types of fracture and these are closed (a simple fracture), in which the bone does not pierce the skin, and open (a compound fracture), in which the bone is exposed by piercing the skin. Open fractures are more serious because of the damage to nerves and blood vessels and the risk of infection.

Fractures are most often caused by an injury such as a twisting movement or impact after falling.

THE BONES OF THE ARM

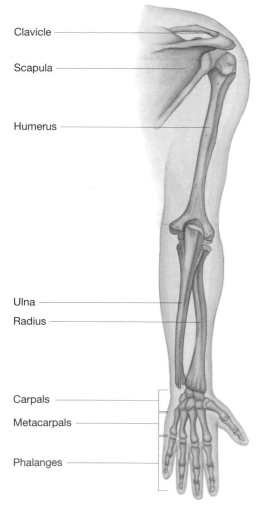

Clavicle

Scapula

Humerus

Ulna

Radius

Carpals

Metacarpals

Phalanges

ARM BONE FRACTURES

If a person trips and puts out a hand, the force that travels up the arm from impact can break any of its bones. There are a number of different fractures of the arm:

- Distal radius (or Colles' fracture) – This fracture, which often occurs in the elderly, takes about six weeks to heal. The end of the radius, near the wrist, breaks and is forced backwards. In children, greenstick fractures are common, but these usually settle within three weeks.
- Scaphoid – This fracture, of the small carpal bone in the wrist, most commonly occurs in young adults. Fractures may be slow to show up on an X-ray, so if a doctor suspects a fracture the wrist may plastered and X-rayed ten days later, by which time any fracture should be clear. This fracture heals in about six weeks.
- Radial head – In this fracture, which can happen at any age, the top of the radius, (at the elbow) fractures. It usually heals if the arm is kept still and supported in a sling for a few weeks.
- Base of the humerus (above the elbow) – This fracture occurs in children and as it may be close to a major artery, doctors will check the pulse.
- Shaft of humerus – The midpoint of the humerus can break. An important nerve is close to this bone so the fracture may need to be stabilized surgically. This fracture is most likely occur in the elderly.
- Neck of humerus – The top of the humerus can be smashed in the elderly. The fracture may appear horrific on X-ray images but it heals well with a collar and cuff support after a few weeks.

GREENSTICK FRACTURE TO THE RADIUS OF THE ARM

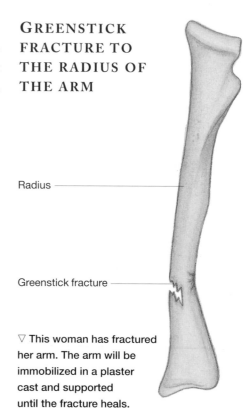

Radius

Greenstick fracture

▽ This woman has fractured her arm. The arm will be immobilized in a plaster cast and supported until the fracture heals.

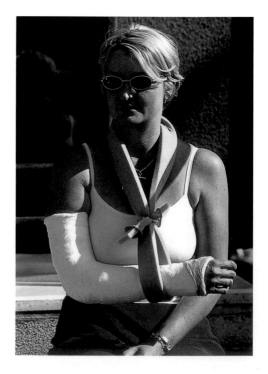

- Clavicle – The middle of the collarbone is easily broken but it heals well with a sling for support.

OTHER COMMON FRACTURES

The commonest fractures caused by a fall from any height are:
- Ankle fractures.
- Fractures of the heel bone.
- Fractures of the tibia and femur around the knee.
- Crush or compression fractures to the vertebrae in the spine.
- Pelvic fractures.
- Fractured neck of femur – This fracture of the top end of the femur (thigh bone) is common in the elderly. It often requires surgery and a half or full hip replacement may be needed. It is a major injury at any age but especially for the elderly, because they have to remain immobile for so long.

Turning over on the ankle produces two main types of fracture:
- Lateral malleolus fracture – The lower

end of the fibula (one of the bones in the lower leg) is broken off and the ankle needs to be put in a cast for six weeks. Sometimes, the lower end of the other shinbone – the tibia – may also break. This usually needs to be fixed with metal screws and plates.
- Base of fifth metatarsal fracture – The end of the fifth toe bone can be snapped off, needing a cast for six weeks.

TREATMENT OPTIONS

Fractures will heal and most need only minimal treatment, which may include:
- Immobilization – Most fractures need to be immobilized to reduce pain. This may be done with a cast or traction. Traction is where the limb is held in place, during bed rest, with weights and pulleys.
- Reduction – Occasionally manipulation under anaesthetic is required to realign the bones.
- Fixation – Some fractures need surgery. Internal fixation involves inserting metal pins and/or plates under the skin to fix the bone. In external fixation, metal pins

are inserted through the skin into the bone. Pins are held in place by a metal frame, the limb can be used in a few days and pins and frame are removed under anaesthetic once the bone has healed.

For all types of fracture, rehabilitation is vital for a return to normal function and physiotherapy sessions will strengthen the weakened joints and muscles.

HOW BONE HEALS ITSELF

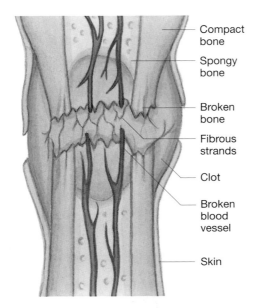

Compact bone
Spongy bone
Broken bone
Fibrous strands
Clot
Broken blood vessel
Skin

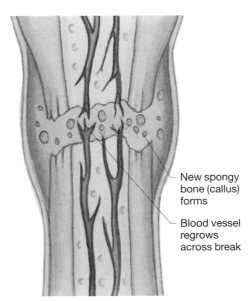

New spongy bone (callus) forms
Blood vessel regrows across break

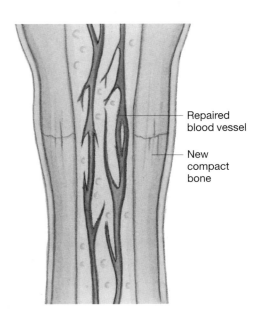

Repaired blood vessel
New compact bone

1 Broken bones have a huge capacity to repair themselves – they must simply be immobilized so that they knit together correctly. First, broken blood vessels heal and a mesh of new fibrous tissue forms.

2 In the second stage of healing, new spongy bone called callus is produced to make a tough temporary fix. Broken blood vessels regrow through the callus, allowing the flow of blood through the new bone.

3 Over the subsequent months and years this temporary repair is gradually replaced by compact bone. Any slight deformity is overlaid with new bone. Finally, it is difficult to tell that a fracture has ever occurred.

Knee injuries and disorders

SEE ALSO

➤ The musculoskeletal system, p106
➤ Osteoarthritis, p112
➤ Joint replacement, p113

The knee is the body's largest joint. The femur joins the tibia and the kneecap (patella) sits over this joint to help protect the knee. The knee is a hinge joint and because it has to bear heavy loads and constant pressure, it risks being twisted out of its plane and damaged. Injuries to the knee are common. They may be caused by activities such as jogging on hard pavements, which stresses the knee and damages cartilage, and skiing, where the constant bending of the knee can tear cartilage and strain the hamstring muscles that allow the knee to flex.

Damage to the knee can cause great pain. Treatments range from ice packs (a bag of frozen vegetables is a useful standby) to anti-inflammatory drugs. Rest followed by special exercises to strengthen the surrounding muscles is vital. Injury to one joint puts pressure on other joints of the body, and assessment of the damage and corrective treatment may be necessary.

TORN OR DAMAGED CARTILAGE

Inside the knee joint are two half-moon-shaped pieces of cartilage called menisci. If you twist awkwardly on a bent knee the menisci can be torn or damaged.

THE KNEE JOINT

▽ This picture shows the inside of the knee joint. Note that the kneecap (patella) has been removed for clarity.

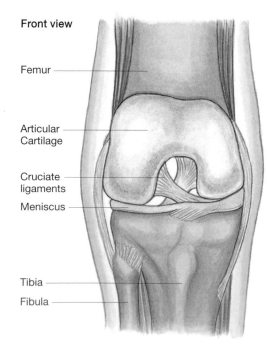

Front view

Femur

Articular Cartilage

Cruciate ligaments

Meniscus

Tibia

Fibula

Tearing the cartilage is extremely painful. The knee often swells up and cannot be straightened fully. The pain and swelling usually settle but can recur even when subjected to very slight trauma.

This condition is usually referred to an orthopaedic surgeon, who will examine and treat the knee via a telescopic viewing device called an arthroscope. This process is performed under a general anaesthetic. The arthroscope is inserted into the joint through a tiny incision in the skin and transmits pictures of the inside of the knee to a screen. Delicate surgery is carried out to shave the surface of the kneecap or remove damaged tissue.

Patients make a good recovery, but the joint may be prone to arthritis in later life.

RECURRENT DISLOCATION OF THE PATELLA

Any dislocation should be treated as an emergency, and medical assistance should be summoned immediately. The foot on the injured leg should be checked for blood flow by monitoring for coldness.

Some people, especially girls, are prone to repeated dislocation of the patella caused by minimal injury. The kneecap usually relocates itself, but it can be painful. Resting the joint in a cast, then exercising to strengthen the thigh muscles can stop the problem, but an operation may be required.

PAIN BEHIND THE KNEE

This condition is common and is usually due to overload of the joint between the kneecap and the femur. The knee is painful

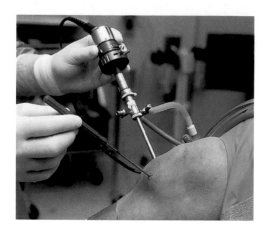

△ Torn cartilage in the knee is treated via an arthroscope. Pictures are transmitted to a monitor while the surgeon corrects the problem.

and may be swollen. Most people recover with rest, painkillers and physiotherapy. Occasionally, the kneecap will not move properly as it slides over the femur while bending the knee, and surgery is required to correct the problem.

CHONDROMALACIA

This condition causes pain in front of the knee and is due to an abnormality of the cartilage at the back of the kneecap. It occurs most commonly in adolescents of either sex and sometimes runs in families.

Chondromalacia can be triggered by a growth spurt, by sports or other injuries, or by putting too much strain on the knee joint while exercising.

The main symptom is pain in the knee when the leg is bent and straightened, for example going up or down stairs. There may be a crackling noise called crepitus when the knee joint is exercised and the joint may get stiff after sitting still.

The doctor may prescribe nonsteroidal anti-inflammatory drugs and advise ice packs for pain relief. Exercises to strengthen the muscles and reduce stress on the joint lessen the risk of developing osteoarthritis in later life. A knee support can provide temporary relief.

BURSITIS

Bursae are fatty sacs found around the joints. They act as cushions to reduce friction as the joint moves. Bursitis is inflammation of the bursae, which become swollen and painful, restricting movement.

The most common form of bursitis is found in the knee and is sometimes known as housemaid's knee, because it may be the result of frequent kneeling. Ice packs will provide some relief and your doctor may prescribe anti-inflammatory painkillers and, if there is a bacterial infection, a course of antibiotics. The condition will usually settle with rest after a few days but if pain and swelling persists, it may be necessary to drain the bursa.

KNEE JOINT REPLACEMENTS

Where damage to the knee joint is severe, through injury or by a condition such as arthritis, a joint may be replaced with an artificial one made of metal or plastic. This involves shaving off damaged bone ends before fitting the new parts.

OSGOOD-SCHLATTER DISEASE

This disease is common in adolescence. It is when the tendon from the muscle on the thigh (quadriceps) pulls on the growing part of the tibia. It causes pain and there may be a tender swelling on the front of the tibia. The pain settles with rest and by avoiding running and cycling. The condition disappears once the teenager stops growing.

LOOSE BODIES

The knee is a large and complex joint and is prone to pieces of bone and cartilage floating freely within it. These usually cause no problems, but if they cause problems they can be removed using an arthroscope.

Sprains

SEE ALSO
➤ Fractures, p120

A sprain occurs when a joint is wrenched, causing stretching or tearing of a ligament. Ligaments are flexible, fibrous connective tissue that attach bones to each other at the joints. Sprains most commonly occur in the ankles, wrists and knees, and can be extremely painful.

Sprains cause intense pain, swelling and discoloration in the affected area. A mild sprain settles with rest in a couple of days, but a more serious ligament tear may require surgery, especially if it has splintering to the bone to which the ligament is attached. An X-ray will confirm whether this is the case.

It is difficult to differentiate between a sprain and a muscular strain. Both involve severe pain, swelling and restricted movement of the limb. Both sprains and strains may recur if not allowed to heal fully. The joints most commonly sprained are:

- Ankles – This sprain occurs when the ankle is twisted, for example by walking on uneven ground.
- Knees – Sporting accidents may tear the ligaments on the inside of the knee.

▷ To avoid sprains while walking and climbing, it is important to wear strong, comfortable boots that provide support around the ankle.

Crutches may be needed to rest the joint.
- Wrists – Commonly sprained when the hand is put out to break a fall.

The ligament should heal in about eight weeks with rest and supportive bandaging – stretchy tubular bandages are easier to put on and are available from pharmacies. In some cases nonsteroidal, anti-inflammatory painkillers are prescribed.

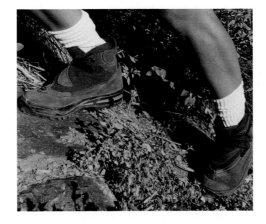

SIMPLE SELF-HELP MEASURES

While waiting to see a doctor, a sprain should be treated with the "RICE" procedure:

➤ Rest – Keep the injured limb still and support it on a cushion or footstool.

➤ Ice – Apply an ice pack (a packet of frozen peas will do) to the affected area for several minutes. This will reduce the swelling and bruising and also helps to relieve pain.

➤ Compression – Wrap the injured limb with a thick padding of cotton wool secured with a bandage wound in a figure of eight.

➤ Elevation – Make sure that the injured limb is supported and raised.

Tendon and muscle injuries

SEE ALSO

➤ The musculoskeletal system, p106

➤ Sprains, p123

Tendons are the tough, fibrous bands that link muscles to bones. They can tear and snap, especially during strenuous sporting activities, or they can be lacerated or cut, as a result of an accident, for example with a knife. Tendons are prone to becoming inflamed. This condition, called tendinitis, usually occurs in conjunction with tenosynovitis, the inflammation of the sheath of tissues that surrounds the tendon. Similar injuries of varying severity can result from overstraining or tearing a muscle, especially as a result of athletic sports or weight-training.

The most common symptoms of tendinitis and tenosynovitis are exacerbated by movement, and include pain, swelling and stiffness, and restricted mobility in the affected area. The skin may be hot and red and there may be a crackling sensation, called crepitus, when the joint is moved.

COMMON TENDON INJURIES

• Snapping of the Achilles tendon – The Achilles tendon links the calf muscle to the heel. It can snap under stress, especially when a middle-aged person does unaccustomed exercise. It causes severe pain around the lower calf and heel. Treatment involves surgical repair of the tendon or wearing a cast for six weeks. In either case, physiotherapy is required to restore mobility.

• Mallet finger – The tendon that is used to straighten the finger can snap off the bone if the end of the finger is bent suddenly. If the finger is splinted for six weeks, it may make a complete recovery.

THE ACHILLES TENDON

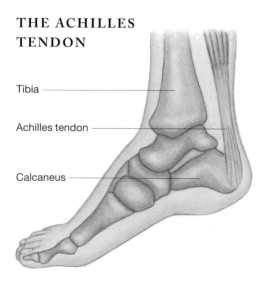

Tibia

Achilles tendon

Calcaneus

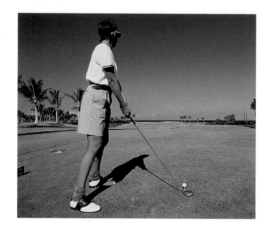

△ The sudden and powerful swing of the wrist involved in a golf stroke can cause golfer's elbow, a common form of tendinitis.

• Cut tendons – Hand lacerations on sharp objects can easily damage the tendons. Urgent surgical repair is needed to preserve their function.

TENDINITIS

All forms of tendinitis need rest and in some cases will heal faster if they are splinted. Physiotherapy is often helpful. Your doctor may prescribe nonsteroidal anti-inflammatory drugs or even an injection of a corticosteroid drug, and these will usually bring fast relief. Types of tendinitis include:

• Achilles tendinitis – Splinting is often recommended to resolve inflammation of this tendon at the back of the heel. Gentle exercises to stretch the tendon may also be helpful.

• Rotator cuff injury – The tendons that lift the arm out to the side can tear, making shoulder movement painful. The pain usually occurs at a certain point as the arm is lifted as the damaged tendon rubs underneath part of the shoulder blade. It is called painful arc syndrome.

• Plantar fasciitis – The flat tendon that covers the sole of the foot becomes inflamed and is painful when standing or walking (also called policeman's heel).

• Golfer's and tennis elbow – This painful condition occurs where the muscles that work the wrist are attached to the elbow – golfer's elbow affects the inner (medial) elbow and tennis elbow affects the outer (lateral) elbow. Rest with ice packs is recommended and for acute pain, a steroid injection can provide relief.

MUSCLE TEARS

Muscle injuries are common at any age, though older people performing unaccustomed movements or exercises and sportspeople are most at risk. Most sports depend on muscle strength and suppleness, and damage can easily be caused by sudden forceful movements or strain when lifting heavy weights. The muscles most often affected are those of the calf (gastrocnemius and soleus), the front of the thigh (quadriceps) and back of the thigh (hamstrings).

On pulling a muscle, you may feel a sharp pain and sometimes a tearing sensation. Bruising later appears and the area will be painful to the touch.

Such injuries usually settle with rest and treatments, such as heat pads or ice packs, over the course of a couple of weeks. Anti-inflammatory painkillers can be especially effective in severe cases. Physiotherapy is occasionally needed.

THE RESPIRATORY SYSTEM

7

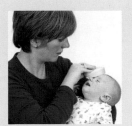

The body fulfils its energy needs by burning up the fuel in food. Like a fire in the grate, this process of combustion (called metabolism) requires a ready supply of oxygen. Supplying this oxygen is the job of the respiratory system. The lungs are rather like a system of bellows, drawing oxygen from the air and delivering it through the blood to each cell in the body. The cells use up the energy in various ways: supplying power to muscles, rebuilding tissue, maintaining body temperature. When the oxygen in each cell is used up, the blood carries the waste – mostly carbon dioxide – back to the lungs, where it is expelled like smoke from a chimney when we breathe out.

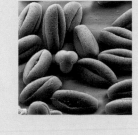

CONTENTS

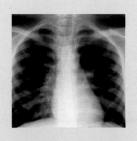

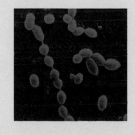

The breathing process

SEE ALSO

➤ The cardiovascular system, p28
➤ Lung cancer, p136
➤ The roles of blood and lymph, p200

Every cell in your body needs a constant supply of oxygen and at the same time needs to get rid of its principal waste product – carbon dioxide. The respiratory system works with the blood circulation system to meet your body's energy demands. The respiratory system delivers oxygen from the air you breathe to the blood system and then transfers carbon dioxide from the blood into the air you breathe out. Your lungs have a network of branching tubes that become ever smaller, maximizing the surface area available for the transfer of oxygen and carbon dioxide.

With every breath, you inhale about 500 ml (roughly 1 pint) of air, and you breathe between 12 and 15 times a minute. The air travels through the upper respiratory tract – first through the mouth or nose, then into the throat and the trachea (windpipe).

From the trachea, air travels down one of the two main bronchi (airways) and into the ever-smaller branches – the bronchioles. At the end of the bronchioles are tiny air sacs called alveoli. The smallest functional units of the lungs, they carry out the sophisticated process of gaseous exchange – exchanging oxygen for carbon dioxide.

GASEOUS EXCHANGE

Each alveolus has a network of tiny blood vessels (capillaries). During gaseous exchange, oxygen from inhaled air diffuses into the walls of the alveolus through the capillaries and binds to haemoglobin

▽ X-rays are often used to diagnose problems in the respiratory system. The lungs are the dark areas at the right and left. They are enclosed and protected by the ribs, which show up here as pale bands.

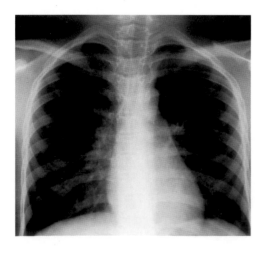

BREATHING IN AND OUT

Breathing is an automatic action controlled by the respiratory centre in a part of the brain called the medulla. The medulla adjusts the rate at which you breathe in response to your body's constantly changing requirements to absorb oxygen and eliminate carbon dioxide.

Receptors in the arteries monitor levels of carbon dioxide in the blood. They relay this information to the brain, which adjusts the rate of inhalation and exhalation to maintain a balance of gases in the body. When you exercise and use up oxygen more quickly, the brain sends out a message to speed up breathing and get more oxygen to the lungs.

The mechanics of breathing are controlled by the intercostal muscles (found between the ribs) and the diaphragm. They work to create different pressures in the chest.

▷ Inhalation – When you breathe in the intercostal muscles contract to lift your ribcage as the diaphragm contracts and flattens. This expands the chest cavity and lowers pressure to draw air into the lungs.

Diaphragm

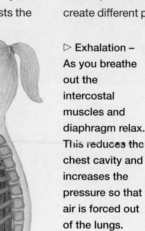

▷ Exhalation – As you breathe out the intercostal muscles and diaphragm relax. This reduces the chest cavity and increases the pressure so that air is forced out of the lungs.

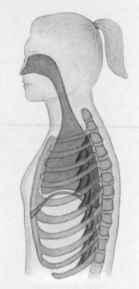

pigment in the red blood cells. This process transports oxygen around the circulation system to power the body's energy-making metabolic processes. At the same time, carbon dioxide, the waste product of the metabolic processes, diffuses from the blood into the alveoli and is expelled from the body during exhalation.

RESPIRATORY DEFENCES

The respiratory tract has different ways to protect itself from infection and irritation:

• Tissue – Protective tissue lines the upper and the lower respiratory tracts. In the upper tract, the protective tissue is concentrated in the tonsils and adenoids, which destroy agents before they can reach the lungs.
• Mucus coating – This sticky, protective coating lines the airways and traps any foreign particles.
• Cilia – These are tiny hair-like projections in the airways, which sweep any foreign particles up and away from the lungs.

HOW THE LUNGS WORK

▷ The unconscious act of breathing sends air down a system of ever-narrower airways and into the bloodstream. The respiratory system is a complex mechanism that also involves the ribcage and various different muscles.

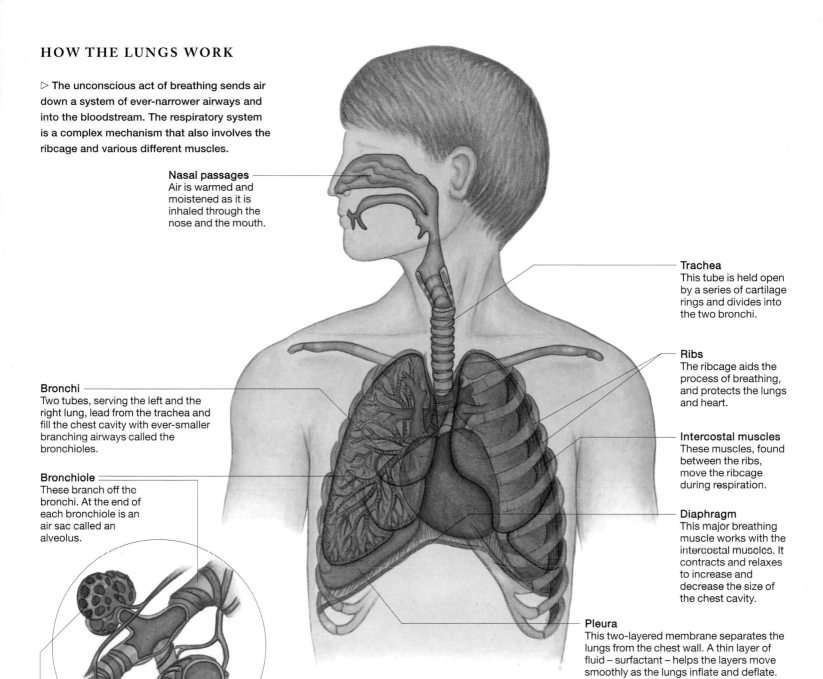

Nasal passages
Air is warmed and moistened as it is inhaled through the nose and the mouth.

Trachea
This tube is held open by a series of cartilage rings and divides into the two bronchi.

Ribs
The ribcage aids the process of breathing, and protects the lungs and heart.

Bronchi
Two tubes, serving the left and the right lung, lead from the trachea and fill the chest cavity with ever-smaller branching airways called the bronchioles.

Intercostal muscles
These muscles, found between the ribs, move the ribcage during respiration.

Bronchiole
These branch off the bronchi. At the end of each bronchiole is an air sac called an alveolus.

Diaphragm
This major breathing muscle works with the intercostal muscles. It contracts and relaxes to increase and decrease the size of the chest cavity.

Pleura
This two-layered membrane separates the lungs from the chest wall. A thin layer of fluid – surfactant – helps the layers move smoothly as the lungs inflate and deflate.

Alveolus
Each alveolus is covered with tiny capillaries to create the maximum surface area for gaseous exchange.

Membranous wall
Alveolar walls allow oxygen from air to diffuse into the haemoglobin in red blood cells. At the same time, carbon dioxide from the red blood cells diffuses into the alveolus and is breathed out.

• Coughing – A cough reflex is triggered by irritation in the airways or the lungs to expel foreign particles from the body before they can do any damage.

INVESTIGATING THE RESPIRATORY TRACT

Your doctor has various ways to diagnose respiratory problems, including:

➤ Listening to you cough and examining your chest.

➤ A chest X-ray can confirm the presence of infections or more serious diseases, such as lung cancer.

➤ A peak-flow meter measures exhalation to give an indication of any obstruction in the airways. It is also used to find out if asthma patients need to make any adjustments to their medication.

A range of investigations may be used by a hospital specialist including:

➤ Lung function tests measure how much air you can inhale or exhale, and how much air your lungs can hold.

➤ Two lung scans are taken to measure blood and air flow through the lungs.

➤ Bronchoscopy – A narrow tube with a camera at its tip is passed through the mouth or nose into the lungs so that the bronchi can be viewed. A local anaesthetic is given.

Colds and flu

Colds and flu (influenza) are viral infections of the upper respiratory tract, and are among the most common reasons for people to visit their doctors. There are more than 200 different viruses that cause the common cold and three main flu types, A, B and C. Approximately half the population catches a cold once a year, most often in the colder months of autumn and winter. Flu affects fewer people and tends to occur in epidemics in winter. The most effective way to fight colds and flu is to ensure that your body is fit and healthy as possible.

Colds and flu are extremely contagious. They are spread by airborne droplets of mucus, expelled when an infected person coughs, sneezes or breathes into the air. The viruses can also be passed on by physical contact if the recipient picks up the virus on their hand and rubs their eyes or nose – which provide entry points for the virus. One infected person can pass on the virus to many others, and you are probably most infectious a day before symptoms develop.

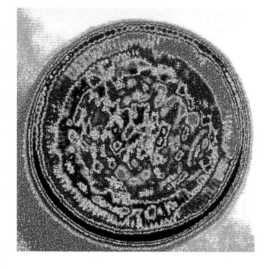

△ The common cold virus, shown here as a computer graphic, is easily spread by airborne droplets and by hand-to-hand contact.

SIGNS AND SYMPTOMS

Both cold and flu produce symptoms a day or two after you've been infected. They share some symptoms but flu symptoms tend to worsen dramatically in a few hours and are more severe.

The usual cold symptoms are:

➤ A runny nose in which the mucus becomes thick and greeny-yellow.

➤ Sneezing.

➤ Sore throat and cough.

➤ Wild fever and headache.

Very often people think they have flu when they have a bad cold. However, flu symptoms sometimes include a blocked nose, a cough and a sore throat but you are more likely to suffer from:

➤ High fever, sweating and chills.

➤ Aching muscles.

➤ Headaches.

➤ Severe exhaustion and weakness.

➤ Loss of appetite.

Since many different viruses can cause the common cold, having one cold does not provide immunity from another. Adults are less susceptible to colds than children because they have developed some immunity to the most common forms, and children spend more time in large groups – at school or in nurseries – where viruses can spread rapidly from child to child.

Flu is principally caused by infection with virus types A or B, particularly the more severe type A virus. However, the flu viruses are continually mutating into new strains. Having one attack of flu will not provide you with immunity against an attack by a new strain. If you are concerned about developing flu, you can be immunized against the strains that are predicted to be most prevalent each year. Immunization is strongly recommended for certain groups of people who are at greater risk of developing complications (see box on flu jabs opposite).

SELF-HELP FOR TREATING COLDS AND FLU

All you can do for a cold or flu is make yourself more comfortable during the worst of the infection. The following may help to soothe the symptoms of a cold or flu:

• Drinking plenty of cool fluids will help to reduce a fever.

▽ A sneeze blasts a jet of tiny droplets into the air, which may be inhaled by anyone close by. This is usually how cold and flu viruses spread.

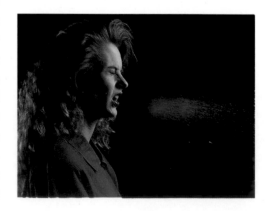

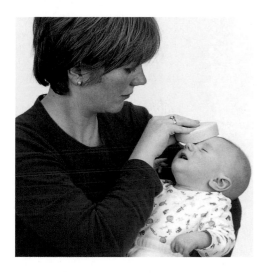

△ The symptoms of a cold can be particularly uncomfortable for a baby so anything you can do to soothe them will be helpful.

- Take painkillers (taking care to follow the directions on the packet) to help to reduce any fever and relieve the pain of a sore throat.
- Keep warm and have plenty of rest.
- Take decongestants to clear a stuffy nose.
- Avoid alcohol and smoking.
- Make sure that rooms are well ventilated and avoid spending time in stuffy, smoky or polluted atmospheres.

COLD AND FLU REMEDIES
A range of medicines are available over the counter and these usually combine a strong painkilling element with various decongestant drugs, caffeine and other ingredients. It is important to check each packet or bottle to find out what the remedy contains (check with your pharmacist if you are doubtful). This is particularly important if you are taking any other medication regularly. Levels of painkiller, especially paracetomol, must be monitored carefully.

Cough medicines simply provide some relief from the pain and irritation of a cough and sore throat. A hot honey and lemon drink contains vitamin C to help the body to fight a cold, and the honey and soothing effect of the hot drink will provide some relief.

A cold should only last a few days but the symptoms of flu can last up to a week. However, the worst symptoms of flu are likely to pass after two to three days, as long as no complications develop. After a bout of flu, you may feel depressed or tired for a while, and a cough may last for a couple of weeks or more.

WHEN TO SEE YOUR DOCTOR
Arrange an appointment with your doctor if you have an infection that seems to be lasting longer than usual or if the symptoms seem to be worse than you would usually expect. Flu can lead to some life-threatening complications and it is important to see your doctor if you suspect that you have a serious infection and if your symptoms are not showing any sign of improvement after two or three days.

WHO IS MOST AT RISK?
Certain individuals are at greater risk of developing complications if they contract flu. These complications include bronchitis, a bacterial infection that affects the airways, and pneumonia, an infection of the lungs. Deaths from pneumonia are common during flu epidemics.

Those most at risk from complications as a result of flu are:
- Newborn babies and infants that were premature or had a low birthweight.
- The elderly.
- Smokers.
- Asthmatics.
- People with weakened immune systems due to, for example, diabetes or AIDS.
- People with poor nutrition and poor general health.

If anyone in the at-risk groups develops the symptoms of flu, they should not be treated at home, but should consult their doctor as soon as any symptoms appear. Antiviral medication is available, but is effective only if taken within the first 36 hours. Your doctor may also prescribe antibiotics as a preventive measure against complications. If complications such as

FLU JABS
People who are at high risk of becoming seriously ill if they contract flu are now recommended to visit their doctor for a flu jab each autumn to protect themselves through the winter months. The immunization is different each year because it targets the strains predicted to be most widespread that winter. Flu jabs are recommended for:

➤ People aged over 65 years.

➤ People with diabetes.

➤ People with asthma.

➤ People suffering from cardio-respiratory disease.

➤ People taking immunosuppressants.

pneumonia are suspected, you may be sent for a chest X-ray to confirm the diagnosis. In very severe cases, you may be admitted to hospital for treatment.

▽ Making sure that you have plenty of rest, keep warm and drink plenty of liquids will enable your body to concentrate its energies on fighting the infection.

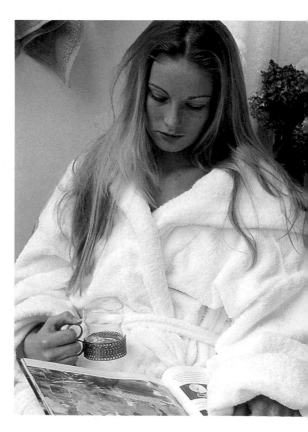

Asthma

Asthma is a condition where intermittent narrowing of the airways results in breathing difficulties. In mild cases, the person may suffer only sporadic bouts of wheezing and shortness of breath, but some people can have disabling and potentially life-threatening attacks almost every day. Asthma has become better recognized over the past two decades and cases are believed to have doubled in that time – although it is thought that this increase may be due to the fact that more people with mild symptoms are classified as asthmatics.

SIGNS AND SYMPTOMS

➤ Wheezing and coughing that is often worse at night, in the early hours of the morning and after exercise.

➤ Tightness in the chest.

➤ Shortness of breath.

➤ Panic and anxiety.

➤ Difficulty breathing out.

Asthma can develop at any age but generally it occurs first in childhood. The condition is often associated with allergies, and common triggers for allergic asthma are house-dust mites, pollen, mould and pet hair. Some of the more common food allergens (see box on asthma triggers) can also trigger an asthmatic attack. Children who are affected by allergic asthma often also develop eczema or hayfever.

Most adults who suffer from asthma first developed the condition as children. However, asthma can also start in adulthood, usually after a respiratory infection. Smoking, polluted or cold air, and stress may all trigger asthma attacks.

MAKING A DIAGNOSIS

Some people suffer only occasional attacks of asthma while others may have frequent and severe attacks in response to a range of triggers. It is not always easy for doctors to diagnose the condition, and the only clue that a child has asthma might be a cough that occurs at night or the fact that their breathing becomes wheezy during or after a bout of activity.

If your doctor suspects that you have asthma, you may be sent to hospital for further investigation. Tests that help with the diagnosis of asthma include spirometry and lung volume tests, which measure and monitor the rate and depth of your breathing. You may also be tested for allergic reactions to different substances, to pinpoint the likely trigger for your attacks. Sometimes, blood tests may be carried out to check the level of oxygen in your blood.

ASTHMA TRIGGERS

In any one individual, it is possible that there is more than one factor that initiates an asthmatic attack. Asthma may be triggered by:

➤ Upper respiratory tract infections, such as colds and flu.

➤ Lower respiratory tract infections, such as pneumonia and bronchitis.

➤ Allergy (allergens include house-dust mites, pollen, hair and saliva from furry animals, such as cats and dogs).

➤ Exposure to cold air.

➤ Dampness and mould.

➤ Anxiety and stress.

➤ Air pollution.

➤ Cigarette smoke.

In rare cases, certain foods – such as milk, eggs, nuts and wheat – prompt an attack. Many people with asthma are sensitive to aspirin and taking tablets can initiate an attack.

CAUSES OF ASTHMA

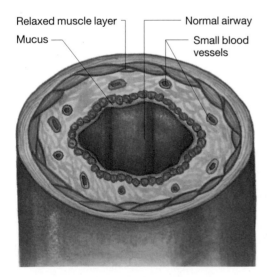

Relaxed muscle layer — Normal airway
Mucus — Small blood vessels

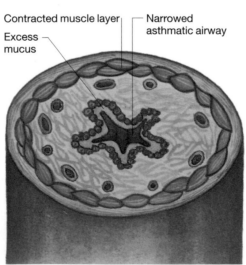

Contracted muscle layer — Narrowed asthmatic airway
Excess mucus

△ In asthma, the muscles in the bronchi constrict, causing them to narrow. At the same time, the mucus that protects the airways from infection is produced in excess and the lining of the airways become inflamed. This means that very little air can get into or out of the lungs.

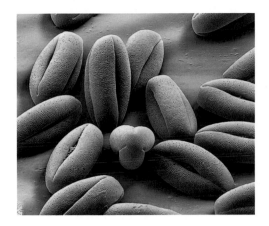

△ This picture shows a magnified image of flowering horse chestnut pollen. Pollen is a common trigger for attacks of allergic asthma.

MANAGEMENT OF ASTHMA

As yet, there is no cure for asthma. However, it can be managed extremely well with both drug therapy and by avoiding triggers – most people with asthma lead normal lives. In addition, many cases of

SEVERE ASTHMA ATTACKS

A severe asthma attack can result in respiratory failure and coma. More than 5000 people a year in the US and nearly 2000 a year in the UK die as a result of an asthma attack. Most of these deaths could be prevented if the severity of the attack had been recognized and treatment had been sought. If an asthma attack becomes severe, you will have some of the following symptoms:

➤ Silent wheezing because breathing is very shallow.

➤ Severe breathlessness.

➤ Blue lips, fingers and toes – due to a lack of oxygen.

➤ Pale, clammy skin.

➤ Exhaustion and confusion.

If your inhaler is not providing any relief, try to keep calm and call for an ambulance. Sit upright in the most comfortable position you can find but do not lie down. Try to slow your breathing, if possible, until medical help arrives.

childhood asthma become less of a problem with age and many cases disappear by the age of 20.

Doctors usually ask people with asthma to monitor their symptoms. Depending on the severity of your condition, you may be asked to perform self-assessment peak-flow measurements every day in the morning and evening. This involves breathing into a peak-flow meter which measures the quantity of air you exhale per minute. Plotting these measurements on a graph helps to show whether you are on the correct dose of drugs and how effectively your asthma is controlled.

Almost all asthma drugs are inhaled in vapour form so that they are taken directly into the lungs and get to work instantly. A "spacer device" can be used to make the lungs take up the vapour even more effectively.

There are two main kinds of inhalers - those that relieve an asthma attack and those that prevent future attacks:

• Reliever inhalers – These inhalers are normally blue in colour and contain drugs called bronchodilators. They relax and widen the airways and provide short-term relief.

• Preventer inhalers – These are usually low-dose corticosteroid devices and are normally brown in colour. They are used twice a day on a regular basis and have a protective effect upon the lungs by reducing any inflammation and the production of mucus.

Corticosteroids may also be prescribed as tablets, usually to relieve severe attacks or for people with long-term severe asthma.

LIVING WITH ASTHMA

If you have asthma, you should always carry your medication with you in case of an attack. You should avoid known triggers, such as smoky or polluted atmospheres or exposure to cold air, and should not keep furry pets if you are allergic to them. Smoking is known to make the condition worse and therefore is not advisable. It is also a good idea to exercise regularly since

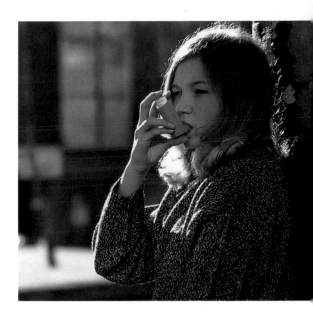

△ Asthma drugs act quickly to widen the airways and relieve symptoms. People with asthma should always carry their inhalers with them so that they can deal with a serious attack.

▽ People with asthma monitor their own condition from an early age. This young girl is breathing into a peak-flow meter, to measure her rate of exhalation.

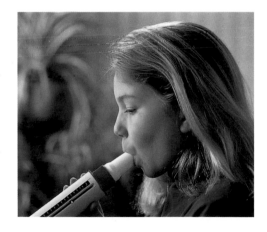

this improves lung capacity and makes breathing easier. You may have to take preventive medicine from an inhaler to make this possible; if in doubt, discuss this with your doctor. Swimming is a particularly good exercise for people with asthma, because of the humid environment, but in theory any sport is possible.

If you find that your asthma is worse when you are stressed, try relaxation techniques or a form of yoga to control levels of stress, which will in turn cut down the risk of an asthma attack.

Chronic obstructive pulmonary disease

Chronic obstructive pulmonary disease (COPD) is a progressive respiratory disease that causes severe shortness of breath and wheezing. The term is used to cover chronic bronchitis and emphysema – bronchitis is the inflammation of the bronchi, the large airways that lead to the lungs, while emphysema means permanent damage to the air sacs (alveoli), which lose their elasticity. People with COPD usually have both conditions, with one being dominant. COPD is almost always caused by smoking and is twice as likely to affect men as women.

COPD is a debilitating condition. As it progresses, people become so short of breath that they are increasingly unable to carry out everyday tasks – eventually they often become housebound.

COPD is almost entirely caused by smoking, although industrial pollutants may exacerbate the damage to the lungs. The condition is often not diagnosed until the damage has been done – many of those affected put early symptoms down to "smoker's cough" and do not seek help. Male smokers who live in industrial areas are most likely to be affected. Some sources estimate that up to one-quarter of all those affected are not diagnosed at all.

SIGNS AND SYMPTOMS

➤ A chronic cough, which is usually worse in the morning.

➤ Gradually increasing production of sputum (phlegm).

➤ Progressive shortness of breath.

➤ Ever-increasing susceptibility to acute lung infections.

➤ Symptoms that get worse in winter.

Some people who have COPD breathe rapidly to get more oxygen into their blood and will often have a rosy glow to their skin. Others can develop a barrel-shaped chest because the lungs have become distended.

If you are a smoker and have any of the above symptoms, it is advisable to make an appointment to see your doctor as soon as possible.

WHAT MIGHT YOUR DOCTOR DO?

If you are a smoker, your doctor is likely to suspect COPD following an initial consultation and examination. In order to determine the extent of lung damage, you may be referred to hospital for specialized tests so that your lung function can be assessed. These specialized tests may include spirometry, in which your rate of inhalation and exhalation is measured, and lung volume tests, which are carried out to measure the volume of air inhaled in one breath and volume of air left in the lungs when you have exhaled.

There is a range of other tests that can confirm the diagnosis, and these may include giving samples of blood in order that the levels of oxygen and carbon dioxide in your blood can be measured. An X-ray may also be taken so that any other underlying causes can be ruled out.

▽ In this spirometry test, a woman blows into a bag connected to a monitor unit, which draws a graph of her rate of exhalation. People affected by bronchitis will have a low rate of exhalation.

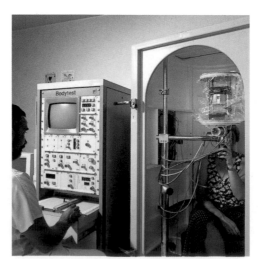

TREATMENT OPTIONS

The first and most important treatment for COPD is for the person to give up smoking immediately since this is the only way of preventing further damage to the lungs.

SELF-HELP MEASURES

➤ Giving up smoking is the only action that can delay the progression of your COPD. Cutting down will have little effect on your lung function. You should also avoid smoky and polluted atmospheres.

➤ Make your home environment free from smoke, dust, pollution, damp and cold – all can exacerbate COPD.

➤ Taking gentle exercise may help to improve your tolerance to exertion.

▽ A GP listens to the sound of the patient's heart and lungs through a stethoscope. This simple procedure can often be enough to make an initial diagnosis of serious lung disorders.

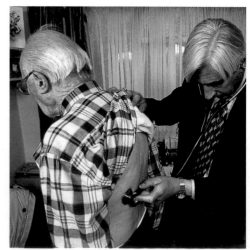

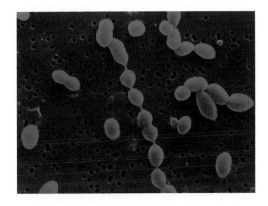

△ *Streptococcus* bacteria, above, are a major cause of pneumonia, which may be fatal in those suffering from COPD.

Unfortunately, it is not possible to reverse the damage that has been caused by COPD. However, there are various drug treatments available that can help to relieve the symptoms.

Your doctor may prescribe any of the following drugs:
• Antibiotics to treat acute infections.
• Bronchodilating inhalers, which help to open up the airways and thus make breathing easier.
• Inhaled steroids to reduce inflammation.
• Diuretics to reduce fluid build-up if you have swollen ankles.
• Continuous low-dose oxygen therapy to raise your blood oxygen levels and reduce the strain on the heart. This treatment is usually given in more advanced cases, and can be organized at home.

In terms of preventive measures, your doctor may recommend a flu jab each winter and another vaccination against *Streptococcus pneumoniae* bacterium. If

someone suffering from COPD develops flu or pneumonia, the consequences can be life-threatening.

THE OUTLOOK

If the illness is diagnosed at an early stage and you give up smoking straight away, you may be able to avoid severe lung damage. However, most people with COPD are not diagnosed until their condition has reached an advanced stage and the damage has been done. If this is the case the outlook is not encouraging – increasing breathlessness and a limited exercise tolerance mean that those affected may find it more and more difficult to carry out everyday activities. Heart and respiratory failure may ultimately result. In most cases, those affected are unlikely to live longer than ten years.

Acute bronchitis

SEE ALSO
➤ Colds and flu, p128

Acute bronchitis is a short-term infection of the larger airways, the bronchi. It occurs either in young adults, when it is usually the result of a viral infection, or as a complication of chronic obstructive pulmonary disease, when the cause is usually bacterial.

Bronchitis often occurs as a complication of a respiratory infection, such as a common cold that has spread into the bronchi from the nose, throat or sinuses. People who smoke or those who are exposed to high levels of pollutants in the air are more susceptible to attacks of bronchitis. People with existing COPD may experience several bouts of acute bronchitis during the winter. The inflammation resulting from the infection produces excessive amounts of mucus, which triggers the cough reflex to remove it from the lungs.

HOW IS IT TREATED?

An otherwise healthy adult will expect to make a complete recovery within a week or so. In such cases, simple supportive treatment is all that is required – that is, plenty of fluids, rest and over-the-counter painkillers such as paracetamol. If you smoke, you should stop immediately.

Older people with COPD or those who have suffered a particularly severe attack of bronchitis will normally require a course of

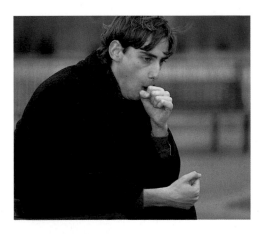

△ An irritating cough is one of the main symptoms of acute bronchitis, which is often associated with smoking.

antibiotics to aid recovery. More severe cases may require hospitalization. If the condition persists for longer than two weeks, you may need to have a chest X-ray to check for any underlying cause.

SIGNS AND SYMPTOMS

The symptoms of bronchitis tend to develop rapidly in one to two days, and may include:

➤ An irritating cough that may produce clear sputum (phlegm).

➤ Chest pain.

➤ Wheezing and tightness in the chest.

➤ Breathlessness.

➤ Mild fever.

Pneumonia

Pneumonia is a serious chest infection that affects the air sacs (alveoli) in the lung, causing them to become inflamed. Because oxygen needs to pass through the walls of the alveoli in order to reach the bloodstream, this is a potentially life-threatening condition – especially if both lungs are affected. Pneumonia is the most common form of fatal infection acquired in hospital and is particularly dangerous for the elderly. In most cases, however, effective treatment with antibiotics leads to a full recovery with no lasting effects.

SIGNS AND SYMPTOMS

Pneumonia may develop gradually, particularly if the cause is viral. Bacterial pneumonia usually develops rapidly over the course of several hours. Symptoms of pneumonia are:

➤ A cough with mucus, which may be bloody.

➤ High fever.

➤ Breathlessness even when resting.

➤ Chest pain on breathing in (inspiration).

➤ Delirium and/or confusion.

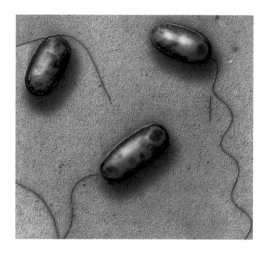

△ These bacteria, *Legionella pneumophila*, cause Legionnaire's disease, a form of pneumonia which can be fatal.

Pneumonia occurs most frequently among the very young and the very old, although it can occur at any age. The offending micro-organism can be a virus, a bacterium or a fungus – but in the majority of cases of pneumonia the cause is bacterial.

Certain factors make a person more likely to develop pneumonia – these include smoking, being malnourished or drinking excessive quantities of alcohol over a long period. People who are suffering from a long-term disorder such as diabetes are more at risk, as are those who have impaired immunity as a result of AIDS or because they are undergoing treatments such as chemotherapy or taking immunosuppression drugs.

Pneumonia used to be a common cause of death but effective antibiotics mean that most people now make a full recovery. But despite the best medical attention, the disease can still be fatal, particularly among the elderly and those already suffering from another serious disease.

TREATMENT FOR PNEUMONIA

Otherwise fit and healthy adults are often treated at home with a course of antibiotics. Painkillers help to lower fever and control pain, and plenty of fluids are required.

Children, elderly people and adults who rapidly become severely ill will normally be referred to hospital for immediate treatment. There they receive intravenous fluids and antibiotics. Sometimes, they need oxygen via an oxygen mask. Occasionally someone affected by pneumonia will need to be connected to a ventilator to maintain adequate levels of oxygen until they recover.

WHAT IS THE OUTLOOK?

People usually recover within a few weeks, although young children often make a full recovery much more quickly. However,

pneumonia is associated with a number of complications. The pleura may become inflamed, leading to pleurisy. In some severe cases, the danger is that the infection may enter the bloodstream, causing septicaemia. And in the elderly and those with weakened immunity, the infection can spread deep into the lungs, causing respiratory failure.

HOW IS IT DIAGNOSED?

Your doctor may suspect pneumonia from your medical history and a chest examination. You may be referred to the hospital for a chest X-ray, and a blood test. A sputum (phlegm) sample may be sent for analysis to establish the cause.

▽ A chest X-ray will show the extent of infection. In this coloured X-ray, the infection shows up as a red patch at the base of the blue lung on the right.

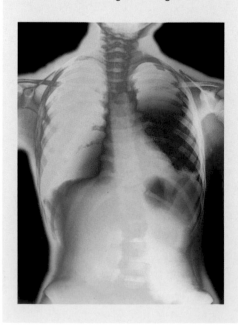

Pleurisy

SEE ALSO
➤ Colds and flu, p128
➤ Pneumonia, p134

Pleurisy is an inflammation of the pleura – the double-layered membrane that surrounds the lungs and separates them from the chest wall. When you are in good health, the two pleural layers slide smoothly over one another as you breathe in and out, which in turn allows the lungs to inflate and deflate. In pleurisy, the inflammation prevents this smooth movement and the layers rub over one another causing intense pain when you breathe in. Pleurisy usually occurs as a complication of other diseases, such as pneumonia.

SIGNS AND SYMPTOMS
Symptoms appear gradually and include:

➤ A sharp pain in the chest, usually located to one side or the other, made worse by breathing in deeply.

➤ A frightening feeling of being unable to breathe.

Pleurisy may be caused by a viral infection such as flu, but is usually due to pneumonia that has spread from the lung tissue. You should seek medical advice within 24 hours if you suspect you have pleurisy. Doctors can often diagnose pleurisy by using a stethoscope to listen for the sound of the pleura rubbing together. A chest X-ray will usually reveal the underlying cause.

TREATMENT OPTIONS
Any underlying cause is treated first and then doctors will want to control the symptoms of the pleurisy itself. This may involve taking an antibiotic to treat any infection in the lung as well as anti-inflammatory drugs to relieve pain and reduce the pleural inflammation. Most cases of pleurisy clear up within a week to ten days of the start of treatment.

HEALTHY AND INFLAMED MEMBRANES

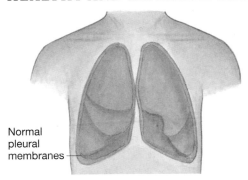

Normal pleural membranes

△ The pleura is a double-layered membrane surrounding the lungs. Fluid between the layers helps them move smoothly as you breathe.

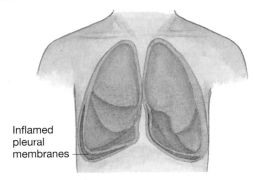

Inflamed pleural membranes

△ Inflamed pleural membranes rub together, causing pain. A pleural effusion is when the space between the layers fills with excess fluid.

Pneumothorax

SEE ALSO
➤ COPD, p132

Pneumothorax occurs when air enters the space between the pleural layers which surround the lungs. The underlying lung may then collapse.

A pneumothorax is generally a medical emergency and may be fatal if not treated quickly. Usually only one lung is affected.

SIGNS AND SYMPTOMS
➤ Shortness of breath, which may be very severe.

➤ Tightness across the chest.

A pneumothorax is when the lung is collapsed and it can occur as the result of a rupture of a small bubble of tissue (bulla) on the surface of the lung. This may occur during a bout of exercise but may have no apparent cause. A pneumothorax may be a complication of lung disease, such as chronic obstructive pulmonary disease. A fractured rib piercing the lung or any chest injury that allows air to pass from outside the body can also result in a pneumothorax.

TREATING A PNEUMOTHORAX
Most mild cases disappear without treatment. However, a larger pneumothorax needs to be treated urgently in hospital. Doctors insert a hollow tube into the affected side of the chest to release excess air and to allow the lung to reinflate. Most people recover fully, but the condition recurs in about 20 per cent of cases.

Lung cancer

Lung cancer is the second most common form of the disease (after skin cancer) and the most common cause of cancer deaths. It is most likely to affect people who are aged between 50 and 70. Lung cancer is largely preventable – the main risk factor is smoking. It has always been more common in men but in recent years the gap has closed as more women have taken up smoking. People who spend a lot of time in a smoky atmosphere – bar staff, for example – are also at risk of developing lung cancer through passive smoking.

SIGNS AND SYMPTOMS

➤ A chronic (persistent) cough, sometimes containing sputum (phlegm) streaked with blood.

➤ Shortness of breath.

➤ Unexplained weight loss.

➤ Chest pain.

➤ Wheezing.

➤ Episodes of bronchitis or pneumonia.

Some forms of lung cancer produce no symptoms until they are well advanced.

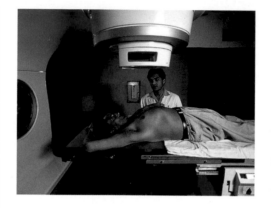

△ This man is about to receive radiotherapy treatment. The machine is being set up so that the X-rays target the affected area in his lung.

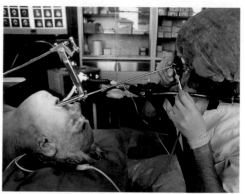

△ A bronchoscope is passed into the lungs under general anaesthetic to enable the doctor to view the airways and remove a tissue sample.

Lung cancer can develop very slowly, taking many years to produce symptoms. Also, some types of lung cancer do not cause any symptoms until they are in the final stages. As a result, lung cancer may be diagnosed only when it is well advanced, when treatment options are limited.

If your doctor suspects that you have lung cancer, you will be sent for a chest X-ray – an abnormal shadow on the lung may confirm the diagnosis. Your doctor may want to send a sputum (phlegm) sample for analysis, so that it can be checked for the presence of cancerous cells, or refer you for a bronchoscopy. In this procedure, a tube is passed through the mouth into the lungs to view the bronchi.

TREATMENT OPTIONS

There are three kinds of treatment and the nature and extent of the cancer will govern which one is used:

• Surgery – A tumour can be removed surgically only if the cancer has not spread to other organs. If there isn't any spread, surgeons will remove all of one lung or a major part of it.

• Chemotherapy – A course of chemotherapy drugs usually follows any surgery to remove a tumour, and it is also used to target highly malignant tumours.

• Radiation therapy – This treatment slows down the growth of a tumour but does not destroy it completely. It is often used to treat the tiny tumours – metastases – that have spread from the lungs to the brain, bones and liver. An initial course of radiotherapy is often followed by a course of chemotherapy.

THE LONG-TERM OUTLOOK

The prognosis is best for those whose cancer is detected early – people can and do survive lung cancer. But overall the outlook is poor: as few as one person in twenty survives longer than five years after treatment. In cases where the disease has spread, active treatment usually achieves only symptom control and improved quality of life, but may not extend life expectancy.

PREVENTING LUNG CANCER

Giving up smoking substantially reduces your risk of lung cancer. Research has shown that ex-smokers are only slightly more at risk of developing the disease than non-smokers.

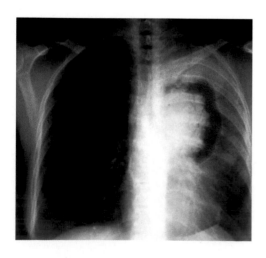

◁ This chest X-ray shows a large cancerous tumour in the lung of a 50-year-old woman. The tumour has been highlighted in red.

8

THE URINARY SYSTEM

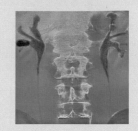

The urinary system, also known as the urinary tract, is a complex filter and drainage unit. This system separates useful by-products in the blood, which it keeps and reabsorbs, from unwanted waste substances, which it passes out of the body in the form of urine. Urine, which is mainly composed of water, is stored in the bladder until it can be passed out of the body. The fact that the urinary tract passes waste out of the body makes it vulnerable to attack by infection. Disease or infection in the kidneys and other parts of the urinary tract can result in a range of problems, from mild cystitis to chronic renal failure, so it is vital to keep this system in good working order.

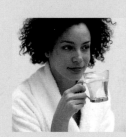

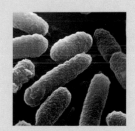

CONTENTS

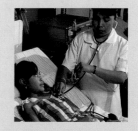

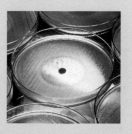

The urinary organs

SEE ALSO
➤ Urinary tract
  infections, p142
➤ Urinary incontinence,
  p144
➤ The roles of blood
  and lymph, p200

The urinary system is a sophisticated filtration unit which maintains fluid and chemical balance within the body. Many chemical reactions occurring in cells all over the body produce unwanted by-products and the kidneys filter these from the blood and excrete them in the form of urine. The urinary system is made up of a pair of kidneys, two ureters, a bladder and a urethra. As well as their important excretory function, the kidneys also produce hormones that control red blood cell production and help to regulate blood pressure.

The kidneys are the main organs of the urinary system, with many vital functions:
• Removing toxic waste products from the blood and excreting them as urine.
• Returning useful substances to the body's circulation.
• Regulating water balance. Your kidneys conserve water at times of relative dehydration and eliminate any surplus.

THE KIDNEY IN DETAIL
Your kidneys are about 12 cm (5 in) long and 6 cm (2.5 in) wide and are at the back of your abdomen, just in front of your spine. The kidney has several regions, each with a different function:
• The cortex – This outer layer houses filtering units called nephrons.

• The medulla – The next inner layer is full of cone-shaped urine-collecting ducts.
• The renal pelvis – This is at the heart of the kidney and is where urine collects before passing on to the bladder.

FILTERING THE BLOOD
Blood is transported to each kidney through the renal arteries. These blood vessels stem from the body's main artery, the aorta, and carry a rich blood supply that accounts for a quarter of the blood pumped by the heart.

Blood passes from these arteries through a sophisticated filtration system. The principal unit of the system is the nephron, which is made up of a glomerulus and a renal tubule.

URINARY CONTROL
The muscular wall of the bladder has an extensive nerve supply, which allows you to control when it is emptied. As your bladder fills your brain receives impulses from the nerves in the bladder wall. When your bladder is full your brain instructs it to contract and, at the same time, your bladder relaxes a ring of muscle at it's lower opening to control the release of urine through the urethra. This process requires a mature nervous system and such voluntary control of urination is not acquired until a few years after birth. Loss of this voluntary control can occur for various reasons in adults and is known as incontinence.

THE STRUCTURE OF A KIDNEY

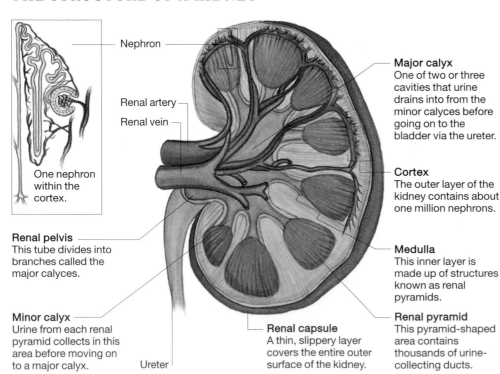

Nephron

One nephron within the cortex.

Renal artery

Renal vein

Renal pelvis
This tube divides into branches called the major calyces.

Minor calyx
Urine from each renal pyramid collects in this area before moving on to a major calyx.

Ureter

Renal capsule
A thin, slippery layer covers the entire outer surface of the kidney.

Major calyx
One of two or three cavities that urine drains into from the minor calyces before going on to the bladder via the ureter.

Cortex
The outer layer of the kidney contains about one million nephrons.

Medulla
This inner layer is made up of structures known as renal pyramids.

Renal pyramid
This pyramid-shaped area contains thousands of urine-collecting ducts.

The glomerulus is a collection of tiny capillaries that allow small molecules to pass into the renal tubules. Only fluid in the blood is filtered, blood cells are not able to cross the membrane. The fluid (filtrate) passes through the tubules and useful substances, such as glucose and sodium, are reabsorbed into the bloodstream while harmful ones, such as urea, are retained.

The renal tubules have three sections:
• Proximal convoluted tubule – Most of the water and nutrients are reabsorbed here; unwanted substances are also secreted into the fluid at this point.
• Loop of Henle – More water and salts are reabsorbed in this section and waste products are secreted into the fluid here.
• Distal convoluted tubule – Fine-tuning of the water content of the urine is performed here.

THE FEMALE URINARY SYSTEM

▽ The bladder and the urethra in the male and female urinary systems have a different structure but apart from these differences the two urinary systems are the same.

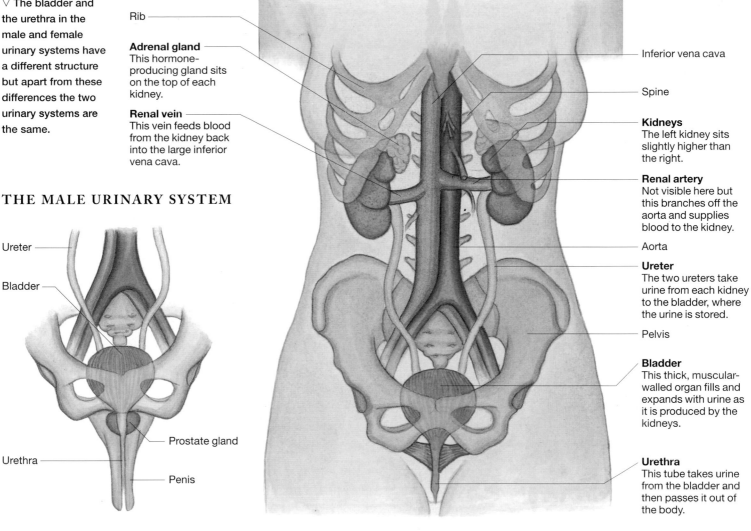

Rib

Adrenal gland
This hormone-producing gland sits on the top of each kidney.

Renal vein
This vein feeds blood from the kidney back into the large inferior vena cava.

Inferior vena cava

Spine

Kidneys
The left kidney sits slightly higher than the right.

Renal artery
Not visible here but this branches off the aorta and supplies blood to the kidney.

Aorta

Ureter
The two ureters take urine from each kidney to the bladder, where the urine is stored.

Pelvis

Bladder
This thick, muscular-walled organ fills and expands with urine as it is produced by the kidneys.

Urethra
This tube takes urine from the bladder and then passes it out of the body.

THE MALE URINARY SYSTEM

Ureter

Bladder

Urethra

Prostate gland

Penis

THE STRUCTURE OF A NEPHRON

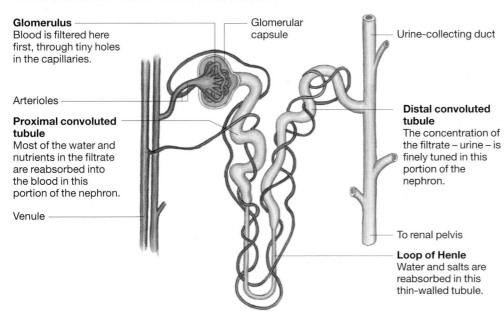

Glomerulus
Blood is filtered here first, through tiny holes in the capillaries.

Glomerular capsule

Urine-collecting duct

Arterioles

Proximal convoluted tubule
Most of the water and nutrients in the filtrate are reabsorbed into the blood in this portion of the nephron.

Venule

Distal convoluted tubule
The concentration of the filtrate – urine – is finely tuned in this portion of the nephron.

To renal pelvis

Loop of Henle
Water and salts are reabsorbed in this thin-walled tubule.

△ The nephron is part of the filtration unit through which the blood passes in the kidneys. Through this filtration system useful substances are reabsorbed into the bloodstream, and waste substances become urine, which is eventually passed from the kidneys by the ureter.

PASSAGE OF URINE

Once fluid reaches the end of the renal tubule it is urine. Urine from the nephrons travels via collecting ducts in the kidney's medulla to storage areas that feed into the renal pelvis. Each kidney is drained by a ureter, which is a thin muscular tube about 30 cm (12 in) long. Ureters carry urine to the bladder, which stores the urine until it is emptied. The bladder has a highly folded lining that smooths out as it expands and fills with urine. A healthy adult excretes 0.5–2 litres (1–3 pints) of urine every day.

WHAT IS URINE?
Urine is 95 per cent water and 5 per cent uric acid, urea, salts (such as sodium, potassium and chloride) and creatinine.

Kidney stones

SEE ALSO
➤ Eat healthily, p14
➤ The urinary organs, p138

Normally, waste products from the body pass out in the urine, which is produced in the kidneys. If the urine becomes saturated with waste chemicals, these can crystallize and form stone-like deposits in the kidneys. Kidney stones come in varying sizes: small ones may travel down the urinary tract and simply pass out in the urine; larger stones tend to stay within the kidney but can move into the ureter, where they can lodge and cause severe pain. Half of all people affected by kidney stones will develop further stones within seven years.

Kidney stones occur more frequently in young to middle-aged men. People living in a hot climate have a higher chance of developing kidney stones if they don't drink enough fluid to replace that lost through sweating. Some individuals may inherit a predisposition towards the condition.

HOW IS IT DIAGNOSED?

Your doctor may suspect kidney stones after taking your medical history. Then you may be referred for further investigations, including a plain X-ray and/or intravenous urography, to identify the presence and

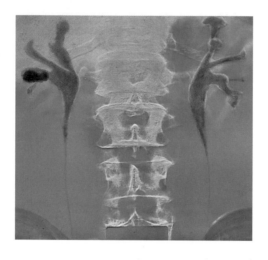

△ An intravenous pyelogram (IVP) image, which shows drainage of urine from the kidneys. Here, a stone can be seen in the right kidney (coloured orange, on the left of the picture).

SIGNS AND SYMPTOMS

Small stones may cause no symptoms whatsoever. However, larger stones are usually very painful because they cause the ureter to go into acute spasm. This is known as renal colic and the symptoms of renal colic are:

➤ Intense pain that radiates from the back (usually on one side) to the groin. Sometimes it can be felt in the genitals as well.

➤ Frequent, painful urination.

➤ Blood in the urine.

➤ Nausea and vomiting.

Renal colic subsides as soon as the offending stone is passed. An episode of renal colic may be an isolated incident, but some people are more prone to the condition and they may experience repeated attacks of kidney stones and renal colic.

location of stones. Some kidney stones are made from calcium salts and show up well on X-ray images. Other stones, made from oxalate, phosphate or uric acid, can be more difficult to see. More tests may be done on urine to check for secondary infection, any presence of blood in the urine and to measure kidney function.

TREATING KIDNEY STONES

Treatment for the condition depends on the size of the stone.

• Small stones may pass with rest, plenty of fluids and some appropriate pain relief. Occasionally smaller stones may become lodged in the ureter, and these can be removed during examination with an instrument called a cystoscope.

• Larger stones can cause more problems. They may not pass spontaneously and are more likely to become lodged in the kidney. These stones are usually treated

PREVENTING KIDNEY STONES

➤ Drink plenty of fluids, approximately 2–3 litres (3½–5 pints) a day.

➤ Increase your fluid intake during hot weather and after exercise.

➤ Avoid too much rhubarb, spinach and asparagus, as these promote the formation of oxalate stones.

➤ Check with your doctor in case you should limit your intake of calcium-rich substances, such as dairy products or calcium-based antacids.

▽ People who are prone to kidney stones may be advised to avoid, or reduce their consumption of, dairy products such as butter and cheese.

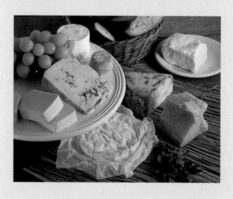

through a process known as lithotripsy. This method uses high-energy shock waves to break the stones down into a powder, which can then be expelled in the urine.

• In some cases, stones have to be removed surgically, although this is rare and generally only used as a last resort.

Kidney failure

SEE ALSO
➤ High blood pressure, p30
➤ Diabetes, p66
➤ Enlarged prostate gland, p160

In kidney failure, the kidneys are no longer able to carry out their normal function of filtering the body's by-products from the blood. As a result, waste products and excessive fluid build up in the body. Kidney failure may happen very suddenly (acute renal failure) but more commonly the kidneys fail gradually over a period of many months, sometimes years – this is known as chronic renal failure. The degree of kidney failure depends on its cause in each individual. The main text here will focus on kidney failure of the chronic kind.

SIGNS AND SYMPTOMS OF CHRONIC RENAL FAILURE

Apart from a general tiredness and malaise, symptoms can include:

➤ Infrequent passage of urine.

➤ Shortness of breath.

➤ Nausea.

➤ Muscle cramps.

➤ Back pain.

Chronic renal failure develops gradually and symptoms may not appear for many months. It can be caused by:
• Acute renal failure (see box, right).
• Any chronic kidney disease that impairs function, e.g. polycystic kidney disease.
• High blood pressure.
• Diabetes mellitus.
• Prolonged urinary-tract obstruction, e.g. one caused by an enlarged prostate gland.

WHAT MIGHT YOUR DOCTOR DO?

Your doctor will probably ask for a sample of urine for testing. Other tests may need referral to a hospital specialist and include intravenous urography, ultrasound scanning, cytoscopy and kidney biopsy.

TREATMENT OPTIONS

Chronic renal failure may progress slowly. Renal failure can be limited by treating causative factors. Good management of patients with diabetes, high blood pressure and/or prostate disease is vital, and is carried out by a team of specialists.

When deterioration in kidney function is progressive and advanced, a person may consider dialysis or a kidney transplant.

There are two types of dialysis, peritoneal dialysis and haemodialysis, used to treat acute and chronic renal failure.
• In peritoneal dialysis, the peritoneum (a membrane that surrounds the abdominal organs) acts as a filter, instead of the kidneys. It can be carried out anywhere several times a day and the fluid is changed every four to six hours.
• In haemodialysis a machine does the work of the kidneys. Blood is taken from a vein in the arm to the dialysis machine, where waste is removed. The blood is returned via a cannula (a plastic or metal tube used to withdraw or introduce fluids). Patients are attached for up to four hours at a time, about three times a week.

PERITONEAL CATHETER

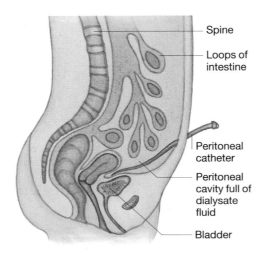

Spine

Loops of intestine

Peritoneal catheter

Peritoneal cavity full of dialysate fluid

Bladder

△ Peritoneal dialysis uses the peritoneum (a two-layered membrane lining the abdominal cavity) as a filter. The blood passes through the membranes, which allows waste such as urea to pass out, but keeps proteins in the system.

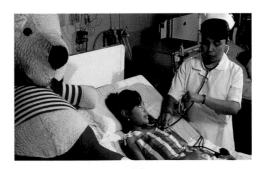

△ In some cases of kidney failure, renal dialysis is used. This is where a machine performs the function of the kidneys, filtering waste products and returning purified blood to the system.

ACUTE RENAL FAILURE

Acute renal failure is a medical emergency that can be fatal without immediate attention. It can be caused by:

➤ A dramatic fall in blood pressure due to severe infection, blood loss or heart attack.

➤ Acute disorders of the kidney.

➤ Drugs that are toxic to the kidney.

➤ Acute obstruction of the urinary tract.

Symptoms include:

➤ Dramatically reduced urine output.

➤ Vomiting.

➤ Drowsiness and headaches.

As long as the damage to the kidneys is reversible and causative conditions are managed, normal kidney function can return within several weeks. If the kidneys have sustained irreversible damage, they may not recover and the condition may progress to chronic renal failure.

Urinary tract infections (UTIs)

The urinary tract includes the kidneys, ureters, bladder and urethra, and the most common infection is cystitis, which affects the bladder. The bacteria most likely to cause a urinary tract infection are *Escherichia coli* (*E. coli*), normally found in the bowel. If a large number of *E. coli* get into the urethra, parts of the urinary tract can be infected. If the infection remains in the urethra it is called urethritis, and if it spreads to the kidneys it is pyelonephritis. Infection can take hold in a number of ways, including poor toilet hygiene, sexual intercourse and childbirth.

Urinary tract infections are less common in men and in childhood. Urinary tract infections more commonly affect women, and this is partly because a woman's urethra is shorter and nearer the anus and so is more vulnerable to infection.

CAUSES OF UTIs

Normally, urine is sterile – it contains no bacteria or fungi. However, sometimes bacteria from the digestive tract can find their way into the opening of the urethra, where they start to multiply. This causes infection and inflammation. These bacteria are usually *Escherichia coli* (*E. coli*) organisms, normally found in the bowel, where they are harmless. Occasionally, bacteria can make their way even further up the urinary tract and travel up the ureters into the kidneys, where they cause an infection known as pyelonephritis. Other organisms can be

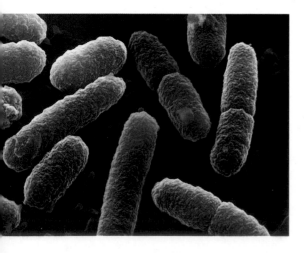

▽ E. coli bacteria are normally found in the human intestine and are generally harmless. Sometimes, however, they increase in number and find their way into the urinary tract, where they cause infections such as cystitis.

responsible for causing cystitis and other urinary tract infections, such as those acquired during sexual intercourse, for example chlamydia and mycoplasma.

Generally, the urinary unit works to prevent infection, stopping urine from backing up to the kidneys and washing bacteria out of the system through urination. Urinating immediately after sexual intercourse can prevent infection.

THOSE AT RISK

Groups that are at risk from urinary tract infections include the following:

• Postmenopausal women – Women who have been through the menopause are more prone to cystitis because the lack of oestrogen in their bodies causes the lining of the urethra to become thinner, making it vulnerable to bacterial attack.
• Someone with an abnormality of the urinary tract – An example would be a man with an enlarged prostate gland, which increases the risk of infection.
• People who are more prone to infections in general – Older people, those with diabetes and anyone taking drugs to suppress the immune system.

CYSTITIS

Your doctor will probably ask for a sample of your urine so that it can be tested for a variety of substances – white bloods cells, red blood cells and protein. Such tests are usually done quickly and simply using different dipsticks, and the results are usually available immediately.

Your doctor may want to send the sample to a laboratory to determine which

RECURRENT CYSTITIS

Recurrent episodes of infection in a woman or a single episode in a man or young child need further investigation. Your doctor will probably arrange for blood tests to check kidney function, an ultrasound scan, a cystoscopy (in which the bladder is viewed directly) and an intravenous urogram. You will probably be referred to a specialist known as a urologist. Such investigations aim to identify structural abnormalities that predispose to infection and assess the functional capacity of the bladder and how effectively it empties, because this affects its susceptibility to infection.

types of bacteria are growing and which antibiotics will be most effective. As this process takes a minimum of 48 hours, your doctor may decide to prescribe an appropriate antibiotic immediately rather

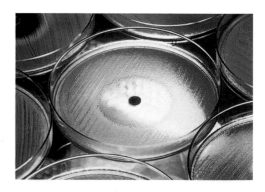

△ This picture shows how antibiotics are tested to find out how effective they are against different bacteria. The clear area around the antibiotic in this dish shows that it is killing the bacteria. Antibiotics are usually the most effective way of treating urinary tract infections.

▽ Drinking plenty of fluids throughout the day is always a good idea, and it is also an effective way of avoiding cystitis and halting it at an early stage.

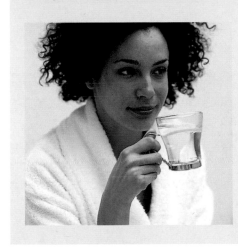

than wait for the results. The antibiotic can be changed once the bacteria's identity and sensitivity are known.

If an infection does not clear up within a few days, your doctor may recommend a test known as an intravenous pyelogram (IVP), a form of X-ray that shows the bladder, kidneys and ureters.

PYELONEPHRITIS

This is an infection that affects the kidney and it has similar symptoms to cystitis. These symptoms include difficulty in urinating accompanied by a burning sensation, and a pain in the back and below the ribs which may also spread to the abdomen. In extreme cases, it causes vomiting and high fever. The infection causes inflammation in the part of the kidney that collects urine, the renal pelvis, often accompanied by abscesses. It can be treated with antibiotics, but your doctor may advise further investigation to ensure there are no other underlying causes. If pyelonephritis is not treated, it may turn into a more serious condition called pyonephrosis or a larger kidney abscess. Both may require surgery to correct them.

In pyonephrosis, the kidney fills with pus and enlarges, causing great pain and a swelling that can be seen in your side. The infection can be a result of untreated pyelonephritis or hydronephrosis – distension of the kidney because of an obstruction in the ureter, which prevents urine flowing to the bladder; it can also be caused by kidney stones.

TREATMENT OPTIONS FOR UTIs

Infections of the urinary system can become worse very quickly, causing great discomfort and other potentially severe problems, so never hold back on seeking advice – especially if you are pregnant, suffer from

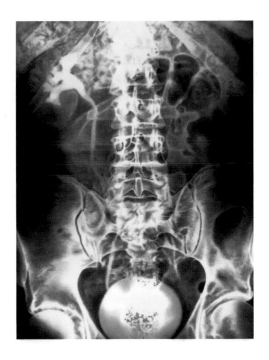

△ This X-ray shows a full bladder plus the ureters and the kidneys' branched collecting ducts. Images like this are produced by injecting a substance that shows up on X-rays into the blood. The kidneys automatically perform their filtering function and filter this substance from the blood – at which point the image is taken.

diabetes, or have high blood presssure or kidney disease. Treatment is often very straightforward. With cystitis, for example, it is vital to drink a great deal of extra fluid as soon as an episode starts. Many women find that cranberry juice eases discomfort, and simple painkillers and anti-inflammatory drugs are often effective in reducing any fever and dulling the pain. A mild cystitis episode may pass off quickly with a high fluid intake, but if the condition does not settle within 24 hours or if it worsens at all (and also if it recurs regularly), help should be sought. The infection will usually respond well to a short course of antibiotics.

Apart from cystitis, infections caused by other organisms, such as chlamydia and mycoplasma, will probably require a longer course of treatment. Your doctor may perform a urinalysis at the end of the course of drugs to ensure that the system is free from infection. The patient may feel better, but there is a chance that the infection may not be fully cleared up.

Urinary incontinence

SEE ALSO

➤ Diabetes, p66
➤ Stroke, p80
➤ Dementia, p90
➤ Pregnancy and health, p148

There are four main types of urinary incontinence – stress, urge, overflow and total. The most common type is stress incontinence, in which small amounts of urine are expelled during exertion, coughing, sneezing or laughing. Urge incontinence is involuntary contractions of the bladder, which release large amounts of urine suddenly and without control. Overflow is a continual dribble of urine caused by the bladder's inability to empty properly, causing it to overflow. Total incontinence is the total loss of control over bladder function.

Complete or partial loss of control over bladder function can be an extremely distressing condition. Incontinence becomes more common in older age and occurs more frequently in women. It is also caused by:

• Any condition affecting the muscles at the neck of the bladder, such as those caused by a difficult labour and delivery.

• Weakness of the urethra and pelvic floor muscles, common during and after pregnancy and after the menopause; also caused by gynaecological conditions such as a prolapsed uterus.

• Bladder outlet obstruction, such as an enlarged prostate or bladder stones.

• Excessive bladder irritability, which may occur as a result of recurrent infection, nervous disease and/or anxiety.

• Abnormalities of nervous control, because of diabetes, spinal injury or spina bifida.

• Abnormalities of brain function, due to a stroke or dementia.

MANAGEMENT OF INCONTINENCE

There are several ways to manage incontinence. Bladder muscle problems may respond to pelvic floor exercises (see chart), physiotherapy or surgery aimed at restoring

INVESTIGATING INCONTINENCE

Urodynamic studies are used to investigate problems with bladder control, such as incontinence. These tests take place in a hospital outpatient clinic using X-ray monitoring and electronic probes to measure bladder filling and emptying.

HEALTHY AND POOR BLADDER CONTROL

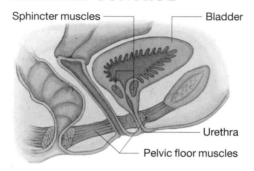

Sphincter muscles — Bladder

Urethra

Pelvic floor muscles

△ A healthy bladder has a firm pelvic floor and strong sphincter muscles.

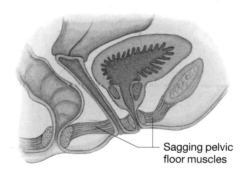

Sagging pelvic floor muscles

△ This picture shows how a sagging pelvic floor means that the neck of the bladder drops. This causes loss of bladder control.

bladder control. Hormone replacement therapy may help postmenopausal women to counteract any loss in pelvic floor muscle tone. Sometimes, however, the only options are to drain the bladder using a catheter (a long, thin tube) on an intermittent or permanent basis.

Where the incontinence is caused by a neurological problem, treatment can be much more problematic. Anticholinergic drugs are often used to help relax the muscles situated in the bladder wall and reduce the urge to urinate.

EXERCISES TO STRENGTHEN THE PELVIC FLOOR

Identify your pelvic floor muscles by imagining that you are urinating and that you have to suddenly stop the flow.

Feel the muscles tighten around your vagina, urethra and rectum. Then contract these muscles again and hold for ten seconds.

Relax the muscles slowly and then repeat. This exercise will be most effective if you repeat it five times, preferably two or three times a day.

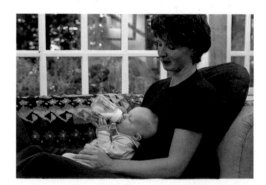

△ Incontinence can sometimes develop as a result of pregnancy and childbirth, because the pelvic floor is weakened. Exercises can be done to strengthen these muscles.

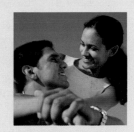

9

THE REPRODUCTIVE SYSTEM

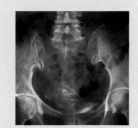

The reproductive system is one of the most intricate areas of the male and female body, with all of the different parts – ovaries, Fallopian tubes, uterus and vagina in women; testes, prostate gland and penis in men – cleverly designed to function together towards the ultimate goal of reproduction. Understanding how the system works is crucial to coping with the various problems men and women can experience at particular times of their lives: from painful periods to prostate cancer, from puberty to menopause.

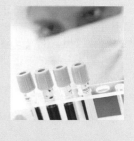

CONTENTS

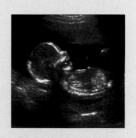

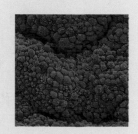

The reproductive organs

SEE ALSO
➤ Pregnancy and health, p148
➤ Menopausal complaints, p151
➤ Sexually transmitted infections, p163

The body's reproductive organs are developed in babies before they are even born. In fact, a baby girl is born with all the ova (eggs) that she will release during her adult life. Puberty is the major developmental stage for the reproductive systems of both genders. It is at this time that hormonal changes in the body bring great physical and mental changes, readying the reproductive systems for their adult role. Both the male and female systems are perfectly designed for their unique ultimate functions – sexual activity and reproduction.

THE FEMALE REPRODUCTIVE SYSTEM

The female reproductive organs are situated in the pelvic cavity and so are enclosed and protected by the pelvic bones. The ovaries are central to the female reproductive system because they hold all the female ova (eggs). The ovaries release one egg during the process of ovulation, and this happens first at puberty. Once released, the egg passes along the Fallopian tube to the uterus (womb) a hollow, muscular organ capable of considerable expansion to accommodate a growing fetus during pregnancy. The neck of the uterus, known as the cervix, projects in to the vagina. The vagina is a muscular organ that is able to expand greatly during sexual intercourse and childbirth.

HORMONES AND THE MENSTRUAL CYCLE

The ovaries produce two hormones – oestrogen and progesterone. These two hormones are controlled by the pituitary gland, which produces follicle-stimulating hormone (FSH) and luteinizing hormone (LH), which regulate the menstrual cycle.

During the first half of the menstrual cycle the pituitary produces FSH, which causes an egg to mature within the ovary in preparation for release. Towards the middle of the cycle, LH levels start to rise and trigger the release of the egg (this usually occurs about 14 days before the onset of menstruation). The hormone progesterone causes the uterine lining to thicken during the second half of the menstrual cycle, in preparation for possible implantation of a fertilized egg, should fertilization take place. Whenever fertilization does not occur, the uterine lining is expelled – menstrual bleeding.

When a woman's ovaries stop responding to the effects of FSH and LH (usually between the ages of 45 and 55), she starts to produce less oestrogen and progesterone; this is the start of the menopause, when menstruation gradually fades out and fertility ceases.

THE FEMALE REPRODUCTIVE ORGANS

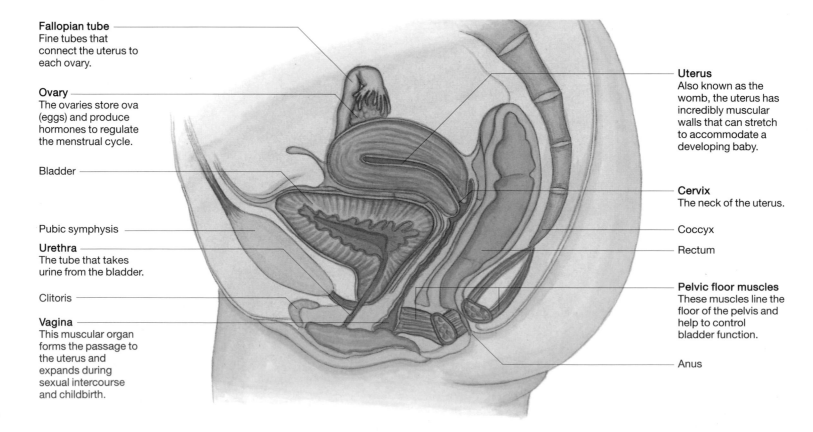

Fallopian tube
Fine tubes that connect the uterus to each ovary.

Ovary
The ovaries store ova (eggs) and produce hormones to regulate the menstrual cycle.

Bladder

Pubic symphysis

Urethra
The tube that takes urine from the bladder.

Clitoris

Vagina
This muscular organ forms the passage to the uterus and expands during sexual intercourse and childbirth.

Uterus
Also known as the womb, the uterus has incredibly muscular walls that can stretch to accommodate a developing baby.

Cervix
The neck of the uterus.

Coccyx

Rectum

Pelvic floor muscles
These muscles line the floor of the pelvis and help to control bladder function.

Anus

THE MALE REPRODUCTIVE SYSTEM

The testes are located in the scrotum, which hangs outside the body where the temperature is more suitable for efficient sperm production. The testes are responsible for the production of sperm and the release of the male hormone testosterone. Testosterone controls the development of male secondary sexual characteristics at puberty, such as deepening of the voice, facial hair, changes in the penis and testicles and the production of sperm.

After a boy reaches puberty, his testes create sperm at a rate of approximately 125 million sperm a day. These gather in the testes and then move on to the coiled tubular system known as the epididymis, where they mature. The epididymis drains first into the vas deferens and from there into the ejaculatory ducts. During sexual activity, these ducts contract and push sperm through the urethra during the process of ejaculation.

Sperm are carried in fluid produced by the seminal vesicles and the prostate gland. This fluid, which is known as semen, is rich in nutrients and provides an effective medium within which sperm can stay alive. For about 20 minutes after ejaculation, the sperm hardly move at all, remaining in the gel-like substance. After this, the semen liquefies, and the sperm swim towards their ultimate goal – a female ovum (egg). It is here that fertilization takes place.

Other elements of the male reproductive system are related to the penis and include the urethra, the foreskin and the glans penis. The urethra is the tube through which semen is ejaculated during sexual activity and it is also the tube through which urine passes.

The glans penis is the conical swelling at the tip of the penis. In uncircumcised men, the glans is enclosed by the foreskin, which is attached at the neck of the penis. After about three years of age, the foreskin, or prepuce, usually becomes retractable so that the glans may be exposed; up until this time it sticks to the glans. The inside of the foreskin is covered with sebaceous glands that secrete a substance known as smegma, and this should be removed by regular, careful cleaning of the penis.

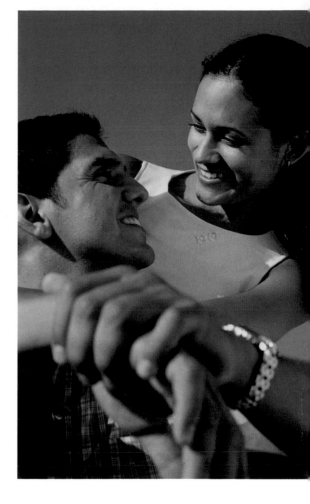

△ It is hormonal changes in the male and female bodies during puberty that prepares them for their ultimate purpose: sexual activity and reproduction.

THE MALE REPRODUCTIVE ORGANS

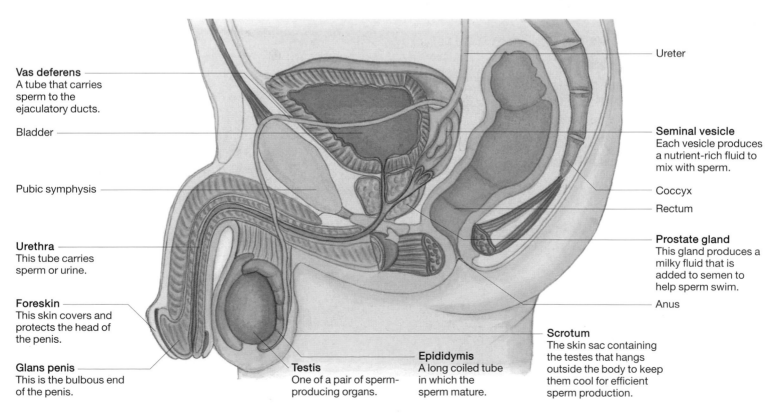

Vas deferens
A tube that carries sperm to the ejaculatory ducts.

Bladder

Pubic symphysis

Urethra
This tube carries sperm or urine.

Foreskin
This skin covers and protects the head of the penis.

Glans penis
This is the bulbous end of the penis.

Testis
One of a pair of sperm-producing organs.

Epididymis
A long coiled tube in which the sperm mature.

Ureter

Seminal vesicle
Each vesicle produces a nutrient-rich fluid to mix with sperm.

Coccyx

Rectum

Prostate gland
This gland produces a milky fluid that is added to semen to help sperm swim.

Anus

Scrotum
The skin sac containing the testes that hangs outside the body to keep them cool for efficient sperm production.

Pregnancy and health

SEE ALSO
➤ Smoking and your health, p20
➤ Routine health checks, p24
➤ High blood pressure, p30

Pregnancy is a time of great excitement and joy for parents-to-be, but the major physical changes experienced by the mother can cause some discomfort and may be stressful. Close contact with your healthcare team is the best way to protect both your own and your baby's wellbeing. The team will also be able to answer any questions that you have and reassure you that your pregnancy is progressing normally. Although most women feel anxious at some stage, it is important to remember that the vast majority of pregnancies end with a healthy baby.

Once you suspect that you might be pregnant, you should visit your doctor. (Over-the-counter pregnancy testing kits are fairly accurate and will test positive around the time of the first missed period or soon after.) By medical convention, pregnancies are dated from the first day of the last period. Most routine antenatal care will be undertaken by a midwife, who will usually be based at your doctor's surgery.

Your doctor will refer you to a specialist obstetric unit based at a hospital but you will probably only see the consultant once in early pregnancy and a short time before delivery. You will also visit the hospital for ultrasound scans.

Your first antenatal visit will usually involve taking a medical history, followed by an examination. You will have to give a sample of blood and urine for a series of

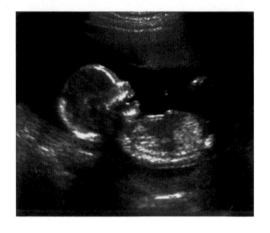

△ An ultrasound scan is vital for checking on the baby's position and development, and is usually carried out at 12 weeks and 20 weeks.

routine tests. At this stage, all tests are designed to pick up any significant risk factors that may complicate the pregnancy as it progresses.

PREGNANCY HEALTH CHECKS

Most women are seen at regular intervals throughout pregnancy. From 20 to 32 weeks, women are checked every 4 weeks. They are then reviewed every 2 weeks until 36 weeks, and at weekly intervals thereafter. At each visit, there is an opportunity for your healthcare team to:
• Carry out routine health checks and answer any questions you have.
• Check the baby's growth and position.
• Listen to the baby's heart.

EATING WELL IN PREGNANCY

A healthy, balanced diet is extremely important during pregnancy in order to maintain your health and nurture your baby. It is usually only in the last couple of months, when your baby is growing rapidly, that you may need to eat more.

The following foods should be avoided:
• Raw or undercooked eggs.
• Mussels and other shellfish.
• Liver pâté.
• Unpasteurized cheeses, such as brie.

Doctors advise all women trying to conceive, and pregnant women during their first 12 weeks, to take folic acid to prevent spina bifida.

EXERCISE AND PREGNANCY

If you exercised before you were pregnant it is a good idea to continue. If you remain fit, you may experience less backache and your pushes during labour are likely to be stronger. You should avoid situations with a risk of falls – such as horse-riding – and should not push yourself too hard.

As your pregnancy progresses, your increasing weight, size and tiredness will limit the type and amount of exercise you can do. Swimming and yoga may be more appealing than other forms of exercise.

▽ There is an increased risk of high blood pressure during pregnancy, so regular health checks are essential to ensure that any changes are picked up as soon as possible.

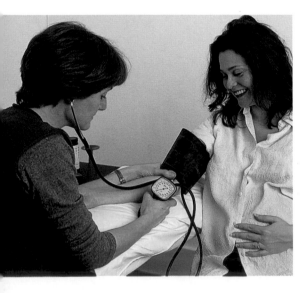

SMOKING AND ALCOHOL
Smoking harms your baby. Smokers should stop while pregnant as they could affect fetal growth, predispose their baby to asthma and increase their baby's chances of cardiovascular disease in later life. If you have trouble stopping, ask your doctor for help. Avoid alcohol for the first 12 weeks (it may be unpleasant to take at this time in any case). After this, try to stick to the occasional tipple only.

THE MAIN STAGES OF PREGNANCY

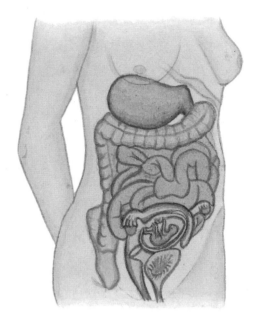

△ **At 12 weeks**
Although still tiny, the fetus is baby-shaped, with fingers, toes, genitalia and facial features.

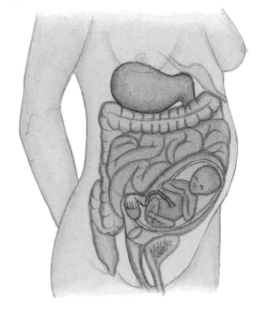

△ **At 18 weeks**
The fetal organs begin to function and bones start to harden at this stage.

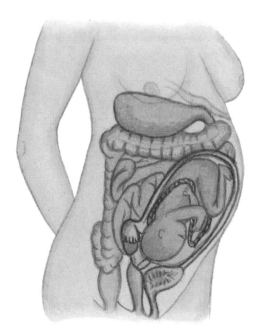

△ **At 24 weeks**
The growth of the fetus begins to place pressure on internal organs.

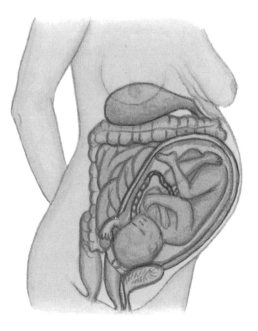

△ **At 36 weeks**
The head sinks down into the pelvis ready for the birth; this is known as "lightening".

AFTER THE BIRTH

It is vital that you continue to look after your health after the birth. Make sure that you eat well and rest as much as possible.

Many women will experience some depression after childbirth, which may be due to the the sudden decline in levels of oestrogen and progesterone once the baby is born. In about 10 per cent of women, this is severe and lasts for months (postnatal depression). Symptoms include persistent low mood, difficulty in relating to the baby, feelings of inadequacy and anxiety and, in some cases, panic attacks. Your healthcare team can provide useful advice, and treatment may not be necessary. However, your doctor may prescribe antidepressants, which help many women.

Irregular menstrual periods

SEE ALSO

➤ Diseases of the thyroid gland, p68
➤ Endometriosis, p155
➤ Ovarian cysts, p156
➤ Polycystic ovary syndrome, p156

The average menstrual cycle lasts for 28 days, and a period can last anything between two and seven days. There are, however, considerable variations between individuals: periods may occur as frequently as every 21 days and as infrequently as 35 days. Irregular menstrual periods are not necessarily cause for alarm and can arise for many reasons. However, it is a good idea to seek advice if your menstrual cycle suddenly changes because it may be a symptom of an underlying problem such as stress, or of other more serious conditions.

Menstrual irregularity occurs most frequently just after puberty and in the years leading up to the menopause, due to hormonal fluctuations at these times.

Where an irregular pattern is the result of stress, anxiety or a recent illness, the problem usually corrects itself. Similarly, any irregularities that occur during teenage years also tend to diminish gradually.

If you have a persistently irregular bleeding pattern with no easily identifiable cause, your doctor may investigate. Blood tests and pelvic ultrasound scans are commonly used testing procedures.

For persistent irregularities in younger women, the contraceptive pill may be used to regulate the cycle. Older women nearing the menopause may be offered hormone replacement therapy (HRT).

POSSIBLE CAUSES

Menstrual irregularity may be a symptom of another condition, such as:

➤ Ovarian cysts and polycystic ovary syndrome.

➤ Endometriosis.

➤ Disorders of the thyroid gland.

➤ Unsuspected pregnancy.

➤ Cancer.

Or it may be caused by factors such as:

➤ Stress and anxiety.

➤ Periods of depression or of general physical ill health.

➤ Fluctuating weight.

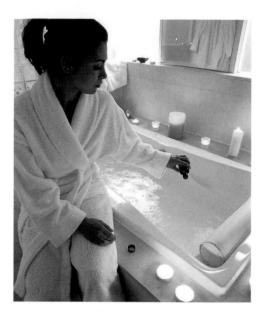

△ Taking time to relax in a warm, soothing environment can help to tackle feelings of stress and anxiety, which may be the underlying cause of menstrual irregularity.

Painful periods (dysmenorrhoea)

SEE ALSO

➤ Endometriosis, p155

Painful periods are extremely common and affect most women at some stage of their lives, to varying degrees. Many women can be quite incapacitated by this problem. Pain is usually most apparent on the day before a period starts and during the first 48 hours of a period.

Painful periods are most common during adolescence and when a woman is in her 20s; the problem often subsides later in life. If you normally have little pain with your periods and suddenly start experiencing unusual levels of discomfort, seek medical advice. Your doctor may want to rule out any gynaecological problems and carry out further investigations.

TREATMENT OPTIONS

Anti-inflammatory drugs are often effective, ideally taken before severe pain takes hold. The combined contraceptive pill can also be taken. This eases painful periods by suppressing ovulation.

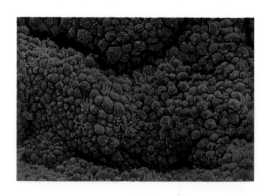

▷ This coloured scan shows the thickening in the endometrium, the lining of the uterus, that occurs during the second half of the menstrual cycle.

Premenstrual syndrome (PMS)

SEE ALSO

➤ Depression, p98
➤ Irregular menstrual periods, p150
➤ Painful periods (dysmenorrhoea), p150

Premenstrual syndrome is a very common problem that affects up to a third of all menstruating women at some point in their lives, and is particularly prevalent in women over 30. Although some people question the existence of PMS, many doctors now believe it is due to an imbalance of sex hormones in the body just before menstruation. The results can be debilitating, even though the problem usually lasts for only one or two days just before or at the beginning of the period. Symptoms range from headaches to severe anger or depression.

SIGNS AND SYMPTOMS
Classic symptoms of PMS are:

➤ Irritability, depression and mood changes.

➤ Tiredness and headache.

➤ Fluid retention and abdominal bloating.

➤ Breast tenderness.

➤ Backache and muscular pains.

If you find that fluid retention is a particularly troublesome symptom then your doctor may prescribe a diuretic to be taken as needed. You might be able to relieve muscular aches and headaches using simple painkillers and anti-inflammatory drugs. Mood changes and depression may respond to antidepressants, which are taken during the second half of the menstrual cycle or on a regular basis. A variety of progesterone preparations have also been tried with varying degrees of success.

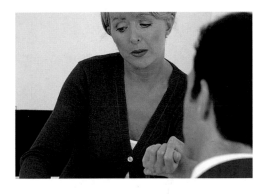

△ Your doctor may prescribe antidepressants to alleviate depression and control the mood swings that can occur in premenstrual syndrome.

Menopausal complaints

SEE ALSO

➤ Osteoporosis, p108

The menopause is the time in a woman's life, typically between 45 and 55, when her periods gradually stop. Hormone replacement therapy can help treat the symptoms associated with the menopause, although it should be discussed carefully with your doctor.

SIGNS AND SYMPTOMS
Many women have only mild symptoms attributable to the menopause. Some, however, experience a range of problems, including:

➤ Hot flushes and excessive sweating.

➤ Mood changes that may include anxiety and depression.

➤ Tiredness and loss of libido.

➤ Vaginal dryness.

➤ An increased susceptibility to urinary tract infection.

Almost all menopause-related symptoms can be treated with hormone replacement therapy (HRT). Here, small amounts of oestrogen and progesterone are given – just enough to minimize the natural oestrogen withdrawal of the menopause. HRT is usually taken for a few years in pill or skin patch form, but may also be given as under-the-skin implants. Women on HRT are periodically assessed for weight, blood pressure and general state of health.

THE LONG-TERM OUTLOOK
There are some advantages in taking HRT on a long-term basis, principally that oestrogen tends to protect bones from osteoporosis. There may also be a small reduction of heart disease among women on HRT. There are also certain health risks associated with HRT, including a slight increase in the risk of breast cancer in women who have taken HRT for more than seven years.

POSTMENOPAUSAL RISKS
Oestrogen protects against heart disease so after the menopause, the risk of cardiovascular problems rises. The decline in oestrogen levels also means you may be more prone to osteoporosis.

Breast pain and lumpiness

SEE ALSO

➤ Pregnancy and health, p148
➤ Premenstrual syndrome, p151
➤ Menopausal complaints, p151

Many women notice a generalized lumpiness and pain that occurs in their breasts at particular stages of their menstrual cycle. This is most apparent in the days immediately before a period, and during puberty and pregnancy. Breast tissue changes as it is affected by female sex hormone fluctuations that occur throughout menstrual life. There are several methods that can help reduce breast pain, but you should always seek advice from your doctor if symptoms persist or you are concerned about any unusual lumps or pain.

Lumps in the breast may often be accompanied by cyclical occurrences of breast pain. Postmenopausal woman often experience this less, although it may be more persistent in women on hormone replacement therapy.

Some simple self-help measures may be helpful for painful and lumpy breasts:
• Taking daily oil of evening primrose.
• Relaxation exercises.

WHAT MIGHT YOUR DOCTOR DO?

Lumpy breasts that are not painful do not usually require any specific treatment. However, your doctor may refer you to a breast specialist for further investigation if:

• Lumpiness is persistent and not affected by your menstrual cycle.
• There is a specific area of lumpy tissue.
• A definite lump can be felt, which may turn out to be either a fibroadenoma or a cancerous tumour.

THE STRUCTURE OF THE BREAST

▷ The breasts are made of fatty tissue, milk-producing lobules and a system of ducts designed to carry milk to the nipple. Breast tissue is subject to constant hormonal stimulation, allowing it to prepare for pregnancy and lactation (milk production) whenever the need arises. As a result, the tissues of the breast are undergoing continual change.

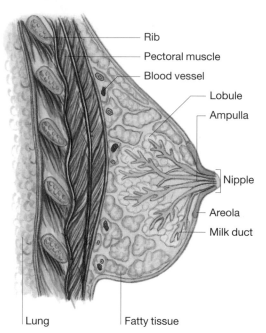

Rib
Pectoral muscle
Blood vessel
Lobule
Ampulla
Nipple
Areola
Milk duct
Lung
Fatty tissue

Fibroadenoma

SEE ALSO

➤ Breast cysts, p153

This non-cancerous (benign) breast lump tends to develop in women aged between 20 and 30. Doctors believe that fibroadenomas may arise because of the effects of oestrogen on breast tissue. They may develop at a number of different sites within the breast.

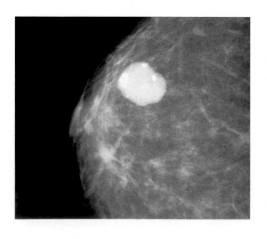

Fibroadenomas are the most common reason for lumps in the breast. They grow very slowly, sometimes over a number of years, and are generally harmless. However, they can be difficult to distinguish from cancerous lumps so you should always seek

◁ Mammographs are X-rays that clearly reveal the soft tissue of the breast. A fibroadenoma (seen here as a white mass) is a small tumour of fibrous tissue; although usually benign, these can become malignant if left untreated.

medical advice if you find an unusual lump. Your doctor will refer you to a breast unit where specialist staff will scan the breast, using ultrasound, and perform a biopsy – taking a sample of tissue from the lump that can be tested to confirm the diagnosis.

Small fibroadenomas can be safely left untreated. They often diminish in size and may disappear completely in time. If the lump is large or growing, it may be appropriate to remove it surgically.

Breast cysts

SEE ALSO
➤ Fibroadenoma, p152
➤ Breast cancer, below
➤ Ovarian cysts, p156

Breast cysts are small, fluid-filled lumps that can develop in the breasts, most commonly in women between the ages of 30 and 50. These lumps are simply lobules that have filled with fluid and they are generally harmless. Occasionally, however, a cyst may contain cancerous cells, so your doctor should investigate any breast cyst to make absolutely sure that it is not malignant. Half of the women affected by cysts find that they have more than one, or that they affect both breasts; recurrence of breast cysts is also not uncommon.

Although breast cysts are usually harmless, as with any lump in the breast it should be checked out to rule out the possibility of breast cancer. Your doctor will normally refer you to a breast unit for specialized scanning and to get the cyst drained (aspiration). A sample of the fluid from the cyst is sent for laboratory analysis to check for signs of cancer.

Aspiration may be the only treatment that is required. Women who suffer from recurrent cysts may need to have them removed surgically.

BREAST ASPIRATION

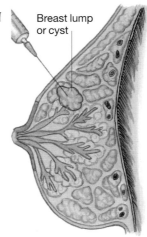

Breast lump or cyst

▷ A breast cyst can be treated by aspiration, where a doctor uses a needle syringe to draw fluid from the lump.

SCREENING AND SCANNING
Although breast cysts are usually harmless, in rare cases they may contain cancerous cells. Specialized scanning can identify the nature of the lump and catch the disease at an earlier, more treatable, stage. Many countries now have screening programmes for older women, between the ages of 50 and 65, who are more susceptible to breast cancer and HRT is thought to be a causative factor.

Breast cancer

SEE ALSO
➤ Lymphomas, p210

Breast cancer is the most common female cancer. Most often seen in women over 50, it also occurs in younger women. Particular factors put women at higher risk of breast cancer and these include aging, a family history of the condition, obesity and being on HRT.

SIGNS AND SYMPTOMS
Breast cancer may not produce any symptoms in the early stages but when signs do appear they include:

➤ A painless lump in the breast.

➤ Blood-stained discharge from the nipple.

➤ "Orange-peel" dimpling of the skin around the lump.

➤ Inversion of the nipple.

If your doctor suspects breast cancer you may be referred to a specialist breast unit. Your breast will be scanned and a sample of the lump will be taken and its fluid drained; cells will be sent for analysis. Only about one in twenty breast lumps turns out to be cancerous. If cancer is confirmed, you may have other scans to determine whether it has spread to other parts of the body.

TREATMENT OPTIONS
Breast cancer is treated with varying combinations of surgery, radiotherapy, chemotherapy and hormone treatment.

• Small tumours are surgically removed (lumpectomy) while large tumours usually involve removing a greater amount of breast tissue. Sometimes the whole breast is removed (mastectomy). Some lymph nodes are removed from the area to check if the cancer has spread.

• Radiotherapy is now used routinely for six weeks after the removal of all lumps.

• Where the cancer has already spread to other organs, chemotherapy is used in conjunction with other treatment.

• Oestrogen-blocking drugs shrink some tumours or impede their growth.

Fibroids

Fibroids are non-cancerous growths that develop within the walls of the uterus (womb). They are very common and may be found in up to a third of all women during their childbearing years. Fibroids occur most frequently in women between the ages of 35 and 55. It is believed that they arise from stimulation of uterine tissue by the female sex hormones, resulting in some pain and unusually heavy menstrual periods. Although these tumours are non-cancerous, they can cause infertility. Treatments vary according to the size and severity of the fibroids.

SIGNS AND SYMPTOMS

A bigger fibroid tends to produce a range of symptoms, including:

➤ Prolonged and heavy menstrual bleeding.

➤ Severe pain during menstruation.

➤ Infertility.

➤ An increased risk of miscarriage.

Fibroids are non-malignant tumours, formed from muscular tissue, which develop in the uterine wall. Fibroids vary in both size and the symptoms that they produce. Some fibroids are very small and produce no symptoms whatsoever, while others grow to the size of a grapefruit. Sometimes fibroids occur in multiples.

They can cause heavy periods and some pain. If they grow to a substantial size, they may even cause infertility or miscarriage.

DIAGNOSING FIBROIDS

Fibroids can sometimes be diagnosed during a pelvic examination. Once your doctor suspects fibroids you may be referred for a pelvic ultrasound scan, which will confirm the diagnosis.

TREATMENT OPTIONS

Smaller fibroids that display no symptoms can safely be left untreated. For larger growths that are causing problems, drugs may be used to try to reduce them in size, but if this is not successful they may need to be removed. This can be done in a number of ways:

• Hysteroscopy – Small fibroids growing on the inner uterine wall may be removed

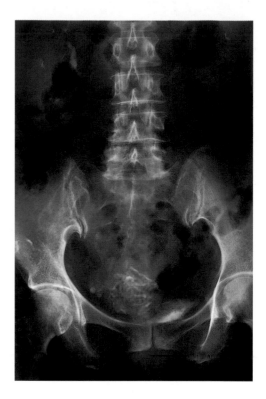

△ On this X-ray of a uterus, a fibroid shows up as an orange lump in the centre of the image. Fibroids are benign tumours formed from fibrous and muscular tissue.

during this procedure, in which a small telescopic instrument is passed into the uterus so that your doctor can see inside your abdomen to locate and then remove the fibroids.

• Abdominal surgery – Larger fibroids can be removed using an abdominal incision in order to gain access to the uterus.

• Hysterectomy – If fibroids are causing a number of serious problems and their size and location means they are difficult to remove, a hysterectomy may be considered. However, this procedure is only used in cases where the fibroids are causing severe pain or discomfort.

WHERE FIBROIDS ARE FOUND

▷ Fibroids are formed from muscular tissue that builds up in the wall of the uterus. There may be just one, which is relatively unusual, or several may develop at the same time.

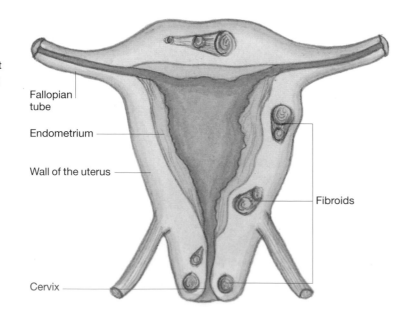

Fallopian tube

Endometrium

Wall of the uterus

Fibroids

Cervix

Endometriosis

SEE ALSO
➤ UTIs, p142
➤ Irregular menstrual periods, p150
➤ Ovarian cysts, p156
➤ Female genital infections, p159

The endometrium is the lining of the uterus. This lining is shed once a month during menstruation, and then regrows. The condition known as endometriosis occurs when endometrial tissue starts to develop in other organs within the pelvis (such as the ovaries or Fallopian tubes), usually because it has been affected by hormones released during the menstrual cycle. Endometriosis may also develop outside the pelvis – the intestines are sometimes affected and the condition can reach as far as the abdominal cavity or even the lungs.

SIGNS AND SYMPTOMS

Typical symptoms of pelvic endometriosis include the following:

➤ Painful, heavy and irregular periods.

➤ Deep pain during sexual intercourse.

➤ Urinary discomfort.

➤ Infertility.

Doctors do not know what causes this condition but it is common in women who have their first child over the age of 30 and in those who remain childless.

When endometriosis develops outside the pelvis, the symptoms depend on which organs are affected. Intestinal endometriosis, for example, tends to cause a change in bowel habit, abdominal pain and sometimes rectal bleeding.

TREATING ENDOMETRIOSIS

Hormone therapy may be used to suppress the menstrual cycle in order to reduce production of the oestrogen on which endometrial tissue depends. Such treatment may be used for up to one year, after which the condition may subside.

Doctors can destroy small areas of endometriosis during a laparoscopy – a minimally invasive procedure where rigid viewing devices are inserted through the abdomen to illuminate, examine and treat organs. If the patient is an older women, or the condition is extremely severe, a total hysterectomy may be considered.

Endometriosis sometimes resolves with pregnancy but may recur afterwards.

▽ This shows the surface of an endometriotic cyst. It has formed where fragments of uterine lining have attached to an ovary.

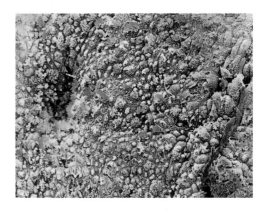

Uterine cancer

SEE ALSO
➤ Ovarian cancer, p157

Cancer of the uterus is most common in women between the ages of 55 and 65. It occurs more frequently in women that have had no children and in those who have had a late menopause. The specific cause of the cancer is not known, but early diagnosis and treatment is essential.

SIGNS AND SYMPTOMS

Common symptoms include:

➤ Heavy menstrual bleeding.

➤ Bleeding after sexual intercourse.

➤ Vaginal "spotting" after the menopause.

Uterine cancer usually causes unusual patterns of vaginal bleeding. If your doctor suspects cancer from your symptoms you may be urgently referred to a gynaecologist, who will take tissue samples from your uterus. This can be done easily using a procedure known as a hysteroscopy. If a cancer is diagnosed, a range of other tests are carried out to determine whether or not the cancer has spread to any other organs.

HOW IS IT TREATED?

This cancer is usually treated by removing all the pelvic organs by means of a total hysterectomy. Cancer that has spread beyond the uterus is usually treated with chemotherapy and hormonal treatment.

After treatment, the outlook is good if the tumour has been diagnosed at an early stage, with at least 80 per cent of women surviving for five years or longer.

Ovarian cysts

SEE ALSO

➤ Irregular menstrual periods, p150

➤ Fibroids, p154

➤ Endometriosis, p155

➤ Female genital infections, p159

Ovarian cysts – fluid-filled sacs that develop within the ovary – are very common during a woman's reproductive years. These cysts may be very small or grow to considerable size and there may be just one or several (the latter is called polycystic ovary syndrome). Ovarian cysts are usually non-cancerous but some have cancerous potential. For this reason your doctor will normally refer you to a specialist for further investigation. It can be difficult to diagnose ovarian cysts as they do not necessarily present symptoms, and the symptoms can come and go.

SIGNS AND SYMPTOMS

Most cysts do not cause symptoms, and many will develop and disappear spontaneously without a woman being aware of their existence. Larger, persistent cysts may produce symptoms, and these include:

➤ Abdominal pain, which may be felt on the same side as the affected ovary.

➤ Abdominal distension or bloating.

➤ Deep pain during sexual intercourse.

➤ Menstrual irregularities.

The presence of a cyst might be obvious from your symptoms, and your doctor may be able to feel the cyst during a pelvic examination. For confirmation, your doctor may refer you for an ultrasound examination. A blood test may also be done to check for the presence of tumour markers, which are proteins produced by tumours that can be measured in the blood. Where a cyst is large, persistent or problematic, a gynaecologist will assess the situation by monitoring the cyst for a while.

▷ **This inside view of a woman's abdomen has been taken with a device called a laparoscope. The round, fluid-filled swelling seen left of centre is an ovarian cyst.**

This is to determine whether it is growing or starting to regress naturally. Large cysts require draining or removal. A cyst is removed surgically if there are cancerous changes within it, but as much of the ovary is conserved as possible.

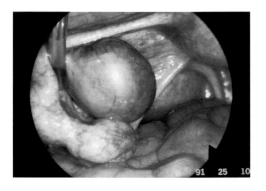

Polycystic ovary syndrome

SEE ALSO

➤ Diabetes, p66

This common syndrome, caused by a relative excess of luteinizing hormone and testosterone, is characterized by multiple fluid-filled ovarian cysts. Women with this condition are at greater risk of developing diabetes and high blood pressure, and of suffering ovulatory failure.

SIGNS AND SYMPTOMS

➤ Irregular, scanty or absent periods.

➤ Excess body hair.

➤ Ovulatory failure.

This condition may result in infertility, so a correct diagnosis and prompt treatment is very important. If your doctor suspects this condition from your symptoms, you may be referred for a pelvic ultrasound to identify the multiple ovarian cysts that form part of this syndrome. Blood tests carried out to measure levels of luteinizing hormone and testosterone may reveal a hormonal imbalance.

Treatment depends on the severity of the condition and whether you want to have children. Fertility drugs may be given to stimulate ovulation, and irregular menstrual patterns may be controlled by prescribing the combined contraceptive pill.

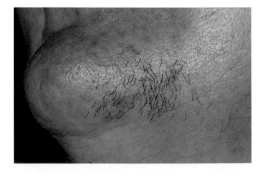

△ **Excessive body hair (this shows a woman's chin) may indicate polycystic ovary syndrome, caused by an excess of particular hormones.**

Ovarian cancer

Cancer of the ovary causes many thousands of deaths worldwide each year. This cancer is often difficult to diagnose because many patients show no symptoms until a relatively late stage of the disease. By the time any symptoms become apparent, the tumour may have already spread beyond the ovary. For this reason it is essential to seek advice if you are demonstrating any of the symptoms listed below, especially if you fall into any of the high-risk groups for this disease. At present, there is no effective way of screening for this form of cancer.

SIGNS AND SYMPTOMS

The possible symptoms of ovarian cancer include:

➤ Abdominal pain and distension.

➤ Frequent urination.

➤ Abnormal menstrual patterns.

➤ General malaise and weight loss.

Certain groups of women have been identified as more likely to develop ovarian cancer. These at-risk groups include:
• Childless women.
• Women who have a late menopause.
• Women who have family members affected by the disease.

SURGICAL TREATMENT

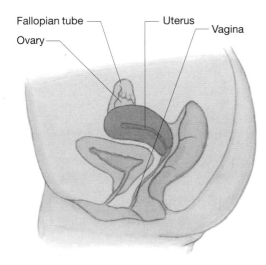

Fallopian tube — — Uterus
Ovary — — Vagina

△ If the cancerous tumour has spread beyond the ovary a hysterectomy may be necessary. This surgery involves the removal of the uterus, Fallopian tubes and ovaries, the top part of the vagina and the lymph nodes.

Ovarian cancer can affect women of any age, although there are more cases diagnosed between the ages of 50 and 60 than any other age-group. Also, women who have taken oral contraceptives appear to be less likely to develop the disease.

HOW IS IT DIAGNOSED?

If there is any question about the possibility of cancer, you will be urgently referred to a gynaecologist for further investigation. Tests include a pelvic ultrasound scan, blood tests to look for tumour markers and keyhole surgery (diagnostic laparoscopy) to inspect the ovary and take a sample of tissue for analysis. If cancer is confirmed, you may need to undergo a series of other scans to determine whether or not the cancer has spread to other internal organs, such as the liver or lungs.

TREATMENT OPTIONS

If the cancer is limited to one ovary and the woman still wants to have children, every effort will be made to avoid performing a full hysterectomy. In these cases, surgery will be limited to the removal of the affected ovary and Fallopian tube.

Where the tumour has spread from the ovary to other parts of the pelvis, or in cases where child-bearing is not an issue, a total hysterectomy is recommended as the safest method of removing all cancerous material from the area. During the hysterectomy operation, the uterus, both ovaries and both Fallopian tubes will be removed, along with some other tissue. In most cases, this surgical treatment is followed by a course of chemotherapy and possibly radiotherapy.

The best prognosis for ovarian cancer occurs when the cancer has been diagnosed in its earliest stages, preferably when it is confined to just one ovary. However, the greatest difficulty in diagnosing this cancer lies in the fact that it can be "silent" (not show any symptoms) until the more advanced stages of the disease, and may then continue to present no symptoms until the tumour has already spread to other parts of the pelvis. Currently, three-quarters of women are diagnosed with ovarian cancer after the disease has already spread to other parts of the body.

There is currently considerable research being undertaken to develop an effective screening test for this disease, although no widespread programmes are in use at the present time. Until screening is available, any symptoms should be taken seriously and investigated without delay.

▽ A viewing device called a laparoscope may be used to diagnose ovarian cancer. During this procedure, several small incisions are made in the abdomen to insert a fibre-optic video camera, along with tools that are used to carry out an examination of the ovaries.

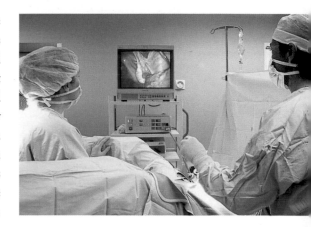

Cervical dysplasia

SEE ALSO

➤ Smoking and your health, p20

➤ Cancer of the cervix, below

➤ Sexually transmitted infections, p163

The cells of the cervix may change from normal to cancerous over a period of many years. Between the extremes of normal and cancerous cells are a range of cellular abnormalities commonly referred to as cervical dysplasia. Doctors can detect cervical dysplasia by taking a cervical smear, which all women should have at least every three years. During an internal examination, cells from the cervix are collected using a spatula or brush. These cells can then be examined microscopically for any evidence of significant cellular change.

The exact cause of this condition is not known but it is associated with the sexually transmitted papilloma virus. Therefore, one risk factor is unprotected sex, and a greater number of sexual partners increases the risk of coming into contact with this virus. People who smoke are more likely to develop cervical dysplasia and cancer, as are people who take immunosuppressant drugs.

TREATMENT OPTIONS

Mild cervical dysplasia requires no specific treatment but you will usually be asked to go for a repeat smear six months after the initial diagnosis. If mild dysplasia persists, or if there is moderate or severe dysplasia, preventative treatment identifies and removes the abnormal cervical cells. During a painless procedure called a colposcopy, a magnifying instrument is used to examine your cervix closely and so identify any abnormalities. Areas of dysplasia (abnormal tissue) can be removed with laser treatment.

After a colposcopy, smears are taken at intervals to ensure that there are no further signs of dysplasia. As the cervical tissue returns to normal, the intervals between smears are lengthened.

TYPES OF CERVICAL DYSPLASIA

There are three grades of dysplasia – mild, moderate and severe. Mild dysplasia may disappear without treatment, whereas moderate and severe types may develop slowly, sometimes over several years, in to cancer if not treated. The chance of a good outcome is improved if abnormalities are caught early and any cancer is treated before it starts spreading through the pelvis.

Cancer of the cervix

SEE ALSO

➤ Uterine cancer, p155

Cervical cancer is a common female cancer. Fortunately, it is one of the few cancers that can be prevented by regular screening. Most developed countries have national screening programmes that detect precancerous changes in the cervix years before cancer develops.

Once cancerous cells have been detected in the cervix, further tests will be carried out to discover how far the tumour has spread. If the tumour is confined to the cervix, doctors may be able to remove the affected area without harming a woman's ability to conceive and bear children.

Where child-bearing is not an issue, a hysterectomy may be considered to remove the cervix and uterus, but the ovaries will usually be conserved. If the cancer has already spread to the uterus, a total hysterectomy will be necessary. If the cancer has spread to other parts of the body, chemotherapy and/or radiotherapy is used to try to contain the disease.

SIGNS AND SYMPTOMS

Cervical cancer may cause few symptoms initially. Symptoms that may develop include:

➤ Vaginal bleeding.

➤ Deep pain during sexual intercourse.

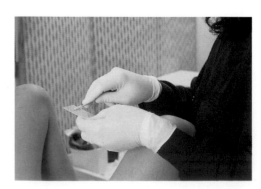

▷ Regular screening by cervical smear tests is widely available in developed countries. This test involves cells being scraped from the cervix (the neck of the womb). The cells are then checked for abnormalities so that cancer can be detected in the very early stages.

Female genital infections

Most women will experience inflammation and itching in the vaginal area at some point in their lives. This may simply be a reaction to using perfumed soaps or bath products. However, this condition also commonly arises from infection by the *Candida albicans* fungus (thrush), or by sexually transmitted micro-organisms such as *Trichomoniasis vaginalis* (trichomoniasis). Most genital infections clear up quickly when treated, but some may spread up into the pelvis, causing pelvic inflammatory disease. This is a major cause of infertility among women.

SIGNS AND SYMPTOMS OF VAGINAL INFECTION

See your doctor if you experience any of the following symptoms:

➤ Itchiness, irritation or soreness in or around the vagina.

➤ An abnormal vaginal discharge, which may or may not have a strong odour.

➤ A burning sensation experienced on passing urine.

➤ Discomfort during sexual intercourse.

Many women feel embarrassed about visiting their doctor with vaginal irritation (known medically as vaginitis). However, vaginitis has many different causes, including serious infection, so it is essential that you have the condition investigated.

If your doctor suspects that you have an infection, vaginal swabs of any discharge may be taken and sent for testing. In most cases, the problem clears up once the infecting micro-organism is identified and the correct treatment given. You should usually abstain from sexual intercourse until the inflammation and irritation has gone. In many cases, your sexual partner should also be treated.

THRUSH

Thrush causes severe itching and a thick white discharge. Many women suffer repeated bouts of thrush, and the infection often seems to be related to general stress and fatigue. Pregnant women, those suffering from diabetes and people on a course of antibiotics or immunosuppressive drugs are particularly prone to thrush.

Antifungal pessaries and creams normally relieve symptoms and clear up the infection. Single doses of oral antifungal drugs are also available, and are safe and effective to use.

If you suffer from recurrent thrush, your doctor may suggest further tests to ensure that the diagnosis is correct. You may find it helpful to lower your intake of dietary sugars and eat *acidophilus* bacteria in the form of live natural yoghurt or acidophilus tablets. Male partners should also be treated as they may carry fungal infection and re-infect you after treatment.

BACTERIAL VAGINOSIS

Bacterial vaginosis causes an off-white vaginal discharge with a fishy odour. It occurs when normally harmless bacteria living in the vagina start to multiply excessively. The usual causes are *Gardnerella vaginalis* or *Mycoplasma hominis*. The condition can be effectively treated with a course of antibiotics.

TRICHOMONIASIS

Trichomoniasis is a sexually transmitted infection, causing severe itching, pain on passing urine and an unpleasant-smelling yellow discharge. The condition clears up quickly if the correct antibiotics are taken.

Men can carry the disease without having symptoms, but they may develop non-specific urethritis (inflammation of the urethra). If a woman has trichomoniasis, her sexual partner should be treated, too.

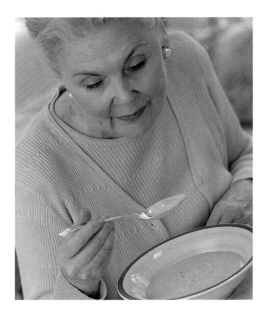

△ A simple self-help option for thrush is eating live natural yoghurt which contains helpful *acidophilus* bacteria.

PELVIC INFLAMMATORY DISEASE (PID)

PID is the largest single cause of female infertility. It starts as an infection in the vagina – usually chlamydia or gonorrhoea, which are sexually transmitted. The infection spreads up from the vagina to infect the Fallopian tubes and other pelvic organs.

Pelvic pain, pain during sex and fever can all be signs of PID, but it often causes no symptoms, with the result that many women are unaware that they have the condition. If PID is treated promptly with antibiotics, most women recover completely. However, if it is untreated, the Fallopian tubes may become damaged, which will affect fertility.

Enlarged prostate gland

Prostate gland enlargement occurs naturally with age and becomes more apparent from the age of 50 onwards, but it can also arise as a result of bacterial infection. Doctors refer to the condition as prostatism (benign prostatic hypertrophy). Whether or not symptoms occur depends on the degree of enlargement. As the gland enlarges, it squeezes the urethra and starts to prevent adequate emptying of the bladder, and so one of the key symptoms is a frequent desire to urinate. Avoiding consumption of certain fluids can help control the symptoms.

SIGNS AND SYMPTOMS

Typical symptoms are:

➤ A frequent need to urinate.

➤ A sensation that the bladder is not completely empty after urination.

➤ Dribbling after urine has been passed.

➤ A need to get up at night to pass urine.

➤ A poor stream of urine.

If untreated, urine can collect in the bladder and cause urinary tract infection.

Inflammation of the prostate gland is commonly caused by bacterial infection. It causes pain when passing urine, the need to urinate frequently (causing disruption to sleep patterns because of the need to get up during the night), pain on ejaculation, blood in semen, pain at the base of the penis and in the testes, fever and general malaise. Sometimes the prostate gland may become inflamed (prostatitis) during episodes of infection and is prone to cancerous change in middle-aged and older men. The symptoms of prostate cancer are similar to those experienced by someone suffering from an enlarged prostate gland but there may be some back or hip pain as well.

Your doctor will base diagnosis on your medical history and an examination. The prostate can be felt and its size assessed by a finger inserted into the rectum. An ultrasound can be done to assess to what degree bladder emptying has been impaired.

THE POSITION OF THE PROSTATE GLAND

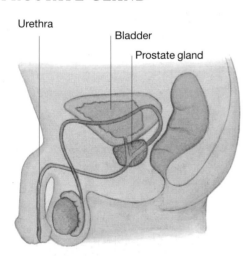

Urethra

Bladder

Prostate gland

△ The prostate gland is a chestnut-sized organ located at the base of a man's bladder. It is wrapped around the urethra as it exits the bladder. The prostate gland produces secretions that are added to semen during the process of ejaculation.

DRUG TREATMENT

When your condition starts to affect your quality of life, it can be treated. It may be possible to control the condition using drugs – alpha-blockers (which make it easier to pass urine), antiandrogens (which shrink the prostate over time) and oral antibiotics (to treat an infection).

SURGICAL MANAGEMENT

If symptoms become progressively worse and drugs have failed to control the condition, there are a number of surgical options and these include:

• Partial transurethral prostatectomy – This is the most common procedure, during which an operating telescope is passed along the urethra to reach the prostate gland. A heated wire is then

MONITORING FLUID CONSUMPTION

Mild symptoms may not significantly interfere with lifestyle. It may be possible to control symptoms of an enlarged prostate by ensuring that you do not drink too much fluid during the evening and by avoiding fluids that stimulate the desire to pass urine, such as caffeine-containing drinks and alcohol.

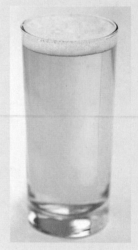

◁ Alcoholic drinks tend to over-stimulate the need to pass urine.

introduced and used to cut away some prostate tissue. As the operation removes only part of the prostate it may need to be repeated. Some men become impotent following this operation.

• Total prostatectomy – If the prostate gland is extremely large, it may be removed completely. This operation may result in infertility and impotence.

Research into new treatments is ongoing and new procedures that are currently being evaluated include prostate laser surgery.

Prostate cancer

SEE ALSO

➤ Routine health checks, p24

➤ Enlarged prostate gland, p160

➤ Testicular problems, p162

Cancer of the prostate gland is most common in men over 50, and especially in those over 65. This tumour generally grows slowly and may not cause significant symptoms for many years. When the tumour is confined to the prostate gland, 90 per cent of men survive for at least five years after diagnosis and many live much longer. As with all cancers, early diagnosis and the right treatment is essential for recovery. Treatments vary according to the size and spread of the cancer. Screening can pre-empt development of the disease, but is not widespread at present.

SIGNS AND SYMPTOMS

Prostate cancer often produces no symptoms at all. If symptoms do become apparent, they include:

➤ A poor stream of urine.

➤ A need to pass urine frequently.

➤ Rarely, blood in the urine.

If prostate cancer is suspected, your doctor will perform a rectal examination to assess the size and regularity of the prostate gland. At the same time, a blood sample will be taken to check the level of prostate-specific antigen (PSA), which may give an indication of cancerous change.

▽ Blood samples are sent away for testing but this only shows changes in the blood that might indicate cancer, and other tests will be needed.

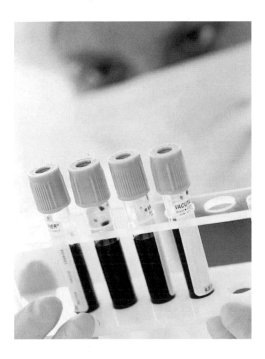

Your doctor will refer you to a specialist (urologist). Further tests include a prostate scan, in which some samples of prostate tissue are removed for microscopic analysis. Other scans to determine cancer spread will be done if cancer is diagnosed. PSA readings can be used to monitor cancer.

HOW IS IT TREATED?

If the cancer is confined to the prostate gland, the general approach is:

• Regular check-ups.

• Hormone therapy to reduce testosterone which can stimulate prostate cancer.

• A radical prostatectomy.

• Radiotherapy.

In elderly men with localized prostate cancer and no symptoms, the best approach is usually to monitor the condition as it is likely that the disease will not progress.

When prostate cancer develops in a younger man, however, there is a greater chance that the cancer may spread. In many cases, the cancer will be treated surgically, although radiotherapy may be offered as an alternative option. Possible treatment options include:

• Surgery – A radical prostatectomy removes the whole prostate gland. This operation, however, results in high levels of postoperative impotence and some urinary incontinence.

• Radiotherapy – The delivery of radiotherapy is now more sophisticated so it is possible to implant radioactive seeds into the prostate gland. This allows a lower total dose of radiation to be delivered more accurately.

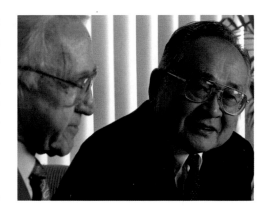

△ Prostate cancer usually occurs in men over the age of 50. In many cases, the cancer remains in the prostate and does not spread. The appearance of this cancer in a younger man indicates that it is particularly malignant and may spread more quickly, so surgery is often the best form of treatment.

SCREENING FOR PROSTATE CANCER

There is much scientific debate regarding prostate cancer screening. A blood test can measure prostate-specific antigen (PSA), which is secreted by the prostate. The levels of PSA can rise during infection, gland enlargement, trauma and cancer. A raised PSA level can indicate cancerous change requiring investigation but is not indicative of cancer. Similarly, a normal reading does not exclude cancer.

Although used routinely in the United States, screening for prostate cancer is not carried out worldwide. This is because the test is not foolproof. Also, there is debate as to which treatements are effective and all the treatments available have the potential to cause serious side effects.

Testicular problems

SEE ALSO

➤ The reproductive organs, p146
➤ Routine health checks, p24

Several testicular-related problems can occur in men, from harmless cysts to cancer. Regular self-examination is key to identifying changes in the testicular region, and medical advice should be sought promptly if any inexplicable symptoms are found. Like many harmless tumours and cysts, conditions such as epididymal cysts may be very worrying when first discovered as they can be mistaken for cancerous growths. Although testicular cancer is relatively rare, any abnormality should be investigated by a doctor, if only to set your mind at rest.

EPIDIDYMAL CYSTS

Small, harmless cysts commonly form in the epididymis – the coiled tubules that conduct semen from the testes. These cysts are very common in men over 40.

DIAGNOSIS AND TREATMENT

Your doctor can identify a cyst by simple manual examination and may confirm the diagnosis by ultrasound examination. Treatment depends on the size of the cyst – small cysts may be safely left alone but larger cysts must be surgically removed, as they may cause considerable discomfort.

TESTICULAR CANCER

Cancer of the testis is rare but is one of the most common cancers in young men between the ages of 20 and 40. This cancer is relatively easy to pick up by regular self-examination and is one of the few completely curable cancers.

WHEN TO SEE YOUR DOCTOR

It is advisable that you report any lump in a testicle to your doctor immediately. Many lumps turn out to be harmless cysts, but if there is any doubt your doctor will refer you to a specialist. Further investigations may include an ultrasound scan and a biopsy where a sample of tissue is taken for testing. If cancer is diagnosed, further scans are done to determine whether or not the tumour has spread to other organs.

HOW IS IT TREATED?

If the tumour is confined to one testicle, the testicle can be removed and it is likely that there will be no need for further treatment.

SIGNS AND SYMPTOMS OF TESTICULAR CANCER

➤ A hard, pea-sized lump, which is usually painless, in a testicle.
➤ Changes in the skin of the scrotum and a dull ache.

If the cancer has already spread, treatment involving a combination of surgery and sessions of chemotherapy or radiotherapy may still be successful.

VARICOCELE

A varicocele is a collection of varicose veins in the scrotum. This condition is not uncommon and is due to faulty valves within the testicular venous system.

WHAT MIGHT YOUR DOCTOR DO?

Your doctor will be able to feel the varicocele – it feels rather like a bag of worms. The treatment given will then depend on the degree of discomfort that the condition is causing. Very mild cases can usually be left alone quite safely as they may not progress any further. More advanced cases, however, will require surgical intervention in which the affected veins are carefully dissected and removed.

SIGNS AND SYMPTOMS OF VARICOCELE

➤ Pain in the testicle or scrotum.
➤ A dragging sensation on the affected side of the scrotum.

HYDROCELE

A hydrocele is a collection of fluid that gathers between the two-layered membrane that surrounds the testicles. It results in a soft swelling in the scrotum and is common in infants and older men. There is usually no apparent cause, although a hydrocele may develop in response to testicular infection or injury.

The classic test to confirm the diagnosis is to shine a light from behind the swelling. In a hydrocele the light shines through the fluid.

Some cases subside without treatment. If it becomes painful, your doctor can treat it either by draining the fluid or by removing the membranous sac that contains the fluid.

A HYDROCELE

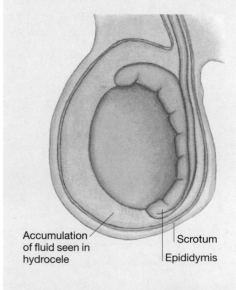

Accumulation of fluid seen in hydrocele

Scrotum
Epididymis

△ A hydrocele literally means a "water hollow". It is a collection of fluid that gathers and causes a swelling in the tissue capsule around the testicle.

Sexually transmitted infections

SEE ALSO
➤ Urinary tract infections, p142
➤ Female genital infections, p159
➤ HIV and AIDS, p220

Sexually transmitted infections (STIs) are passed from one person to another during sexual activity. They are usually transmitted during vaginal and anal intercourse, but some infections may also be transmitted by oral sex. STIs affect both sexes, and can occur in any person that is sexually active, whether young or old. Inevitably, the risk of infection rises among sexually active people who change their partners frequently. Consistent use of an appropriate protective contraception will dramatically reduce the spread of these diseases.

NON-SPECIFIC URETHRITIS (NSU)

A common infection in men.

Symptoms A burning pain when urinating; soreness at tip of penis; penile discharge.

Diagnosis A urethral swab and a urine culture may identify the causative organism.

Treatment One-week course of oral antibiotics. Where chlamydia (see below) is suspected or diagnosed as the cause, it is important that sexual partners are screened.

CHLAMYDIA

A common bacterial infection in sexually active men and women.

Symptoms May show no symptoms. Women may suffer vaginal discharge, urinary frequency, pelvic pain or pain during intercourse. It can cause infertility, pelvic inflammatory disease and ectopic pregnancy.

Diagnosis Chlamydia may be diagnosed by taking a swab from the cervix or urethra.

Treatment Oral antibiotics. Sexual partners should also be treated.

GONNORHOEA

An infection that affects sexually active men and women of any age, and that may be transmitted by oral sex.

Symptoms There may be no symptoms. Pain may develop on passing urine, and there may be penile or vaginal discharge. Women may also have vaginal bleeding.

Diagnosis By taking appropriate swabs. Diagnosis is difficult because a large number of infections have no symptoms.

Treatment Usually responds to oral antibiotics but should be treated early on. If not treated, chronic inflammation in the prostate gland, urethra and epididymis may result. Women risk chronic infection, scarring in the Fallopian tubes, recurrent pelvic inflammatory disease and infertility.

SYPHILIS

A long-term bacterial infection that results in acute genital symptoms. It can spread to other organs if it is not treated early.

Symptoms It has three stages of infection:
- Primary syphilis – Development of a painless ulcer on the penis or vulva and enlarged lymph glands in the groin. The ulcer heals on its own, but secondary syphilis will develop if the condition is not treated at this stage.
- Secondary syphilis – A rash over the whole body. Fever, tiredness and malaise. This may resolve over several weeks. No further symptoms may ever develop but some cases progress (20 or 30 years later).
- Tertiary syphilis – Progressive dementia with confusion, memory disturbance and disorientation. Destruction of the spinal cord resulting in paralysis of the legs.

Diagnosis By taking swabs from the urethra, anus and mouth, and blood tests.

Treatment Primary and secondary syphilis can be treated with injections of penicillin.

GENITAL HERPES

Recurring viral infection that affects both sexes, and can affect a baby during labour and a Caesarean section must be performed.

Symptoms Includes painful, fluid-filled blisters on genitals; tingling and burning sensations in the genitals; fever, aches and pains, tiredness. Symptoms usually subside over a period of two to three weeks.

Diagnosis Usually made from history and examination; can be confirmed by swabs.

Treatment Responds well to antiviral drugs, which reduce the life of infection and degree of infectiousness, but will not eliminate the virus. For recurrent attacks, regular preventative antiviral drugs are advised until the predisposition to recurrent attacks has diminished. The disease often burns itself out over several years.

HEPATITIS

Both hepatitis B and C are viral infections. Hepatitis B virus is transmitted by blood contact and penetrative sex. Hepatitis C virus is transmitted by the blood-borne route, although some cases are believed to be sexually transmitted.

Symptoms These viruses mainly affect the liver. Initial infection is followed by many years of asymptomatic infection and the liver functions normally. Some hepatitis B-positive individuals, and a larger number of hepatitis C-positive individuals, may develop a slowly progressive inflammation of the liver. This may result in liver failure and risk of developing liver cancer.

Diagnosis Blood tests can identify the nature of the virus.

Treatment Increasingly effective antiviral drugs, often used together over a course of about six months. Hepatitis B can be prevented by practising safe sex. People at risk can be immunized against hepatitis B. At-risk groups are gay men, intravenous drug-users, partners of known cases, healthcare workers and workers in long-stay residential units. As yet there is no immunization to prevent hepatitis C.

Impotence

The inability to achieve or sustain an erection is common and affects most men at some time in their lives. The incidence of impotence rises with age and occurs much more frequently among the middle-aged and elderly, although it can affect any man at any age. Occasional impotence is normal and can be caused by a number of factors, including depression or stress. If the problem persists, visit your doctor for further investigation, as more serious diseases may be the root of the problem, including vascular problems or diabetes.

The causes of impotence may be physical, psychological or a combination of the two. Psychological factors often underlie the problem as sexual performance is so closely related to emotional wellbeing. Any man struggling to deal with depression, anxiety, tiredness, relationship problems or a host of other interrelated factors may develop impotence as one physical expression of the stress in his life.

The condition often has physical causes, the most common of which are:
• Vascular disease.
• Drugs (including several used to treat high blood pressure and depression).
• Diabetes.
• Damaged nerves during prostate surgery.
• Liver disease.
• Multiple sclerosis.

Cigarette smoking is known to promote atherosclerosis, which may affect the blood supply to the penis, eventually causing impotence. Heavy and prolonged alcohol consumption may damage the liver and thereby interfere with testosterone production, which affects sex drive and erectile function.

WHAT MIGHT YOUR DOCTOR DO?

Your doctor will want to discuss more easily reversible factors, such as:
• Reducing levels of stress and anxiety.
• Stopping smoking.
• Cutting down alcohol consumption.
• Reviewing regularly taken medication.

To ensure there is no unidentified physical reason, your doctor may examine you and take blood for testing.

PSYCHOLOGICAL COUNSELLING

Psychological factors need to be explored and may require referral to a counsellor. It is very important to have a supportive partner during this process and it is often helpful to agree not to have sexual intercourse for an agreed period of time; this removes pressure of performance and the fear of failure. Attention can then be focused on addressing relevant emotional issues within a relationship.

DRUG THERAPY

The advent of sildenafil, better known as Viagra, has revolutionized the drug treatment of impotence. It works by dilating the small arteries that supply the penis, allowing more blood to flow into the organ and resulting in an erection. Viagra starts to work about one hour after it is swallowed. Some medications used for certain heart disorders may prohibit the use

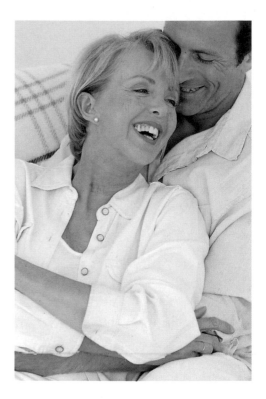

△ Impotence is extremely common and affects most men at some point in their lives. A supportive partner plays a vital role in dealing with the possible causes.

of Viagra, so it is very important that you only obtain such drugs from your doctor.

A number of alternative drugs have been or are in the process of being developed. These include:
• Apomorphine hydrochloride (Uprima), which has recently become available, stimulates the brain into activating the genital areas. It works more quickly than Viagra and achieves erection within 20 minutes of being taken.
• Alprostadil is a drug that is inserted into the penis using a small applicator. It works by acting on the blood supply to produce an erection.

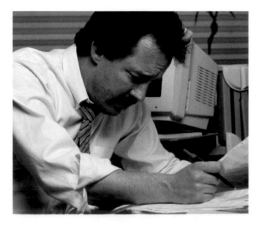

▽ Impotence can be caused by stress, anxiety and overwork. Addressing these psychological factors may well alleviate the problem.

THE EARS, NOSE AND THROAT

10

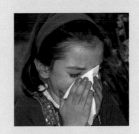

The ears, nose and throat are exposed to the air, and are therefore vulnerable to attack by harmful micro-organisms and foreign bodies. However, these potential invaders have to get past the body's defensive devices. The nose is lined with tiny hairs which serve to trap foreign bodies and prevent them from entering the airway. Protective immune tissue lies at the top of the throat, stopping infection from spreading into the lungs. The outer part of the ears contains cells that produce wax, which traps and expels foreign bodies. When these front-line defences fail, infection, inflammation and blockage may follow.

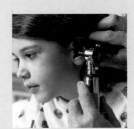

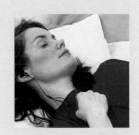

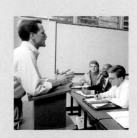

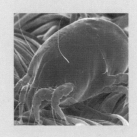

The function of the ears, nose and throat

SEE ALSO
► The breathing process, p126
► Colds and flu, p128
► The roles of blood and lymph, p200

In medicine, the ears, nose and throat are treated as one speciality, which is known as ENT. This is because all are located within the head and neck, and are directly linked by a passageway called the Eustachian tube. The body has a range of ways to repel infection and protect these vulnerable organs, and to prevent micro-organisms from spreading into internal organs such as the lungs. However, because infection can pass easily from one hollow organ to another, sore throats, sinusitis and ear infections are very common.

The ears, nose and throat are vital to our senses of smell, taste and hearing as well as our ability to balance and to breathe.

THE EARS

Organs in the ear are responsible for our hearing and balance. The three parts of the ear – the outer ear, middle ear and inner ear – all play a part in processing sound and transmitting it as nerve impulses to the brain. Our hearing provides the brain with information about our surroundings, and helps us to communicate through the medium of language.

THE NOSE

The nose is part of the respiratory system and is also responsible for smell. Receptors in the nose are stimulated by odours and these then send nerve impulses to the brain.

HOW WE CAN HEAR

Sounds are heard in the ears as a series of air pressure waves. The outer ear acts like an ear trumpet, collecting and focusing sound on to the eardrum, causing it to vibrate. These vibrations then pass to the middle ear, where three connected bones – the malleus, incus and stapes – transmit the sounds to the inner ear, amplifying the sounds as they do so. Sounds enter the inner ear at a junction called the oval window and travel to a specialized hearing organ called the cochlea. The spiral cochlea converts sound waves into nervous impulses, which it then transmits to the brain via the cochlear nerve.

HOW WE BALANCE

Your sense of balance is vital to your ability to remain upright and to move without falling over. The inner ear contains a structure called the vestibular apparatus, which helps with balance by detecting the position of the head and which way it is moving. The vestibular apparatus comprises three semicircular canals, which move when the head rotates, and the vestibule, which senses the head's position. Once the brain knows where the head is in space and how it is moving, it can use information from the joints to work out the positions of other parts of the body, and adjust them as necessary.

The human sense of smell is not as acute and well used as that of animals, but we can distinguish more than 10,000 odours.

Our sense of smell is responsible for most of our sense of taste. Your tongue detects only the tastes of salt, sweet, sour and bitter, and the aromas from the foods you eat help to build on these four basic variants. The role of the nose in tasting food becomes obvious if your nose is blocked, when your sense of taste diminishes.

The lining of your nose is packed with small blood vessels, which warm the air as you inhale. Tiny hairs lining the nose help to trap foreign bodies, preventing them from entering the lungs. You breathe with one nostril at a time – the nostrils shut down in rotation to allow the lining to recover from the drying effects of air passing in and out during breathing.

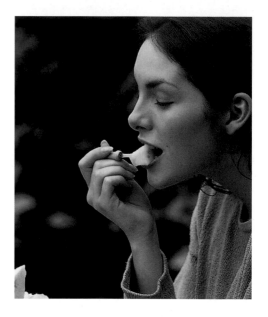

△ Our sense of smell is crucial to our sense of taste – helping us to distinguish tiny differences in flavours.

THE THROAT

A ring of immune system tissue sits at the back of the nose and throat, which helps prevent infection moving into the lungs. This ring – known as Waldeyer's ring – is formed by the tonsils, adenoids and lymph nodes at the back of the tongue. The airway and oesophagus meet in the throat (pharynx), so food and drink, and air, pass through it. During swallowing, a flap of cartilage known as the epiglottis closes over the airway, so that food does not enter the respiratory system.

The larynx ("voice box") acts as a valve, to divert food from the airway, and has the role of producing speech and other sounds. Vocal cords within the larynx vibrate to produce sounds, which are modified by the tongue and the lips to produce the elements of comprehensible speech.

THE STRUCTURE OF THE EARS, NOSE AND THROAT

▷ The structures of the ears, nose and throat are closely linked, which is why medicine groups them together. A problem in one of these three areas often affects the others.

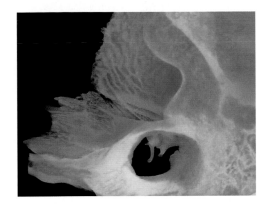

△ The middle ear bones transmit sound waves from the eardrum towards the inner ear, where vibrations are turned into nerve impulses.

These artworks have been designed to show the location of different parts of the ear, nose and throat clearly, and are therefore not to scale.

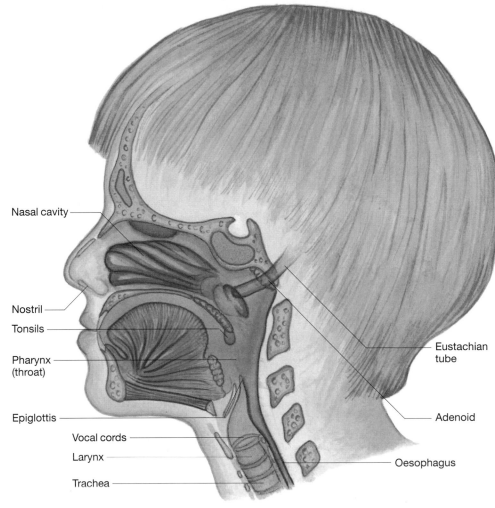

Nasal cavity

Nostril

Tonsils

Pharynx (throat)

Epiglottis

Vocal cords

Larynx

Trachea

Eustachian tube

Adenoid

Oesophagus

INSIDE THE EAR

Pinna
This flap of cartilage is perfectly shaped to funnel sound into the ears.

Auditory canal
Ears are self-cleaning. Cells lining the outer ear produce wax and move out from the eardrum, carrying foreign bodies.

The outer ear
This comprises the external ear – or pinna – and the auditory canal, leading down to the eardrum.
The middle ear
This contains three small bones – the malleus, incus and stapes (the smallest bone in the body).
The inner ear
This fluid-filled part of the ear contains the cochlea, the semicircular canals and the vestibule.

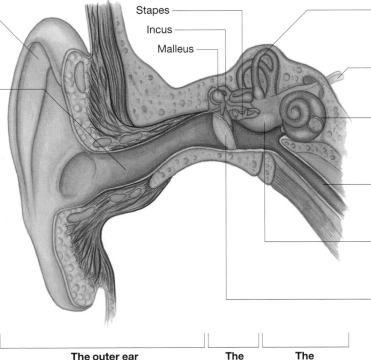

Stapes

Incus

Malleus

The outer ear

The middle ear

The inner ear

Semicircular canals
These fluid-filled canals, at right angles to each other, are responsible for balance and detect rotational movements of the head.

Cochlear and vestibular nerves
These nerves take data on sound (from the cochlea) and balance (from the vestibule) to the brain.

Cochlea
This spiral organ is full of sensitive hair cells, each tuned to a different frequency of sound. Movement in the hairs triggers nervous signals to the brain.

Eustachian tube
This links the middle ear to the back of the nose and aids the equalizing of air pressure on either side of the eardrum.

Vestibule
Two devices in this part of the inner ear send information about linear movement – travelling up or down – and static position – which way is up.

Eardrum
This vibrating membrane, known as the tympanic membrane, separates the outer and middle ears.

Earache

SEE ALSO
➤ Routine health checks, p24
➤ Hearing loss and deafness, p169
➤ Earache in children, p226

Pain in the ear can be distressing, particularly for young children. It is often due to an infection in the middle or outer ear, but can also be caused by an injury or the build-up of wax. Diseases of the ear, jaw or anywhere within the head and neck can also cause pain in the ear. It is advisable to consult your doctor if you have an earache that lasts longer than 24 hours, since an untreated infection could damage your hearing. Antibiotics are usually necessary if there is a bacterial infection, and most causes of earache can be sorted out within days or weeks.

Earache can be painful and debilitating but it usually has a straightforward cause, and usual causes include:

- Inflammation or infection in the ear canal – also known as otitis externa. The skin becomes red and inflamed, and there may be pus discharge from the ear.
- Inflammation or infection in the middle ear – otitis media. In this condition, the middle ear can fill with fluid or pus, leading to partial hearing loss.
- Pressure changes causing damage or pain in the middle ear – barotrauma. This is usually the result of scuba diving or travelling by air. It should correct itself without treatment, but see your doctor if it persists for more than a few hours.
- Jaw or teeth-related problems such as temporomandibular joint disorder. The temporomandibular joint is just in front of your ears. It can become inflamed, often as a result of poor or loosely fitting teeth or dentures, causing severe pain near your ears.

WHAT MIGHT YOUR DOCTOR DO?

If you have pain in your ear, your doctor will look into the outer ear canal using an instrument called an otoscope. Any ruptures of the eardrum, wax blockages or pus collections will be visible. The treatment depends on the cause.

- Otitis externa – Ear drops or sprays with a steroid antifungal agent and antibiotics usually settle the problem in a few days.
- Otitis media – Most cases are caused by a viral infection and usually clear up without treatment. However, if the cause

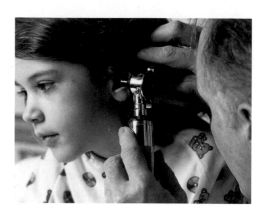

△ A doctor examines his patient using an otoscope, which comprises lenses, a light and a funnel-shaped tip which is inserted into the ear.

is bacterial, antibiotics are usually given.

- Temporomandibular joint disorder is often eased by dental treatment. Stress can play a part in some cases, so relaxation techniques may be advised.

Noises in the ear (tinnitus)

SEE ALSO
➤ Anaemia, p202

Tinnitus can be alarming. It results from sounds generated within the ear itself and affects up to 15 per cent of us at some time in our lives. The noises are usually high-pitched and vary from ringing to hissing or whistling. People notice it most when it is quiet, so it disturbs sleep.

Tinnitus can affect people on and off, as brief episodes, or almost non-stop. Some of those affected hear noises only when they concentrate on them, while for others it is persistently intrusive and disruptive.

Many cases of tinnitus relate to the aging process while others are related to conditions such as anaemia and an overactive thyroid gland. Symptoms similar to tinnitus may be experienced if the ears are blocked with wax. Both ears tend to be affected and noises that occur in one ear only could be due to other causes.

COPING WITH TINNITUS

After an examination to exclude any other cause, your doctor may discuss strategies for managing tinnitus. These include:

- Using a masker – This is a device, similar to a hearing aid, which produces sounds in order to mask the tinnitus. Some people find having a radio under their pillow at night can be helpful.
- Drug therapy – Occasionally, if tinnitus is causing severe disruption and upset, your doctor may prescribe sedatives and antidepressants.

Hearing loss and deafness

SEE ALSO
➤ Routine health checks, p24
➤ The function of the ears, nose and throat, p166

About one in five adults has some form of hearing impairment, ranging from mild hearing loss to complete deafness. The first thing people notice is difficulty listening to conversations, which may be particularly troublesome if there is background noise. There are different types of deafness and your doctor will be able to diagnose the exact type by an examination of your ears and eardrums, together with a series of tests with tuning forks. If hearing loss is permanent, hearing aids can usually enable you to participate in normal daily life.

Doctors categorize hearing loss into types:
- Conductive – This is where there is a problem conveying sound often caused by a blockage or an infection. As the nerves are intact, treatment is usually successful.
- Sensorineural – The most common type, where the sound-detecting hair cells of the inner ear, or the nerves taking messages to the brain, are damaged.
- Combined sensorineural and conductive.

CONDUCTIVE LOSS

Hearing is usually restored once the cause is treated, and causes include:
- Wax – This common cause can treated with wax softening ear drops which can

THE STRUCTURE OF A COCHLEAR IMPLANT

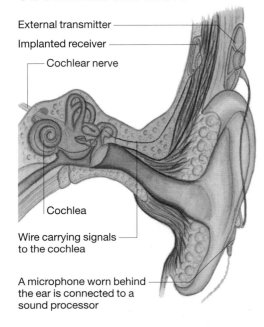

External transmitter
Implanted receiver
Cochlear nerve
Cochlea
Wire carrying signals to the cochlea
A microphone worn behind the ear is connected to a sound processor

△ In a cochlear implant (hearing aid), sound impulses are picked up by a receiver under the skin, then sent along a wire to tiny electrodes implanted in the cochlea.

HEARING AIDS

Initially, wearing a hearing aid can be disappointing since all noise, including background noise, is amplified. With perseverance, however, hearing usually improves. Hearing can be better if both ears are fitted with an aid. There are several types:

➤ Behind-the-ear-aids are widely used. A battery, microphone, amplifier and speaker are housed in a case worn behind the ear, and a transmission tube is passed into the ear canal.

➤ In-the-ear aids are smaller. All the components are contained in a case, which fits neatly into the ear canal.

➤ Newer hearing aids can be anchored directly into the bones of the skull.

➤ Cochlear implants can be used for profoundly deaf people. They create an impression of sound which, combined with lip-reading, can help profoundly deaf people to understand speech.

be purchased in pharmacies, or in severe cases by gently syringing your ears.
- Otitis externa – In which the ear canal is filled with skin debris. A spray or drops containing antibiotic and an antifungal agent usually clears up the problem.
- Otitis media (glue ear) – In which pus and fluid prevent the three bones of the middle ear vibrating. The condition may respond to antibiotics but if not it needs draining surgically via grommets.
- Perforated eardrum – It often follows an infection and can heal without treatment in a few weeks, but can require surgery.
- Otosclerosis – In which the bones of the middle ear fuse. It usually affects older people and does not respond to drugs. Possible treatments are surgery to replace the stapes bone or a hearing aid.

SENSORINEURAL LOSS

This is hard to treat, but a hearing aid can help. Some causes include:
- Noise trauma – Regular exposure to loud noise, or exposure to one very loud noise, can destroy the hair cells of the inner ear.
- Exposure to very high air pressure.
- Increasing age – Inner ear function declines as you get older.
- Drugs – Inform your doctor of any drugs being taken because this can be a factor.
- Skull fracture.
- Viral infections such as mumps.
- Labyrinthitis – An inner ear infection.

▽ Listening to loud music on a personal stereo can put you at risk of hearing loss.

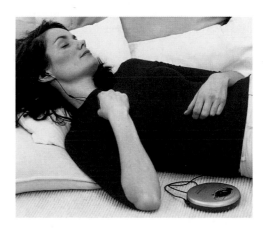

Vertigo

SEE ALSO

➤ High blood pressure, p30
➤ Stroke, p80
➤ Cervical spondylosis, p112

Vertigo is the unpleasant sensation of spinning: the person feels that either they or their surroundings are moving when in fact they are still. This distressing feeling develops suddenly and may last from a few minutes to several days. It is commonly due to problems in the ear and is often associated with nausea and vomiting. Occasionally there is a more serious underlying cause, so if you experience any such symptoms you should see your doctor urgently. Vertigo usually clears up by itself or once the underlying cause has been treated.

Vertigo is often the result of a problem in the inner ear, which contains the organs that control balance. The causes include:

• Acute labyrinthitis – This is an inflammation of the labyrinth, part of the vestibule in the inner ear. The condition can be extremely unpleasant and there may be associated nausea and vomiting. A simple viral infection is the most common cause. The problem usually settles in a few days and antiemetic drugs can help control the sickness.

• Chronic labyrinthitis – In this condition vertigo lasts for a few minutes, but recurs over weeks and months. It can be due to a long-term bacterial infection in the middle ear (otitis media) or to deposits of crystal in the balance mechanisms, which cause dizziness when the head moves.

• Ménière's disease – This is a rare disorder of the inner ear, in which the balance mechanism becomes filled with fluid. The symptoms can be severe and include recurrent bouts of vertigo, deafness, tinnitus and pain in the ears.

• Acoustic neuroma – This rare tumour affects the nerve connecting the inner ear to the brain. It is non-cancerous but can press on the nerve or part of the brain, causing dizziness and balance problems.

Non-ear-related problems such as a stroke can also cause vertigo. In these cases, the person affected may have difficulty in speaking or seeing and may experience weakness in the limbs, and medical treatment should be sought as a matter of urgency. Some people develop vertigo as a result of high blood pressure or arthritis in the neck (cervical spondylosis). Older people are most likely to be affected but either condition can occur at any age.

WHAT SHOULD I DO?

A bout of vertigo is usually relieved if you lie down and keep the head still for a few minutes. However, if the vertigo persists or if you suffer from repeated attacks, you should see your doctor to rule out any serious underlying cause.

INVESTIGATING VERTIGO

Your doctor will examine your eyes, ears and neck, and check your blood pressure. Antiemetic drugs may be prescribed to relieve symptoms. Vertigo can often clear up on its own, but you may need treatment for the underlying cause. For example, antibiotics will be necessary if you have a bacterial infection in the middle ear.

MOTION SICKNESS

Also called travel sickness, this condition causes the same spinning sensation as vertigo. It affects almost everyone at some point in their lives and most often occurs during travel. The problem arises when the brain receives conflicting messages from the balance organs in the inner ear and the eyes. For example, your ears will register the motion of the car even though your body is not actually moving. If you suffer from motion sickness, there are a number of self-help options to try the next time you travel.

➤ Eat only a light meal before you set off on a journey. Fatty foods can aggravate feelings of nausea.

➤ Avoid reading while travelling and keep your eyes on the horizon.

➤ Take an antihistamine drug before the journey, but if you are driving be aware that some cause drowsiness.

➤ Suck ginger-based sweets – ginger can help to soothe nausea.

▽ Medically, vertigo does not mean the fear of heights and the sensation of dizziness that you feel when looking down from a high place. This condition is known as acrophobia.

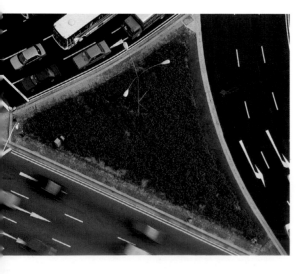

▽ Many people develop motion sickness on a boat, and the spinning sensation can persist for a few hours afterwards.

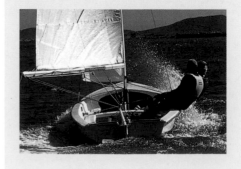

Nosebleeds

The lining of the nose has a plentiful blood supply, with many small blood vessels just beneath the surface. These serve to warm the air as it passes through the nose on its way to the lungs. Unfortunately, they mean that the nose is prone to bleeding. Nosebleeds are particularly common in children. The cause is usually straightforward – for example, damage to the lining caused by a blow or by nose-picking. Occasionally, however, nosebleeds can be a symptom of a serious disorder, so you should consult a doctor if bleeding is persistent.

The commonest cause of a nosebleed is nose-picking, which can damage the fragile blood vessels in the nose lining. Children and some adults habitually pick their nose, some even in their sleep.

Forceful nose-blowing, or inserting a foreign body into the nostril, can also result in a nosebleed. Very rarely, nosebleeds may be a sign of a serious disorder, such as cancer of the nasopharynx (the passage that connects the nose and throat) or a bleeding disorder. It is therefore very important that you seek medical advice for persistent or recurrent bleeding.

The cause of persistent nosebleeds can also be investigated by means of an endoscopy. In this procedure, a flexible narrow tube is passed into each nostril to look for the presence of a tumour or damage to the blood vessels. A sample of tissue can be taken at the same time.

TREATING NOSEBLEEDS

Seek medical advice if a nosebleed lasts longer than 30 minutes but these steps will usually stop a nosebleed in minutes:

➤ Gently squeeze the soft end of the nose. Apply this pressure to the nose for at least ten minutes, breathing through your mouth.

➤ If bleeding persists, apply the pressure for a further ten minutes.

➤ Do not dab, wipe or blow your nose – this just prolongs the nosebleed.

▽ Avoid blowing the nose for three hours after a nosebleed, since this can interrupt clotting and cause further bleeding.

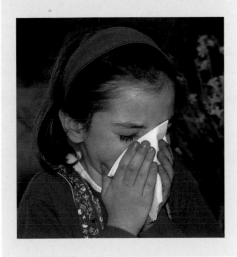

THE SOURCE OF A NOSEBLEED

In almost all cases, the bleeding comes from a patch just inside the nose called Little's area. Applying pressure to the end of the nose (see treating nosebleeds box) usually stops the bleeding.

Bleeding from the back of the nose is less common but may have a more serious cause. It is harder to treat since it is difficult to apply direct pressure, and may therefore lead to significant blood loss.

Anyone with a bleeding disorder (such as haemophilia), or those taking blood-thinning drugs (anticoagulants), tends to bleed for longer.

PERSISTENT NOSEBLEEDS

You should seek urgent medical treatment if a nosebleeds lasts longer than half an hour, or if so much blood is lost that the person feels dizzy or turns pale.

The bleeding may be stemmed either by packing the nose tight with ribbon gauze or by using a urinary catheter (hollow tube). The balloon that normally holds a urinary catheter in the bladder can be blown up inside the nose to apply pressure to the bleeding spot. Another form of treatment is to destroy some tissue just inside the nose using heat or by freezing. You may need such cauterization again if nosebleeds recur.

NASAL POLYPS

Many people develop nasal polyps, non-cancerous fleshy growths that arise from the sinuses. Their cause is unknown, but they are more common in people who suffer from asthma and hayfever. The severity of the symptoms depends on the number of polyps and their size. Symptoms often include:

➤ A blocked nose.

➤ A decreased sense of smell.

➤ A runny nose, in some cases.

Nasal polyps can be shrunk by using a steroid spray, or removed via endoscopic surgery, in which a fine, flexible telescope device is guided up your nose.

▽ A nasal polyp may disappear without treatment, but will usually be removed under general or local anaesthetic.

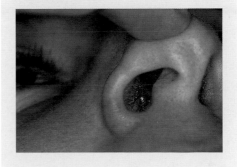

Hayfever and perennial rhinitis

SEE ALSO
➤ Asthma, p130
➤ The function of the ears, nose and throat, p166
➤ Sinusitis, p173

Hayfever is an acute allergic reaction that causes inflammation of the membranes lining the nose and throat and also affects the eyes. It is usually caused by sensitivity to pollens – of grasses, trees, flowers and weeds. Hayfever is a seasonal condition, with symptoms usually occurring in spring and summer. Some people suffer from hayfever-like symptoms all year round, a condition known as perennial rhinitis which is triggered by additional allergens. Symptoms can usually be brought under control by avoiding known triggers (allergens) and using medication.

SIGNS AND SYMPTOMS

The same symptoms occur in both hayfever and perennial rhinitis, but may be more severe in hayfever sufferers. The signs and symptoms include:

➤ A runny nose.

➤ Watery, red and itchy eyes.

➤ A dry and uncomfortable throat.

➤ Frequent sneezing.

➤ A general feeling of irritability and being unwell.

Hayfever or perennial rhinitis can affect anyone but will occur most commonly in people who have other forms of allergic disorder such as asthma. The trigger for hayfever is usually pollen, so symptoms occur in spring and summer when pollen counts are high. Perennial rhinitis can be triggered not only by pollen but by other allergens, such as house-dust mites,

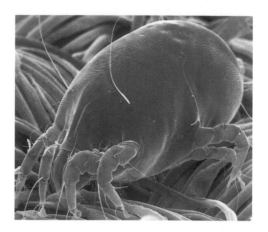

▷ Tiny dust mites (shown magnified in this picture) are common triggers for perennial rhinitis and other allergic disorders.

feathers, animal fur and mould. Symptoms may occur all year, but are often exacerbated during the hayfever season.

TREATMENT OPTIONS

The main treatment for hayfever and perennial rhinitis is the management of symptoms and can include:

• Antihistamines – These drugs are taken orally to treat the acute symptoms of hayfever and allergy. They may be taken as needed for intermittent symptoms or on a regular preventative basis when symptoms are persistent. They are usually taken once a day and have few or no side-effects.

• Nasal sprays and eye drops – These act on a preventative basis and need to be taken at least twice a day to have a beneficial effect. Inhaled steroid sprays often provide good control for individuals with troublesome nasal symptoms.

PREVENTING HAYFEVER AND PERENNIAL RHINITIS

The following can help to reduce the effects of pollen in spring and summer:

➤ Avoid areas with long grass or where grass is being cut.

➤ Stay indoors in late morning and early evening, when pollen counts are high, and keep windows and doors closed.

➤ Wear sunglasses outside to reduce eye irritation.

If you suffer from perennial rhinitis, the following may help to reduce symptoms:

➤ Avoid the provoking allergen where possible. For example, do not keep cats if you are allergic to them.

➤ Keep house dust to a minimum. Have wooden floors rather than carpets, blinds rather than curtains.

➤ Regular vacuuming of the mattress and bedding removes skin scales, which form a dust mite's food.

▽ Swollen eyes are a common symptom of hayfever, and are caused by an allergic response to airborne allergens such as pollen.

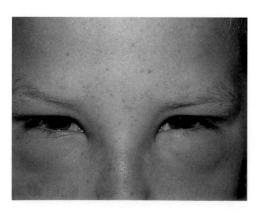

▽ Feather-filled pillows and duvets can trigger allergic disorders such as perennial rhinitis, so foam-filled bedding helps to reduce attacks.

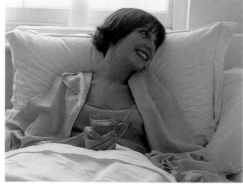

Sinusitis

SEE ALSO

➤ Colds and flu, p128

➤ Hayfever and perennial rhinitis, p172

The sinuses are air-filled cavities around the eyes and nose, within the bones of the skull. Doctors do not know the precise function of our sinuses but it is thought that they may serve to modify the quality of the voice. Inflammation of the sinuses – or sinusitis – is often associated with an infection in the upper respiratory tract, such as a cold or hayfever, and the condition can be both painful and distressing. It often clears up without treatment but may recur with more severe symptoms. In severe cases, bouts of sinusitis can last for several months.

SIGNS AND SYMPTOMS

The usual symptoms of sinusitis include:

➤ Headache.

➤ Fever.

➤ Blocked nose and discoloured nasal discharge.

➤ Pain and tenderness over the affected sinus.

➤ Sometimes, redness around an eye.

THE LOCATION OF THE SINUSES

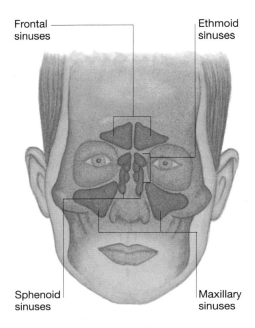

Frontal sinuses

Ethmoid sinuses

Sphenoid sinuses

Maxillary sinuses

△ The different sinuses are named after the bones in which they are found. The maxillary sinuses are located in the cheekbones, the frontal sinuses are in the spaces above the eyebrows, and the ethmoid and sphenoid sinuses lie deep within the skull.

Many people suffer from pain in the sinuses, but some individuals are more prone to regular episodes of sinusitis. Young children rarely suffer from the condition because the sinuses do not develop fully until they are four or five years old.

WHAT CAUSES SINUSITIS?

An attack of sinusitis is usually the result of infection by common cold viruses. The sinuses can block, fill with fluid and cause facial pain. Most symptoms occur between three and ten days after a cold. Simple painkillers and steam inhalation to loosen the discharge are the best treatments, along with rest if you have a fever and feel unwell.

Consult your doctor if your symptoms last longer than three days. You should also seek medical advice if symptoms suddenly recur along with more pain and a fever. This so-called "secondary sickening" is due to an infection by bacteria.

MAKING A DIAGNOSIS

Your doctor will press on your cheeks and forehead to check for tenderness, and may shine a light through your skin to see if your sinuses are clear. If a secondary bacterial infection is likely, you will be prescribed a short course of antibiotics, which usually clears up the problem. Your doctor may also arrange for X-rays of the sinuses if chronic sinusitis is suspected.

SIMPLE SELF-HELP

• Take decongestant tablets which are available from pharmacies.
• Avoid smoky atmospheres and prolonged exposure to dust and irritants.

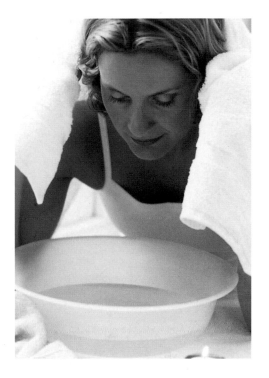

△ Inhaling steam from a bowl of boiling water, for a few minutes at a time, loosens discharge and helps it to drain away more easily.

• Do not blow your nose too forcefully during a cold since this can push the infection up into the sinuses.

CHRONIC SINUSITIS

If short-lived infections occur frequently in the sinuses, they may never seem to clear up. This form of the condition is known as chronic sinusitis. The cause is not known, but smoking and industrial pollution appear to make the condition worse. Symptoms usually improve with steroid nasal sprays, although in some very severe cases the problem may be referred to an ENT specialist, who will wash out and drain the sinuses.

Snoring

SEE ALSO

➤ Weight control, p16
➤ Smoking and your health, p20
➤ Sensible drinking, p22

Breathing noisily during sleep is a common and usually harmless condition. However, it can disturb the snorer's sleep and can also be disturbing to those sleeping near them. The noise is due to vibration of the soft palate (the back of the roof of the mouth) because people often breathe through their mouths when they are asleep. Snoring is common in children, and in adults between 30 and 50 – men are more likely to be affected than women. Loud snoring may be a symptom of a more serious condition called obstructive sleep apnoea.

Snoring can affect anyone, but certain factors are more likely to make you breathe noisily when you are asleep. These include:
• Smoking.
• Drinking alcohol or taking sedatives.
• Being overweight or obese.
• Having a cold or nasal congestion.

Most snoring problems in children are not caused by adenoidal disease, but enlarged adenoids can sometimes cause snoring.

WHAT CAN I DO?

Sleeping on your back promotes snoring so try another sleeping position – sewing a bumpy object into the back of your night clothing can help. You should also give up smoking, lose weight if you are overweight and refrain from drinking alcohol or taking sedatives before bedtime.

Consult your doctor if you have other symptoms, such as daytime drowsiness, as this may suggest sleep apnoea.

HOW SNORING OCCURS

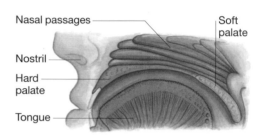

△ Air passes the soft palate on its way to the nasopharynx. If the airway is blocked, the soft palate tissues vibrate, causing snoring.

Obstructive sleep apnoea

SEE ALSO

➤ Heart disease, p34

In obstructive sleep apnoea, the airway is sucked closed, causing you to stop breathing briefly. This interruption in breathing means that less oxygen reaches your lungs and the oxygen level in your blood falls. Low oxygen levels prompt you to wake up and take a deep breath.

SIGNS AND SYMPTOMS

The typical pattern in obstructive sleep apnoea is for a person to snore more and more loudly and then stop breathing for ten seconds or more. Breathing begins with a choke or splutter as the airway reopens. This pattern continues during the night. Other symptoms include:

➤ Daytime sleepiness.

➤ Morning headache.

➤ Reduced libido (sex drive).

➤ Feeling drunk in the morning.

➤ Ankle swelling.

Sleep apnoea usually occurs in middle-aged men but can affect anyone, including children. It is often the result of an obstruction in the airway but may have other causes. It is important to have the sleep apnoea diagnosed since it can contribute to serious disorders such as heart disease or high blood pressure.

WHAT MIGHT A DOCTOR DO?

Your doctor will examine your nose and throat for signs of obstructions, and may arrange for you to have an endoscopy, where a narrow tube is passed through the nostrils to allow a more detailed examination. Sleep tests, in which oxygen levels in the blood and heart rate are measured, can confirm the diagnosis. Treatment is aimed at removing the causes of sleep apnoea. If this fails, a positive pressure device may be used, which involves air being pumped from a compressor to keep the airway open.

CAUSES OF SLEEP APNOEA

Sleep apnoea is usually the result of an obstructed airway, caused by:

➤ Obesity.

➤ Enlarged tonsils or nasal abnormality.

➤ Drugs that decrease breathing or relax the airway, such as alcohol, sedatives and opiate painkillers.

Sore throat and tonsillitis

SEE ALSO
- ➤ Colds and flu, p128
- ➤ The roles of blood and lymph, p200
- ➤ Glandular fever, p219
- ➤ Colds, sore throats and earache, p226

The tonsils are large lymph nodes that are situated either side of the back of the tongue. They are part of the ring of immune tissue around the mouth and nose which serves to intercept any invading viruses or bacteria. Infections and inflammation of the throat and tonsils are common and the vast majority are viral infections that last a few days. Most can be treated at home with simple self-help measures, but you should seek medical advice if your symptoms are particularly severe, if you have any difficulty in breathing, or if symptoms persist.

SIGNS AND SYMPTOMS

A sore throat or tonsillitis causes similar symptoms, such as:

- ➤ Pain and inflammation in the throat.
- ➤ Swollen lymph nodes in the neck.
- ➤ Difficulty in swallowing.
- ➤ A high temperature.

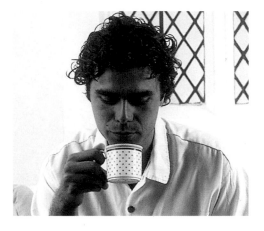

△ Most sore throats clear up quickly with plenty of fluids, painkillers and rest.

Most sore throats are caused by a viral infection and usually clear up in a few days. The only treatments needed are:

- Rest.
- Plenty of fluids.
- Simple painkillers. (Gargling with soluble aspirin can be helpful for a sore throat but you should be very careful that you do not exceed the safe dosage levels for painkillers.)

If symptoms persist, consult your doctor. Glandular fever may have similar symptoms to a sore throat but tends to last

▽ Tonsillitis is usually easy to spot: the tonsils become red and inflamed, with a white coating.

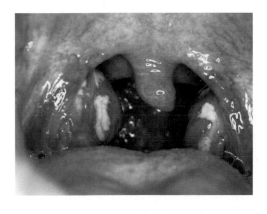

for weeks rather than days. Glandular fever can be easily diagnosed by a blood test.

STREP THROAT

An extremely sore throat can be the result of infection by *Streptococcus* bacteria. This requires treatment with antibiotics.

Distinguishing a viral sore throat from a bacterial infection can be very difficult, and doctors now try to avoid unnecessary use of antibiotics as this contributes to bacteria becoming resistant to antibiotics. In general, a bacterial sore throat will make you feel more unwell than a viral one. You may also have pus and ulcers on your tonsils and throat. To aid diagnosis, a swab may be taken and sent to the laboratory for testing.

RECURRENT TONSILLITIS

Tonsillitis is an infection that is confined to the tonsils. The tonsils are larger in children than adults, which is why so many more children are prone to tonsil infections. In the past, thousands of children had their tonsils surgically removed (tonsillectomy) to prevent recurrent infections. Nowadays, doctors are reluctant to remove the tonsils because they perform a useful function as part of the body's defences, and because there is always a danger that the operation, like any other, can lead to complications.

However, those affected by recurrent tonsillitis – that is, those suffering more than three bouts a year for two years or more – are usually referred to an ear, nose and throat specialist so that surgical treatment can be considered.

PERITONSILLAR ABSCESS

Rarely, the infection causing tonsillitis causes an abscess or a collection of pus to form behind the tonsil – this is called a peritonsillar abscess. This is very painful and can cause severe malaise. An operation to drain the abscess is required as well as a course of antibiotics.

▽ Hot or very cold drinks will help to ease the irritation of a sore throat, and drinking different fruit juices will increase your vitamin intake at the same time.

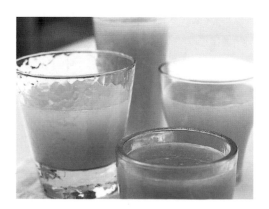

Hoarseness of the voice

SEE ALSO

➤ Smoking and your health, p20

➤ Sensible drinking, p22

➤ Sore throat and tonsillitis, p175

The most common cause of a hoarse voice is a viral infection of the larynx that has led to inflammation. People who put a lot of strain on their voices, such as actors or singers, and people who smoke and drink excessively, may also suffer from temporary hoarseness. It can also be caused by air-conditioned atmospheres, pollution or high pollen levels. In most cases, the hoarseness will settle without treatment if the voice is rested and you refrain from smoking. However, hoarseness can be a sign of serious illness so if it persists it is advisable to seek medical advice.

If you notice a change in your voice that is persistent, it is advisable to visit your doctor. Most causes are relatively simple, and do not result in long-term damage. However, persistent hoarseness can be a symptom of more serious conditions such as cancer.

Any vocal changes lasting over three weeks will be referred to a ear, nose and throat specialist. In this case, your throat will be inspected by means of an angled mirror and a light, or by an endoscope – a flexible telescopic device that is passed through the nostril into the throat. A local anaesthetic may be given. To help with diagnosis, a small sample of tissue may be taken. This procedure is called a biopsy.

WHAT THE LARYNX DOES

▷ The larynx, or voice box, is situated at the back of the tongue, at the start of the airway that leads down into the lungs. The larynx acts as a valve to close off the airway during swallowing, but it also contains the vocal cords, which produce sounds and speech.

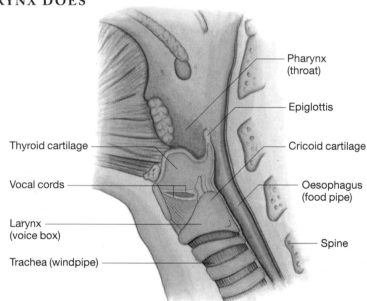

Pharynx (throat)

Epiglottis

Cricoid cartilage

Thyroid cartilage

Vocal cords

Oesophagus (food pipe)

Larynx (voice box)

Spine

Trachea (windpipe)

CAUSES OF HOARSENESS

• Chronic laryngitis – This is a long-standing inflammation of the larynx. It is usually the result of smoking or the persistent overuse of the voice. There is

▽ Teachers and lecturers may suffer from vocal nodules as they regularly strain their voices.

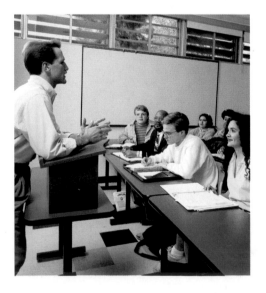

no specific treatment but it usually improves if the voice is rested. If you smoke, you should give up, and you should also reduce alcohol consumption.

• Vocal polyps – These are fleshy, non-cancerous growths on the vocal cords. They are quite common and can easily be removed by a minor surgical procedure.

• Vocal nodules – These thickenings on the vocal cords are caused by overusing the voice. They are most often seen in people such as singers and teachers, but sometimes affect persistently noisy children. In most cases, the nodules disappear if the voice is rested, but they may have to be removed surgically.

• Cancer of the larynx and the pharynx – Cancers of the larynx and of the lower pharynx are more common in smokers and people who regularly drink alcohol to excess, and are also more likely to affect men than women. If caught in the early stages when the tumour is small, radiotherapy can often effect a cure. Larger tumours of the larynx require surgery and these operations can make it difficult or impossible for a person to speak and they may end up with a permanent opening to their airway in the neck (tracheostomy). As with most cancers, the smaller the tumour, the better the prognosis.

PERSISTENT HOARSENESS

Persistent hoarseness can be caused by cancer of the larynx and the pharynx, so seek medical advice if hoarseness persists for over three weeks. Other symptoms might include difficulty in swallowing or a feeling of a lump in the throat. Treatment has a high success rate if the cancer is caught early.

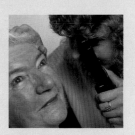

11

THE EYES

It is easy to take sight for granted, but this is one of the most intricate and miraculous senses a human being enjoys. Light bouncing off objects around us enters the eyes and forms images on the retina. These images are translated into electrical impulses which are sent along the optic nerve to the brain, where the information is interpreted. The structure of the eyes and how they function is impressive, and an investigation of the range of disorders and infections that can threaten your sight highlights the importance of protecting the health of these incredible and fragile organs.

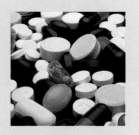

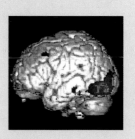

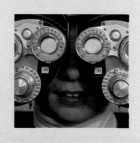

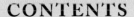

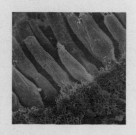

How the eyes function

The human eye is a truly impressive organ and human beings have the most sophisticated light-detection system of any animal on Earth. Of all the senses, sight is perhaps the most important, supplying vast quantities of information about the world in which we live. Our sight allows us to interact with other people, judge speeds and distances, work in bright sunlight or semi-darkness, discern colours and work up close in tiny detail. The eyes are well protected by the skull and the eyelids, and produce tears to keep them lubricated, clean and free of infection.

The eyes perform one of the most important functions in the human body. In conjunction with the brain, they allow you to see, recognize, remember and react to objects and people around you.

THE EYE AS A CAMERA

The eye is similar to a video camera in that visual information from your surroundings streams in continuously. Cameras, in fact, mimic the features of the eye. A series of lenses bends and focuses light rays on to a light-sensitive layer (the film) at the back of the camera. Even the aperture, in SLR cameras, reflects the actions of the pupil of the eye – it expands to let more light in or gets smaller to restrict the amount of light.

In a video camera, the end product is the series of images captured on the film or disk. But in humans, the light rays hitting the back of the eye are registered as images and then are converted to nerve impulses that travel to the brain, where the information is interpreted.

▽ As light hits the eyes, impulses are sent from the retina to the brain, which analyses and interprets this information to form a rounded, colour image of the object you have seen.

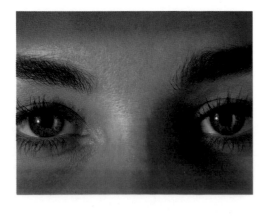

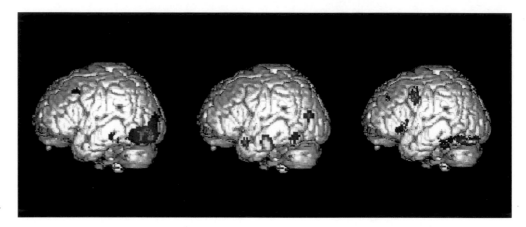

△ These coloured scans of the left side of the human brain show which areas are active while images are processed. The far left scan shows the brain responding as an object is seen, while the middle scan shows part of the temporal lobe lighting up as the object is recognized. The far right scan shows which areas are active when a person speaks to name the object.

The layers (cornea and lens) that bend light in the eye are of a much poorer quality than those in the average camera. However, the human eye compensates for this by having a much more sensitive light-detection system and a truly immense computer (the brain) to analyse and enhance the images. Each eye views objects in a slightly different way, so healthy eyes produce very detailed information for the brain to interpret and use.

HOW THE BRAIN SEES

The visual centres at the back of the brain do much more than receive simple signals from the retina. Most of the processes that produce a sharp, full-colour image in three dimensions occur within the brain. Visual signals are integrated with many other kinds of information in different parts of the brain. The brain also stores detailed information, about people and objects, provided by the eyes.

CONDITIONS AFFECTING THE EYES

Despite being fairly well protected, some outer parts of the eye can become infected, causing styes or conjunctivitis. Most of these conditions are easily treated and, while uncomfortable, do not cause lasting damage. More serious eye conditions occur when the complex inner workings of the eye are affected.

Many people suffer from myopia (short sight) or hypermetropia (long sight, usually in later life). These can be corrected by special lenses (glasses or contact lenses). These days more people are opting for laser

PROTECTING THE EYE
The eye is served by two kinds of protection: eyelids help to keep harmful particles out of the eye, while tears prevent infection, wash away dangerous material and even contain an antiseptic.

THE STRUCTURE OF THE EYE

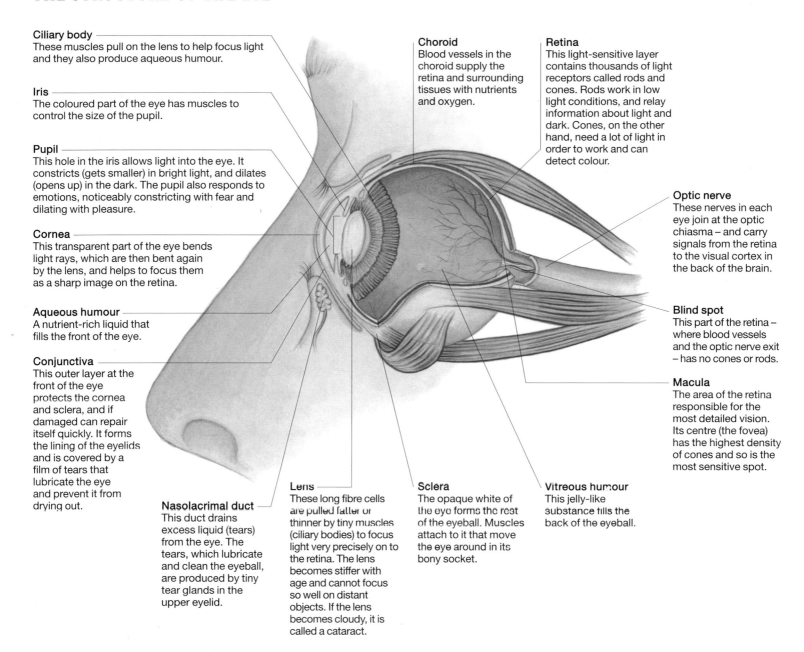

Ciliary body
These muscles pull on the lens to help focus light and they also produce aqueous humour.

Iris
The coloured part of the eye has muscles to control the size of the pupil.

Pupil
This hole in the iris allows light into the eye. It constricts (gets smaller) in bright light, and dilates (opens up) in the dark. The pupil also responds to emotions, noticeably constricting with fear and dilating with pleasure.

Cornea
This transparent part of the eye bends light rays, which are then bent again by the lens, and helps to focus them as a sharp image on the retina.

Aqueous humour
A nutrient-rich liquid that fills the front of the eye.

Conjunctiva
This outer layer at the front of the eye protects the cornea and sclera, and if damaged can repair itself quickly. It forms the lining of the eyelids and is covered by a film of tears that lubricate the eye and prevent it from drying out.

Nasolacrimal duct
This duct drains excess liquid (tears) from the eye. The tears, which lubricate and clean the eyeball, are produced by tiny tear glands in the upper eyelid.

Lens
These long fibre cells are pulled fatter or thinner by tiny muscles (ciliary bodies) to focus light very precisely on to the retina. The lens becomes stiffer with age and cannot focus so well on distant objects. If the lens becomes cloudy, it is called a cataract.

Choroid
Blood vessels in the choroid supply the retina and surrounding tissues with nutrients and oxygen.

Sclera
The opaque white of the eye forms the rest of the eyeball. Muscles attach to it that move the eye around in its bony socket.

Retina
This light-sensitive layer contains thousands of light receptors called rods and cones. Rods work in low light conditions, and relay information about light and dark. Cones, on the other hand, need a lot of light in order to work and can detect colour.

Vitreous humour
This jelly-like substance fills the back of the eyeball.

Optic nerve
These nerves in each eye join at the optic chiasma – and carry signals from the retina to the visual cortex in the back of the brain.

Blind spot
This part of the retina – where blood vessels and the optic nerve exit – has no cones or rods.

Macula
The area of the retina responsible for the most detailed vision. Its centre (the fovea) has the highest density of cones and so is the most sensitive spot.

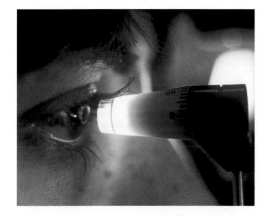

△ This test is used by an ophthalmologist to check for glaucoma. The instrument is an applanation tonometer, it gently presses the eye to give an indication of its internal pressure.

surgery to correct impaired vision caused by these conditions.

Glaucoma can be treated if caught early on, but damage is often irreversible, and treatment focuses on trying to prevent any further deterioration.

OPHTHALMOLOGY

An ophthalmologist should check all parts of the eye: the eyelids and the skin around the eyes, as well as using ophthalmic instruments, such as a slit-lamp microscope, to check for internal disorders. The movement of the eye, the vision fields and the pressure within the eye should also be

checked. A regular check-up will probably involve a vision acuity test to detect signs of long or short sight in either or both eyes.

FIND YOUR BLIND SPOT

With your left eye shut, look at the cross with your right eye and move closer to the page. The dot disappears when its image falls on to your blind spot.

Conjunctivitis

SEE ALSO
➤ Hayfever and perennial rhinitis, p172
➤ Causes of infectious disease, p214
➤ Autoimmune diseases, p211

Conjunctivitis is the name given to an inflammation of the conjunctiva – the thin layer of cells that lines the front of the eye and the inside of the eyelids. This condition can cause a lot of discomfort but is rarely serious and often looks worse than it actually is. Conjunctivitis is usually caused by an infection; other causes include allergies, most notably hayfever, which can produce serious swelling of the conjunctiva. Like any viral infection, viral conjunctivitis does not respond to antibiotic treatment but usually clears up naturally in a few days.

SIGNS AND SYMPTOMS

The first time you notice conjunctivitis symptoms is likely to be when you wake up in the morning. It is usual for both eyes to be affected, with any of the following symptoms:

➤ The whites of the eyes become red and inflamed.

➤ Stinging, itchy or watering eyes.

➤ A gritty or uncomfortable sensation in the eyes.

➤ The eyelids may become stuck together with discharge.

The commonest causes of conjunctivitis are:
• Infection – Bacteria, and more commonly viruses, can cause conjunctivitis.
• Allergy – There are a number of factors that can cause allergic conjunctivitis, the most common being pollen.
• Irritants – Irritant chemicals in make-up, contact lens solution and some eye-drops can inflame the conjunctiva. Other irritants include dust, smoke, pollution and ultraviolet light.

DRY EYE SYNDROME

If your eyes feel dry and gritty, it may be due to decreased tear production. The most common cause is old age, but it can occur in people with autoimmune conditions such as rheumatoid arthritis or SLE. You can restore moisture levels with drops called "artificial tears".

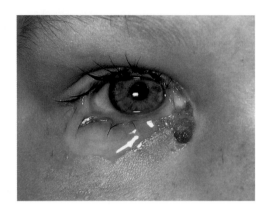

△ Severe bacterial conjunctivitis can cause great discomfort and a heavy discharge of water or pus, as seen here. Bacterial conjunctivitis usually responds well to antibiotic treatment.

The conjunctiva heals quickly, so most problems settle down with treatment or if the causative factor is removed.

MAKING A DIAGNOSIS

Your doctor will examine your eyes and try to establish a cause. If infection is suspected, antibiotic ointment or eye-drops are prescribed; if the likely cause is an allergy, anti-allergy eye-drops will help. Other types usually clear up in 5 to 7 days.

SIMPLE SELF-HELP MEASURES

An infection such as conjunctivitis is easily spread from hand to eye so it is important to pay close attention to hygiene to ensure you do not spread infection or pass it on to someone else:
• Use separate face cloths or towels; do not share them.
• Wash your hands after bathing your eyes or touching them.
• Bathe your eyes with warm water or with artificial tear eye-drops.

CORNEAL ULCERS

The most common cause of this condition is when a foreign body, such as a tiny piece of grit, gets into the eye and scratches the conjunctiva, exposing the underlying cornea. It can be extremely painful but once the foreign body has been removed, the conjunctiva heals itself within a few days. Other possible causes include:

➤ Viral infections, such as herpes simplex or shingles.

➤ Severe blepharitis.

➤ Acids and alkalis can cause large corneal ulcers if accidentally splashed into the eye. The eye must be washed with copious amounts of saline, water or eyewash to minimize damage. Medical help must be sought as a matter of urgency.

People who wear contact lenses are susceptible to these ulcers and should take great care with eye hygiene.

▽ Corneal ulcers affect the outer layer of the cornea. Doctors can identify the affected area by introducing a coloured dye to the eye. A corneal ulcer can be seen, stained green, in the picture below.

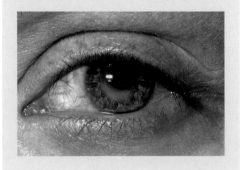

Styes

SEE ALSO
➤ Diabetes, p66
➤ How the eyes function, p178
➤ Blepharitis, below

Common styes are pus-filled swellings (abscesses) of the eyelash hair follicles. They can cause the eyelid to become inflamed and painful, usually because the small head of pus stretches the follicle and the surrounding skin. Most styes are caused by infection with *Staphylococcus aureus* bacteria and can be spread easily to other eyelash follicles. Antibiotic cream usually cures the infection, but recurrent styes can be a sign of general ill-health and occasionally of even more serious conditions such as diabetes, so medical advice should be sought if the problem persists.

SIGNS AND SYMPTOMS

You may first notice a stye as a slight red lump on the edge of your eyelid, but it will then swell up, become very painful and the eyelid will grow red and inflamed.

A stye will usually rupture, drain and heal within a few days. If it persists or becomes worse, then visit your doctor, because some antibiotic eye ointment may be necessary.

SIMPLE SELF-HELP MEASURES

Whether you have a stye or are suffering from blepharitis, there are ways to ease the discomfort and speed up recovery. Doctors offer the following advice:
• Place a clean, warm, damp washcloth on your eye and leave for about 20 minutes. Repeat this cleansing and soothing treatment three or four times a day.
• Avoid spreading infection by not sharing towels or cloths with others, and washing your hands after touching your eyes.

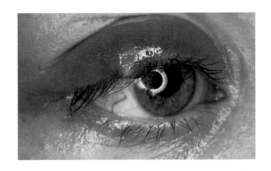

△ Styes are caused by a swelling in the gland at the base of an eyelash hair. A pus-filled abscess develops at the centre of the stye and the whole eyelid is affected.

Blepharitis

SEE ALSO
➤ Styes, above

In this condition, which may affect one or both eyes, the edges of the eyelids become inflamed and sore, and scaly skin may develop at the base of the eyelashes. Blepharitis may be caused by an allergic reaction to make-up, dust or smoke, or by a bacterial infection.

This condition is not easy to get rid of and even with the right treatment it may take many days to show an improvement. The best approach is regular, gentle cleaning of the edges of the eyelid with warm water, to remove the caked-on crusts. Once you have had blepharitis it is likely to recur, so take great care with eye hygiene. People who

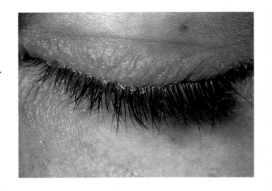

△ Blepharitis is characterized by inflammation of the upper eyelid along with scaly skin at the edges of the lid.

have dandruff and eczema seem to be prone to blepharitis, perhaps because they have dry, sensitive skin.

SIGNS AND SYMPTOMS

Your eye may be sticky and crusts may appear on the lashes. Your eyelids will be swollen, red and itchy, and sometimes a stye may develop at the same time.

EYELID DISORDERS

In entropion, the eyelid turns in so that lashes rub the cornea and conjunctiva, causing irritation and, in severe cases, corneal ulceration. It can be present at birth (but usually clears up after a few months) and it affects older people.

In ectropion, the lower lid turns out and exposes its inner surface, which becomes dry and sore. This condition is most common in older people.

Both conditions risk damaging the cornea and may require minor surgery, to realign the eyelids.

Short sight (myopia)

Myopia sufferers can focus on nearby objects clearly but have difficulty focusing on objects in the distance, so their vision is blurred and fuzzy. The condition is caused by variations in the structure of the eyeball – such as the distance from the cornea to the retina, or the focusing power of the cornea. Short sight can be corrected by wearing concave lenses (see diagram below), in the form of either glasses or contact lenses. It is also – increasingly – corrected by laser surgery, which flattens the curve of the cornea to solve the problem.

Short sight is rare in children under the age of six, but vision will often change very rapidly during the teenage years. It seems to be that the earlier a person develops short sight, the more severe it becomes with age. In cases where sight deteriorates rapidly, the eyes will be tested and glasses may need to be changed every six months.

If you wear glasses, it is essential that you visit an ophthalmologist so your eyes can be checked for symptoms of other conditions. People with myopia are more prone to retinal detachment, glaucoma and macular degeneration, so it is important to tackle these problems as soon as they arise.

RETINAL DETACHMENT

Short-sighted people are more susceptible to this condition which is where the photoreceptor layer of the retina peels away from its blood supply. It can result in partial or complete blindness. If your retina detaches you might notice flashes of light or new "floaters" (tiny marks in your field of vision which everyone experiences to a certain degree).

If you have the impression of a dark curtain or shadow in one eye you should see a doctor as soon as possible.

▽ This is a refractor – a complex piece of equipment used by opticians to measure eye function very precisely and so determine the right lenses to correct any defects.

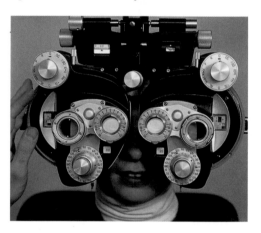

NORMAL FOCUSING

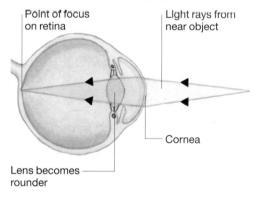

Point of focus on retina

Light rays from near object

Lens becomes rounder

Cornea

Point of focus on retina

Light rays from distant object

The lens is longer and thinner

△ The cornea bends light on to the lens. The lens changes shape to bend light to a greater or lesser degree, depending on the distance of the object, so that a sharp image is formed on the retina.

HOW THE EYE FOCUSES

Light rays are directed on to the retina via the cornea and lens, through a process called accommodation. This is the process by which the ciliary muscles push and pull the lens into different shapes to change the angle of the light rays entering the eye. To focus on distant objects, the lens needs to be long and thin in order to bend light accurately on to the retina; to focus on closer objects, the lens becomes rounder. Focusing depends on the focusing power of the cornea and lens as well as the distance from the cornea to the retina – the length of the eyeball.

LASER EYE SURGERY

Surgery can be carried out to remove a small piece of the cornea, making it flatter, and so can restore vision in people with mild short sight. Laser-assisted in-situ keratomileusis (LASIK) is the most widely used method, but is not suitable for everyone with short sight.

MYOPIC FOCUSING

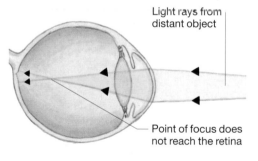

Light rays from distant object

Point of focus does not reach the retina

△ If the distance from cornea to retina is longer than normal, the lens focuses distant objects just short of the retina, causing a blurred image.

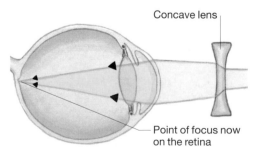

Concave lens

Point of focus now on the retina

△ Concave lenses are used to correct myopia. These lenses bend light outwards and so help to focus the image on the retina, not in front of it.

Long sight (hypermetropia)

SEE ALSO

➤ Routine health checks, p24

➤ High blood pressure, p30

➤ Diabetes, p66

People with long sight, or hypermetropia, are able to focus on distant objects but struggle to focus on those closer to them. Reading can be particularly problematic. The condition is more common in older people, because the elasticity of the lens declines naturally with age.

Hypermetropia can be caused by the shape of a person's eyeball, where the focal length of the eye is too short, or by the ability of the cornea and lens to focus light on to the retina. Convex lenses (see diagram below) are normally used to correct this focusing error.

PRESBYOPIA

This form of long sight is caused by the lens becoming stiffer and less able to focus on near objects. Presbyopia is particularly associated with aging – it affects everyone to some extent as they get older, which is why so many people start to wear reading glasses from around their mid-40s.

▽ The focusing ability of the eyes changes with age, but lenses are able to correct even very severe sight problems.

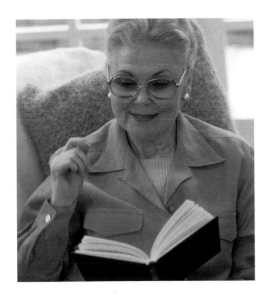

EYE TESTS

Regular eye tests, carried out by a qualified ophthalmic optician or optometrist, are vital for people who already wear glasses, as an incorrect prescription may cause blurred vision, headaches and/or migraines. However, even if you do not wear glasses, it is advisable to have an eye test every couple of years because eyesight deteriorates so gradually. Good vision is especially vital for people who drive regularly.

As well as assessing your sight, your optician checks the general health of your eyes to assess any ongoing conditions.

➤ Sight check – To test how well the eyes work together (sometimes using a Snellen chart and phoropter).

➤ Ocular examination – Using an instrument called an ophthalmoscope, to inspect the optic nerve, retina and lens. Early signs of diabetic retinopathy, damage from high blood pressure or macular degeneration can be picked up during this examination.

➤ Pressure check – Using a tonometer to measure the pressure within the eyeball. Raised pressure can indicate glaucoma, which needs to be treated promptly to avoid further damage to the optic nerve and loss of sight.

➤ Examination of the eyelids, lashes and cornea, using a slit lamp.

➤ Visual field test – To check there are no areas of missing vision.

People with diabetes should have an eye test at least once a year and may need more regular checks and treatments if diabetic changes occur in their eyes. This test usually includes dilating the pupils with a special chemical, so that the optometrist can examine the back of their eyes.

Many problems affecting the eyes can be treated as long as they are detected promptly, so it is a good idea to visit a doctor or optician as soon as you notice any problem with your eyes.

ASTIGMATISM

A normal cornea is curved like the surface of a ball, but sometimes the cornea is not perfectly round and has flat areas. This condition is known as astigmatism, and the abnormal shape of the cornea means that the eyes can focus on either vertical lines or horizontal ones, but not both at the same time. The problem can be corrected totally by wearing the right kind of lenses.

HYPERMETROPIC FOCUSING

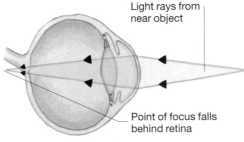

Light rays from near object

Point of focus falls behind retina

△ For someone with long sight (hypermetropia), images of close objects appear blurred. This is because their eyeball is shorter than normal or the cornea is weak.

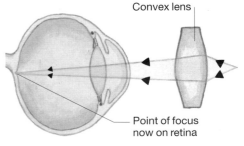

Convex lens

Point of focus now on retina

△ A convex lens can be used to correct long sight. This lens bends light more before it reaches the eye, so that a sharp image is focused on the retina.

Cataracts

SEE ALSO

➤ Smoking and your health, p20
➤ Diabetes, p66
➤ Eye tests, p183
➤ Viral infections, p218

Cataract is the term used when a lens becomes cloudy or opaque, causing blurred vision. In the West, the most common cause of cataracts is aging, as the fibres that make up the lens deteriorate naturally over time. Cataracts are found in 75 per cent of people over 65. It is usual for both eyes to be affected, but one eye will tend to have more severe vision problems than the other. The changes to the lens fibres are irreversible, but cataracts rarely cause total blindness; even in severe cases, sufferers can usually distinguish light from darkness.

SIGNS AND SYMPTOMS

Typical symptoms include the following:

➤ Blurring and gradual loss of vision.

➤ Objects have blurred edges as light is "scattered" by the opaque lens.

➤ Deterioration in colour vision so that dimmer colours are seen.

If you have a cataract in just one eye, you may have difficulty judging distances. Also, cataract-sufferers who wear glasses may find that their prescription keeps changing.

The lens of the eye consists of elongated fibre cells. In a cataract, changes in these cells' proteins cause the normally transparent lens to become cloudy or opaque. The transparency of the lens is crucial in allowing light through it and into the eye. Any cloudiness restricts and scatters light entering the eye and therefore affects how well a person can see.

CAUSES OF CATARACTS

The majority of cataracts are simply a sign of aging, and most sufferers from the condition are over the age of 65. However, there can be other causes for cataracts. These include:

• Diabetes – Diabetes mellitus can cause complications in the eyes and anyone with cataracts will have blood or urine tests to check sugar levels.
• Rubella – If a pregnant woman has rubella (German measles) it can cause cataracts in her baby.
• Eye injury.
• Prolonged exposure to sunlight.
• Ionizing radiation, including X-rays.
• Long-term steroid drug therapy.
• Smoking.

DIAGNOSING CATARACTS

A cataract can affect just one eye, in which case the sufferer may well be aware of a difference between the vision in each of the eyes. If your doctor or optometrist suspects that a variation in vision is caused by a cataract, your eyes will be examined with an ophthalmoscope. An optometrist may also use a slit-lamp microscope and dilate your pupils with eye-drops to allow a more thorough examination.

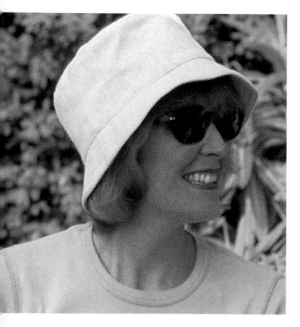

◁ Prolonged exposure to harmful ultraviolet rays in sunlight is one of the causes of cataracts. Wearing sunglasses and a hat will help to protect your eyes.

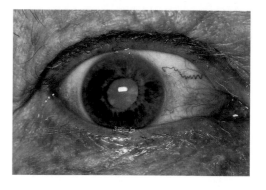

△ Cataracts are usually easy to diagnose – the normally transparent lens of the eye appears clouded or "milky".

HOW ARE CATARACTS TREATED?

Your cataracts may only be treated when the loss of vision seriously disrupts your life, and this obviously varies from person to person. For example, a 50-year-old lorry driver with only minor cloudiness of the lens will need treatment but an 80-year-old who doesn't read much may be relatively unaffected by fairly advanced cataracts.

Currently, no treatment exists for restoring the transparency of the lens once cataracts have appeared. The only treatment available to cure cataracts is an operation to remove the affected lens and replace it with an artificial one. In the most advanced technique – called phako-emulsification – a small incision is made in the cornea and the lens sac. The lens is broken up, using an ultrasound probe, and is sucked out. A replacement soft lens is then positioned within the lens sac. For most people, this operation is done under local anaesthetic as a day-case procedure. You may need to wear glasses for driving or watching television after this operation.

Glaucoma

SEE ALSO

➤ Diabetes, p66
➤ Diseases of the thyroid gland, p68
➤ Parkinson's disease, p92
➤ Short sight, p182

Glaucoma is the name given to conditions in which the optic nerve is damaged at the point where it leaves the retina at the back of the eye. The cause of the damage is usually raised pressure from the fluids within the eyeball. Glaucoma can occur suddenly (acute glaucoma), but it is more usual for the condition to develop gradually over a period of years (chronic glaucoma). Untreated glaucoma is a major cause of blindness, but regular check-ups can detect the condition in its early stages, when it can easily be treated.

SIGNS AND SYMPTOMS

Obvious symptoms tend not to appear until glaucoma is well developed, so regular check-ups are vital. For example, testing may reveal patterns in a person's field of vision that suggest glaucoma, even in the early stages. The individual would not notice this themselves because, initially, areas of visual loss are filled in by the two eyes' overlapping visual fields.

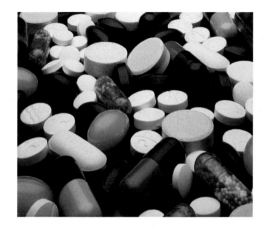

△ Some drugs such as antidepressants or those prescribed for Parkinson's disease may exacerbate an existing glaucoma.

Glaucoma usually affects both eyes, although one eye tends to be worse than the other, and it slowly destroys vision. If glaucoma is left untreated, it causes blindness. In the West, glaucoma affects 1 in 50 people over 40. Chronic glaucoma accounts for 90 per cent of glaucoma cases in the developed world.

HOW PRESSURE BUILDS UP

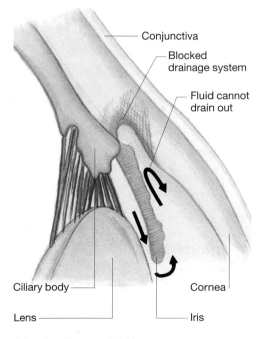

Conjunctiva

Blocked drainage system

Fluid cannot drain out

Ciliary body

Lens

Cornea

Iris

△ In a healthy eye, fluid known as aqueous humour circulates between the cornea and the iris. If a blockage occurs, the fluid cannot circulate. This creates a build-up of pressure, resulting in glaucoma.

CAUSES OF GLAUCOMA

Glaucoma may be due to high pressure in the eye affecting the blood supply to the optic nerves, causing damage to nerve fibres as they leave the eyes. Pressure within the eye is created by the level of a liquid called aqueous humour, which maintains the shape of the eye. This liquid is produced and drained at a certain rate in order to maintain the right pressure. Abnormally high pressure in the eye is caused by blockages or faulty draining of the eye via the trabecular meshwork (drainage system).

WHO IS MOST AT RISK?

Groups that are at risk of developing glaucoma include:

• People with a family history of glaucoma.
• People over 80 years old – One in ten suffer from the condition.
• Short-sighted people.
• Diabetics.
• Thyroid eye disease sufferers.

At-risk groups need to have regular eye checks to monitor their intraocular pressures, the appearance of their optic nerves and visual fields.

TREATMENT OPTIONS

Treatment aims to control the condition by reducing pressure in the eye, which can usually be done simply by using eye-drops. These drops ease the pressure by either improving the circulation of the fluid within the eye or decreasing its rate of production. If these treatments fail, there are surgical or laser options to increase the circulation of the fluid within the eye. There is, however, no cure for the optic nerve damage, which is permanent.

ACUTE GLAUCOMA

This rare form of glaucoma needs urgent treatment to prevent loss of vision. It occurs because of a sudden blockage to the drainage of fluid within the eye. It usually occurs in one eye, which becomes red and painful; the iris may also bulge forwards. Your vision becomes blurred, your pupils may be fixed and dilated, and you may feel sick and see coloured halos around lights. Acute glaucoma tends to occur in middle-aged people with long sight and it affects four times as many women as men.

Macular degeneration

This condition is generally age-related and commonly affects older people, although there is a juvenile form. It is due to degeneration of the light-sensitive cone cells in the macular area of the retina. The macula is the site of your most sensitive vision in terms of detail and colour. In macular degeneration there is a gradual loss of visual details and of the central field of vision (in contrast to glaucoma, where sight at the outer edges of the visual field is lost). It can affect both eyes, but usually one eye is affected a few weeks before the other.

SIGNS AND SYMPTOMS

Macular degeneration may cause:

➤ Difficulty in focusing on the text in a book.

➤ Inability to recognize faces easily.

➤ Problems making out details when watching television.

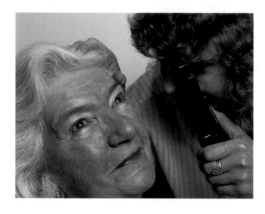

Sandwiched between the choroid and the retina of the eye lies a protective insulating layer. With age, this layer may develop defects that allow some of the eye's fluid to escape into the retina itself. This fluid can then cause progressive damage to the sensitive rods and cones that are key to producing clear, recognizable images – a disorder known as macular degeneration.

WHAT IS THE MACULA?

The macula is a very small but highly sensitive area in the centre of the retina. Its function is specifically to allow you to focus on objects in the centre of your field of vision. Macular degeneration results in increasing loss of sight in this central area, but the outer edges of the field of vision will be relatively unaffected.

SPOTTING THE CONDITION

It is not always easy to spot the signs of macular degeneration, because the deterioration can happen very slowly and gradually over a period of several years. However, if you notice a gap or distortion in your central field of vision you should seek immediate medical advice.

WHAT MIGHT YOUR DOCTOR DO?

Your doctor or optometrist may be able to identify changes in the macular region of the retina when inspecting your eye with

◁ Macular degeneration often occurs as part of the aging process. An ophthalmologist will test for the condition by examining the interior of the eye to check for changes in the macula.

an ophthalmoscope. Further tests are sometimes done to assess the extent of the damage and include a procedure called fluorescein angiography, in which pictures of the blood vessels in the eye are taken.

Laser eye treatment can be helpful in some cases, although it can only halt the progress of the disorder, rather than reversing damage that has already been done. For most people, however, this condition is untreatable.

THE STRUCTURE OF THE RETINA

At the centre of eye function is the light-sensitive layer at the back of the eye called the retina. The retina is made up of specialized cells – called rods and cones – that produce electrical signals when exposed to light. These signals then travel along the optic nerve to the brain, where they are processed.

Rods

These cells are sensitive to light, and several share one connection to the brain. They work in low light conditions and relay information only in black and white. Rods are sensitive to movement, but do not give a very sharp image. They are concentrated at the edges of the retina, hence the ability to see movement out of the corner of your eye.

▷ This picture shows the microscopic light-sensitive cells of the retina – rods (blue) and cones (blue-green).

Cones

These cells respond to colours – red, blue and green – and each cell has its own connection to the brain. They produce sharp colour images but only work well in high light intensities. Cones cluster in the centre of the retina, especially at the point where the lens focuses an image – the macula.

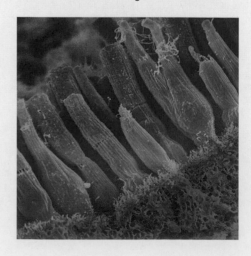

THE SKIN

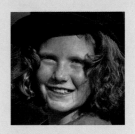

The skin is the largest organ in the human body. Able to heal and renew itself continuously, it also provides an essential heat-regulation system for the body, as well as providing it with a covering and protection from infection. This front-line exposure, however, means that your skin is vulnerable to damage from various outside elements, particularly the sun. Human skin is exceptionally sensitive to both internal and external changes and stimuli. This sensitivity is a wonderful quality in many ways, but any disruption to it can lead to many different kinds of problems, from irritant or allergic reactions to stress-related rashes.

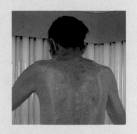

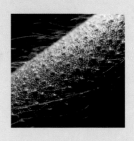

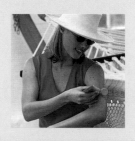

CONTENTS

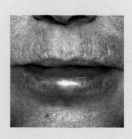

The functions of the skin

SEE ALSO
➤ Travel health and safety, p26
➤ Skin cancers, p194

The skin is the body's largest organ because, on average, it measures an impressive 2 m² (21½ ft²). Your skin cells are constantly growing, dying and replacing themselves so that this organ can keep doing its main job efficiently – keeping out potentially harmful micro-organisms such as bacteria. Kept waterproof and supple by an oily substance called sebum, your skin helps to control body temperature and to shield you from the harmful effects of the sun. Its receptors also give you all kinds of sensory information about the world around you.

The skin is composed of two layers – the epidermis and the dermis.

• Epidermis – This upper layer of your skin is made of sheets of dead cells. Cells at the base of the epidermis continually grow, divide and migrate to the surface. As they travel upwards, they fill with a tough, fibrous protein called keratin, which gives skin its strength and suppleness. (Your hair and nails are also made principally of keratin, and so are considered to be closely allied to skin.) By the time they reach the surface, the skin cells are dead and are then shed as flakes of skin, making way for new skin. The epidermis also contains cells called melanocytes. These make the pigment melanin, which is responsible for filtering ultraviolet (UV) light from the sun (see below) and also gives your skin its colour.

• Dermis – This lower layer is made of strong elastic tissue. The dermis contains all the blood vessels, nerves, lymph vessels, sweat glands, sebaceous glands, hair follicles, muscle fibres and receptors

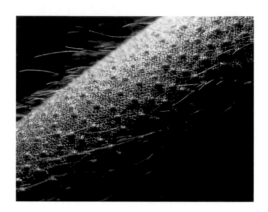

△ This close-up image of the epidermis on the arm shows "goosebumps" and erectile hairs. These hairs trap warm air – part of the skin's way of controlling body temperature.

(sensitive organs that detect touch, pressure, heat and cold) that supply and support the epidermis. The cells that repair any damage are also found here.

CONTROLLING BODY TEMPERATURE

As well as protecting the body's internal organs from the outside world, the skin has another vitally important function – helping to control body temperature. If your body becomes too hot, then the blood vessels in the dermis widen to disperse the heat, and sweat glands release perspiration to cool you down. If the body starts to get too cold, the blood vessels become narrower to hold on to the warm blood, and hairs all over your skin stand on end to trap a layer of warm air around your body.

THE SUN AND YOUR SKIN

Most of us love to be out in the sunshine and the sun does have beneficial effects, but its ultraviolet radiation can also do great damage to the skin. The skin's pigment, melanin, reduces the amount of UV that can reach the dermis, but this is often not enough. Even the indigenous populations of very hot climates, whose dark skin means that they have high levels of filtering melanin, can still suffer from sunburn if over-exposed to the sun. As its name suggests, sunburn can be a serious burn and, apart from being very painful, can cause scarring and premature aging of the skin.

Regularly exposing your skin to the sun with no or insufficient protection can quickly lead to damage that may go much deeper into the skin's layers than you might expect. UV light can trigger a cancer of your skin's pigment-producing cells – called a

▽ Prolonged exposure to the sun can have long-term effects on the skin. It is essential to use sunscreens to protect it from damage – especially if you are fair-skinned.

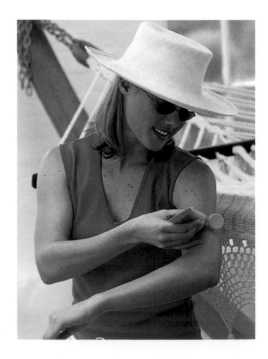

BE SAFE IN THE SUN

It is wise during the summer months to stay out of direct sunlight between the hours of 10 am and 4 pm. If you are out in the sun there are three main ways to avoid damage to your skin:

➤ Wear a T-shirt.

➤ Put on a wide-brimmed hat.

➤ Apply sunscreen regularly.

THE STRUCTURE OF THE SKIN

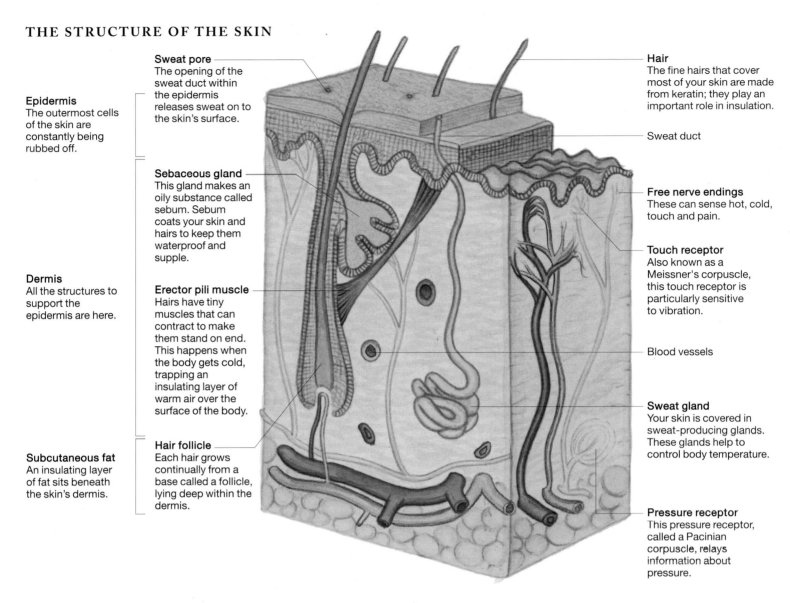

Epidermis
The outermost cells of the skin are constantly being rubbed off.

Dermis
All the structures to support the epidermis are here.

Subcutaneous fat
An insulating layer of fat sits beneath the skin's dermis.

Sweat pore
The opening of the sweat duct within the epidermis releases sweat on to the skin's surface.

Sebaceous gland
This gland makes an oily substance called sebum. Sebum coats your skin and hairs to keep them waterproof and supple.

Erector pili muscle
Hairs have tiny muscles that can contract to make them stand on end. This happens when the body gets cold, trapping an insulating layer of warm air over the surface of the body.

Hair follicle
Each hair grows continually from a base called a follicle, lying deep within the dermis.

Hair
The fine hairs that cover most of your skin are made from keratin; they play an important role in insulation.

Sweat duct

Free nerve endings
These can sense hot, cold, touch and pain.

Touch receptor
Also known as a Meissner's corpuscle, this touch receptor is particularly sensitive to vibration.

Blood vessels

Sweat gland
Your skin is covered in sweat-producing glands. These glands help to control body temperature.

Pressure receptor
This pressure receptor, called a Pacinian corpuscle, relays information about pressure.

malignant melanoma. This cancer is responsible for a large number of deaths worldwide each year. However, it can be cured if it is caught early enough – prompt detection is the key.

The message is simple: Always cover up properly with creams, hats and other clothing in strong or prolonged sun – especially if you are fair. Research has shown that several episodes of serious sunburn in childhood can lead to cancer later in life, so keep babies and children well protected.

UV BENEFITS

UV light does, however, bring some good news. A certain amount of UV is vital to body processes and the UV light that does penetrate the skin is crucial to production of Vitamin D, which is in turn essential for strong bones.

TACKLING SKIN COMPLAINTS

The skin's role as protector of the body from infection and injury means that it is exposed to a wide range of dangers, including viral and bacterial infection and various allergens and irritants. Many skin conditions manifest themselves as rashes or raised red marks and typical symptoms include itchiness and sore or broken skin.

While skin diseases are often distressing and uncomfortable, they are rarely fatal. Most, including the many rashes whose cause is never discovered, can be relieved by topical steroid or antibiotic creams, and sometimes with tablets. The psychological impact of some skin diseases should never be underestimated when devising treatment – an unsightly rash on the face or some other visible part of the body can cause the sufferer great anxiety.

DIAGNOSING SKIN CONDITIONS

Your doctor will ask you about your symptoms and then examine the affected area of skin. A magnifying glass may be used for a detailed examination, and a swab may be taken if there is any weepiness or fluid. The samples will be sent to a laboratory for analysis to try to establish the underlying cause.

Many skin conditions will disappear without treatment over a period of time. It is advisable, however, to seek medical advice if a problem is persistent or is particularly troublesome or painful, as some skin conditions can develop into more serious complaints and are sometimes indicative of more general underlying problems and ill-health.

Eczema (dermatitis)

SEE ALSO

➤ Asthma, p130
➤ Hayfever and perennial rhinitis, p172

Eczema, or dermatitis, refers to a family of diseases that usually inflame the skin, making it dry and itchy; there may also be small blisters. The cause often remains a mystery, although an allergy may be to blame. Infection is common because the skin easily becomes very dry, scaly and cracked, allowing micro-organisms to enter. Eczema can affect any part of the body, but is most commonly found on the hands, legs and feet. Treatment focuses on soothing the itching and preventing scratching – using ointment and perhaps dressings or wearing cotton gloves.

SIGNS AND SYMPTOMS

➤ Dry, scaly and cracked skin.

➤ Red and inflamed skin.

➤ Itchiness and irritation.

➤ Fluid-filled blisters, also known as vesicles, which can burst, causing "weeping".

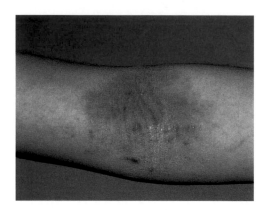

△ Atopic eczema (pictured) can occur without any identifiable cause and often develops in skin creases at joints. It is usually treated with emollient or antibiotic ointments.

There are several different types of eczema:

• Atopic eczema – This usually starts in childhood and is related to other diseases such as hayfever and asthma. It tends to improve as the child gets older, and can usually be managed using emollients (hydrating creams), but persistent cases may need short courses of steroid cream.

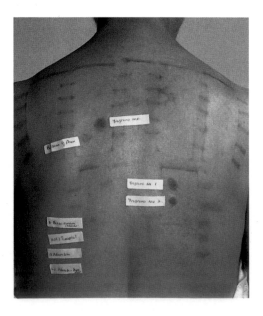

▽ An allergy patch test. Small amounts of common allergy-producing substances are applied to light scratches on the skin, to find out which ones, if any, are causing reactions.

• Irritant-induced eczema – This tends to affect the hands, which can become red, sore and cracked. Detergents, soaps, oils, acids, alkalis and solvents are common causes. If contact with the irritant cannot be avoided, wearing gloves or applying emollient cream will help.

• Allergic contact eczema – With this form, the reaction to an irritant lasts longer and can be triggered by minimum exposure. Common culprits are dyes, nickel (in gold and zips), chromium (in leather), lanolin (in cosmetics), resins and certain plants (such as ragweed). Often, the reaction is restricted to the area in contact with the irritant, for example in a band around a finger under a nickel-containing ring. Patch-testing of the skin may be able to uncover the cause. Avoidance of the irritant is the best solution, although topical steroid creams also work well.

• Seborrhoeic eczema – This affects areas of skin rich in sebaceous glands, such as the face, scalp and joint creases. Steroid creams are useful, but should not be used on the face. Coconut oil is helpful for soothing itchy scalps.

PATCH TESTING

To find out what is triggering your allergic reaction, a dermatologist applies small strips or discs containing allergy-provoking substances to your skin. Two days later, results are assessed. Red, inflamed patches indicate the cause of your eczema.

TREATMENT OPTIONS

The mainstays of treatment are:

➤ Emollients – These help to keep moisture locked into the skin; creams can be used, or special products can be added to the bath.

➤ Corticosteroid (steroid) creams – These are effective in reducing inflammation. However, if used in excess or for too long, they can make the skin thin and fragile. They must be used very sparingly on the face and only if prescribed by a doctor.

➤ Steroid ointments – These moisture-retaining, water-repelling ointments are useful in treating eczema.

➤ Antibiotic creams – These creams may be helpful where there is evidence of infection, particularly if combined with steroid creams.

➤ Steroid drugs – These are needed very rarely and only in the most severe cases of eczema.

Psoriasis

This is a common skin complaint, found all over the world. Psoriasis can strike at any age and the cause remains unknown. The condition produces areas of red, thickened skin known as plaques, which may have a covering of silvery scales and are often itchy and painful. These plaques can occur anywhere, but are most commonly found on the backs of the elbows, on the knees and in the scalp; they may also develop on scar tissue. In affected areas, the epidermis layer of the skin produces new cells at a much faster rate than normal – hence the thickening.

SIGNS AND SYMPTOMS

➤ Areas of red, inflamed, thickened skin.

➤ Flaky skin – often silvery in colour.

➤ Pitted or discoloured nails.

➤ Pain in the joints.

➤ Occasionally the infected area will produce a sterile pus.

Stress, physical injury, infection and some drugs, such as lithium and beta-blockers, can trigger psoriasis, although the precise cause of this skin problem is unknown. Many psoriasis sufferers have a family history of the condition. In some rare cases, the condition can be associated with an arthritis, similar to rheumatoid arthritis, known as psoriatic arthritis.

Although it can be distressing and cause great discomfort, only the most severe cases of psoriasis are life-threatening. If the thickened plaques appear across large areas of skin, then the condition may interfere with the body's all-important heat regulation mechanisms and a potentially dangerous rise in body temperature could occur. Such patients need specialist treatment in hospital, so medical advice should be sought as early as possible if psoriasis seems to be spreading.

As with many skin conditions, cases where the problem is widespread may cause the sufferer a great deal of embarrassment and anxiety – especially if the face is affected in any way. In these instances, the sufferer may well be referred for psychological counselling.

TREATING PSORIASIS

There is no cure, so the various treatments are aimed at controlling the condition:

• Steroid creams rapidly improve psoriasis; unfortunately psoriasis quickly returns once treatment is stopped.

• Coal tar preparations and dithranol (originally from the Indian Goa tree) have formed the backbone of psoriasis treatment for decades and are very effective. The strength of the cream is slowly increased until an effective dose for an individual's psoriasis is found. These preparations can be unpleasant to use and they stain clothing or bedding.

• Vitamin D derivatives have been developed as alternatives to coal tar and are now generally preferred because they do not smell or stain skin or clothes and are usually effective.

▽ This picture shows an area of skin affected by psoriasis. Typical cases cause red, inflamed skin that may also be scaly and itchy. There may be stiffness in joints – knees or elbows are commonly affected by the condition.

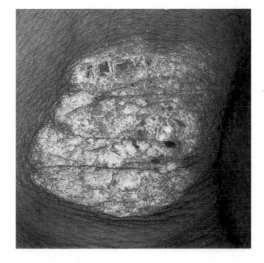

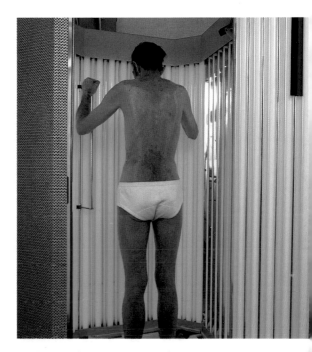

△ Ultraviolet radiation therapy may be used for chronic cases of psoriasis. However, this treatment can prematurely age the skin and studies suggest that it increases the risk of skin cancer, so it is prescribed with caution.

• Ultraviolet (UV) light treatment can be very effective when psoriasis is affecting large areas of the body. However, UV light ages the skin and may increase the risk of skin cancer so this treatment is usually only recommended for people suffering from very severe psoriasis.

• Powerful drugs, such as the anticancer drug methotrexate or the immuno-suppressant cyclosporin, are sometimes prescribed for severe cases of psoriasis. Like UV treatment, however, these drugs can produce various problematic side effects and so patients taking them should always be very closely monitored by their doctor.

Urticaria

SEE ALSO

➤ Learn to manage stress, p12

➤ Eczema (dermatitis), p190

Urticaria, also known as hives or nettle rash, produces itchy red weals, usually caused by an allergic reaction. It may also be provoked by infections and physical stimuli such as cold, pressure, heat or stress. In most cases, no definite cause can be pinpointed. Urticaria tends to develop fast – sometimes within just a few minutes – and can occur anywhere on the body. It can vary in severity, appearing as a small patch or covering the entire surface of the body, and lasting from a few minutes to a few hours. It usually clears up without treatment.

Conditions associated with this skin complaint include dermographism (see below) and angioedema. Angioedema is a sudden and severe swelling of the mouth, eyes and tongue. It may sometimes affect the throat, which in turn can give rise to breathing difficulties that need emergency care, so always seek medical advice urgently. Urticaria is an extension of the allergic response and may occur at the same time as anaphylactic shock (a life-threatening allergic reaction).

WHAT YOUR DOCTOR MIGHT DO

It is often difficult to pinpoint the exact cause of urticaria. Your doctor may arrange a skin-prick test, using potentially allergenic substances, to see if any of these might be the culprit. This is a common diagnostic step for many skin complaints. It should be remembered, however, that this form of testing may yield no positive results.

Urticaria usually disappears on its own within the space of a few hours. Recurrent

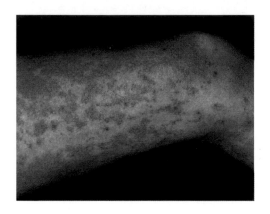

△ The hundreds of small, raised weals on the skin that indicate urticaria are often caused by stress but can also be the result of a severe allergic reaction.

sufferers often find the condition distressing and may be prescribed antihistamine tablets (which can produce side effects such as drowsiness). Prolonged attacks of urticaria may respond well to steroid drugs.

▽ Swelling of the mouth's soft tissue is a typical symptom of angioedema. This condition is similar to urticaria and is usually caused by an allergic reaction to foods or insect bites. It can cause difficulty in breathing, so seek medical help urgently (this usually involves treatment with anti-inflammatory drugs or antihistamines).

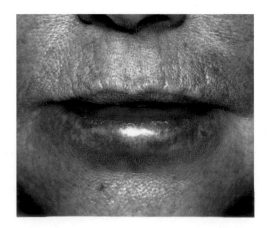

CHRONIC URTICARIA

In some cases, urticaria persists for weeks or months. Such chronic urticaria is very common and it can be impossible to find the cause – to the frustration of the patient and doctor alike. Possible causes include:

➤ Food allergies – fish, eggs, dairy products, chocolate, nuts.

➤ Food additives – tartrazine dyes.

➤ Inhalants – house dust.

LUMPS AND BUMPS

The skin is prone to a whole family of minor skin lumps that tend not to cause problems. You can, however, have some removed, if they become large or develop in an awkward spot.

➤ Lipomas – These are mobile fatty lumps that sit just beneath the skin's surface.

➤ Sebaceous cysts – These blocked sebaceous glands can feel hard and smooth to the touch. They may grow to quite a size and are often susceptible to infection.

➤ Skin tags – These harmless flaps of skin most often occur on the neck, trunk, groin and/or armpit.

DERMOGRAPHISM

Literally meaning "drawing on the skin", dermographism is a highly over-sensitive reaction to pressure. It sometimes develops in people suffering from urticaria. A raised red rash appears on the skin when it is stroked firmly, with the end of a pencil or a finger nail for example; the rash follows the line of pressure. (However, similar reactions may occur in other skin disorders and on exposure to heat, cold or water.)

This extreme sensitivity can be a long-term problem. Doctors are still unsure of the exact cause, although it is thought to be related to a high level of immunoglobin E. It also seems to be particularly prevalent in fair-skinned people and those who suffer from other allergic skin conditions.

Teenage acne (acne vulgaris)

SEE ALSO
➤ The functions of skin, p188
➤ Blepharitis, p181
➤ Bacterial skin infections, p196

This is a common condition that affects 90 per cent of adolescents to some degree. It follows the onset of puberty, and typically affects the face and trunk. These areas are particularly rich in sebaceous glands, which produce the oily sebum that keeps our skin moist. Adolescent acne is more common in boys than girls and can be very upsetting, because it appears at a time when people are especially self-conscious about their appearance. Acne also occurs in adults (acne rosacea), and in contrast to the teenage type affects women more commonly than men.

The root cause of acne is an overproduction of sebum by the sebaceous glands, so sufferers' skin often looks obviously greasy. Instead of flowing on to the skin and hair, the excess sebum blocks the hair follicles and sebaceous glands, giving rise to tiny blackheads. If a plug of keratin forms over the top, bacteria (*Proprionibacterium acnes*) can colonize the area, causing inflammation and pustules of acne. In severe cases, or when spots are picked, prominent scars (keloids) may be left behind when the skin heals.

The overproduction of sebum may be triggered by hormonal changes at puberty. There is no significant evidence that eating fatty foods, chocolate and sweets causes or aggravates acne.

HOW IS IT TREATED?

There is no quick fix for acne, and treatment may last from six to twelve weeks. It is also likely that you will need

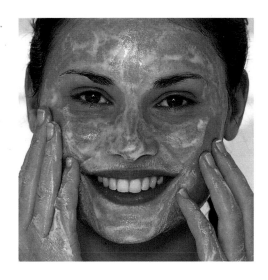

△ Careful cleansing of affected areas can help keep acne at bay and moderate exposure to sunlight can also be beneficial.

repeat treatment in the future. Cases occasionally respond to treatment within two to three weeks, although it normally takes longer than this. Possible treatments include the following:

- To begin with, you may be given creams or gels containing benzoyl peroxide – to combat the acne bacteria.
- If benzoyl peroxide proves ineffective, the next line of attack involves antibiotic creams, or courses of oral antibiotics if the cream alone fails to work.
- For women, certain types of contraceptive pill can be helpful in preventing the occurrence of acne.
- If your acne is particularly severe, you will be seen by a hospital specialist, who may prescribe retinoid drugs. Once you start taking these drugs, you have to be monitored closely as they can cause side effects, including birth defects if given to pregnant women.

ACNE ROSACEA

Also known as adult acne, this tends to affect the face only and usually develops between the ages of 30 and 55. It more commonly affects women, often runs in families, and is possibly caused by overuse of corticosteroid creams. Acne rosacea usually affects the nose, cheeks and forehead. The white- and yellow-headed pimples often itch or sting, and the sebaceous glands may become inflamed and scarred. If the skin of the nose is involved, particularly in cases affecting men, it can become enlarged, red and scarred – a condition known as rhinophyma. Occasionally, an eye condition called blepharitis also develops. There is no known cure, so treatment is aimed at reducing symptoms, and includes antibiotics in the form of creams and capsules.

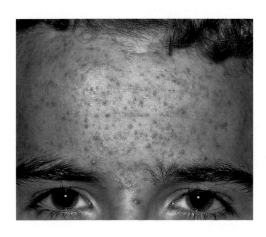

▽ The skin on this 16-year-old's forehead is affected by acne. In this skin disorder, overactive sebaceous glands lead to the infection and blockage of hair follicles, causing blackheads and spots.

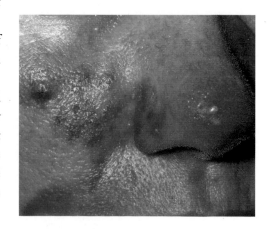

▽ This 36-year-old woman has acne rosacea, a chronic skin disease. It can start as temporary flushing of the skin, and then permanent redness usually develops, often followed by the appearance of large yellow pustules.

Skin cancers

There are several different types of skin cancer. Most are associated with prolonged exposure to the damaging ultraviolet radiation in sunlight and fair-skinned people are most at risk. Skin cancer is very common, affects millions of people around the world and causes a large number of deaths every year. However, most types can be treated successfully if they are detected at an early stage. Most skin cancers grow slowly, confine themselves to the skin and do not spread to other parts of the body. The exception, however, is malignant melanoma.

Skin cancer is one of the most treatable forms of the disease, but like most cancers, it is essential to seek advice if you have any symptoms at all, to make sure that you catch the problem in its earliest stages.

Skin cancer may have no apparent cause, or it may develop as the result of external factors – as in exposure to strong sun. Cancer of the skin can also arise because cancer has spread there from other parts of the body, such as the breast, kidney or lung. This latter type usually forms hard skin nodules, most frequently on the scalp.

▽ People who are fair-skinned are among potential risk-groups for skin cancer, as they are more likely to suffer from sunburn.

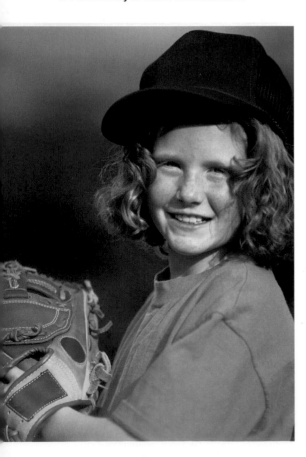

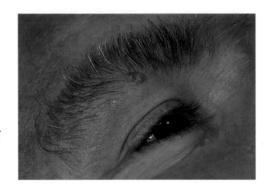

△ This raised lump on the eyebrow is known as a rodent ulcer – one of the most common forms of skin cancer.

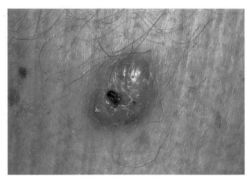

△ Squamous cell carcinomas produce wart-like swellings on the skin. They are most often seen in the fair-skinned and the elderly.

MOLES

The ordinary moles that you have on your skin are also known as non-cancerous melanomas. Most moles are perfectly harmless, but some may develop into malignant melanoma. Moles are typically flat and brown, of differing size, and sometimes hairy. Usually present from birth, more may develop during a person's lifetime. Although cancerous moles are rare, it is wise to keep an eye on them, as changes can indicate malignancy (see signs and symptoms of malignant melanoma box). Remember that hairy moles will very rarely become cancerous.

BASAL CELL CARCINOMAS

Also known as rodent ulcers, these carcinomas look like small pearls with open sores (ulcers) in the centre. Rodent ulcers mainly affect skin that is exposed to the sun, especially around the nose and eyes. They grow slowly and do not spread to other organs (metastasize). However, if not treated,

a basal cell carcinoma can spread, causing tissue damage to other parts of the body local to the skin cancer.

This skin cancer is more common later in life. If your doctor suspects you have a rodent ulcer, the diagnosis can be confirmed by taking a biopsy, where small samples of the tissue are removed and sent to a laboratory for testing. The ulcer can be removed surgically or treated with a course of radiotherapy, or a combination of both, to ensure complete removal of the cancerous cells. Superficial ulcers may be frozen off using a process called cryotherapy. Treatment is likely to be effective – 90 per cent of people with basal cell carcinomas are treated successfully.

SQUAMOUS CELL CARCINOMAS

These cancers look like small nodules with raised hard edges. They occur:

• On sun-exposed areas of the skin.

• In chronic leg ulcers.

• On the lips of smokers.

Any of the following changes to a mole could indicate development of a malignant melanoma. It is advisable to see your doctor as soon as possible if you develop a new skin growth, or if a pre-existing mole changes in any way. The changes to look for include:

➤ Any rapid change in size.

➤ Changes in shape or an irregular border (normal moles have a smooth, regular shape).

➤ Change in colour, especially darkening to blue-black.

➤ Bleeding.

➤ Pain or itching.

➤ A softening of the mole.

➤ Crumbling, or the breaking away of pieces of the mole.

➤ The appearance of new moles around the original one.

Squamous cell carcinomas are similar to rodent ulcers. They start out as small, firm lumps in certain parts of the body and, although they are painless, they can grow quite rapidly. It is rare for them to spread to other parts of the body, but this does happen in some cases. They can also occur

▽ Solar keratosis is a red skin-growth caused by too much exposure to the sun over a number of years. Although not cancerous to begin with, it may develop into skin cancer, so your doctor will always recommend its removal.

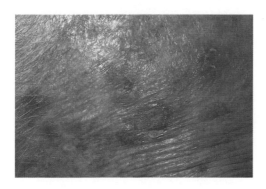

at multiple sites in the body. Squamous cell carcinomas can be very destructive, especially when they occur on the face and if left untreated. They are cured by radiotherapy or are removed surgically.

MALIGNANT MELANOMAS

Malignant melanoma is the most serious form of skin cancer. It affects the melanocytes – the skin's melanin-producing cells – and can strike any part of the body. In women, malignant melanomas are often found on the legs; in men, the back is a common site. Rarely seen in children, these cancers are more usually found in adults of middle age and older, although there have been occurrences in young adolescents.

This cancer is connected with excessive exposure to the sun and so is especially common in fair-skinned people and in countries such as Australia. Incidence has risen because people travel more widely and like having a tan.

About 50 per cent of these cancers develop from moles. They grow quickly and if untreated can spread rapidly to other parts of the body. Melanomas can be cured by surgical removal, but only if caught while small. A first step in treatment is analysing a sample of the cancer. Radiotherapy and/or chemotherapy may be used.

POTENTIALLY CANCEROUS CONDITIONS

There are certain conditions that can change, in rare cases, into skin cancers and these include:

• Bowen's disease – This produces slow-growing, red, scaly patches on the skin. Rarely, these turn into squamous cell carcinomas. Your doctor can diagnose the patches under a microscope and can cure the condition using a drug called 5-FU, surgery or radiotherapy.

• Acitinic (or solar) keratoses – These pinkish red crusts appear on sun-exposed areas of skin and can develop into squamous cell carcinomas. They can be cut out or treated with 5-FU paint.

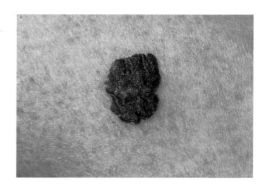

△ This picture shows a malignant melanoma on the skin of the lower leg. Malignant melanomas are more common in people with pale skin because their skin contains less of the pigment melanin, which provides protection against the harmful effects of the sun.

Although most forms of skin cancer are eminently treatable, with a survival rate much higher than most other types of cancer, the signs of skin cancers should be taken seriously. Prevention is better than cure, and taking care in the sun will often stop cancer from developing.

At risk groups include:

➤ People who work outdoors.

➤ People over 50 years old.

➤ People who have had radiation treatment or who are exposed to radiation as part of their job.

➤ People who had severe sunburn regularly in childhood.

It is a good idea to examine yourself every few months for any skin changes, and to check existing moles and the appearance of new ones. Ask a friend or partner to inspect areas you cannot see. If you are familiar with marks on your skin you will notice any change and can bring it to the attention of your doctor.

Changes to look out for include:

➤ New growths or sores that do not heal within four weeks.

➤ Spots or sores that itch, hurt, scab or bleed persistently.

Fungal skin infections

SEE ALSO

➤ Diabetes, p66
➤ Female genital infections, p159
➤ Causes of infectious disease, p214

Millions of fungi, including yeasts, live naturally on your skin. Normally, there is healthy competition in the body between bacteria and fungi. However, if the bacteria are wiped out by a course of antibiotics, the fungi can be free to colonize and infect certain areas. Some people are more prone to fungal infections than others, although there is no known medical reason for this. If fungal infections recur, this can be an indication of diabetes or of other more general disorders, so it is a good idea to contact your doctor as a precautionary measure.

RINGWORM

This is caused by a fungus and not, despite its name, by a worm. The infected skin develops well-defined, scaly patches, which are usually itchy. Ringworm commonly affects the scalp and groin. It disappears quickly with antifungal cream treatment.

ATHLETE'S FOOT

The fungi that cause this itchy rash between the toes thrive in warm, humid conditions. They can also affect the nails, making them brittle and deformed. Wearing certain types of footwear, such as trainers, makes the feet sweat and more likely to develop this infection. The skin rash settles rapidly with antifungal creams, but the nail infection can need extended treatment with antifungal tablets or nail paints.

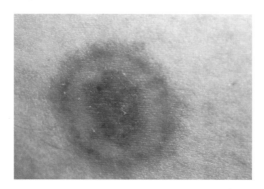

▽ This picture shows ringworm on the skin of a farmworker. The condition may have been picked up from an infected sheep.

ORAL THRUSH

The yeast *Candida albicans*, which lives normally on the skin, can easily infect the mouth and/or vagina (vaginal thrush). With oral thrush, the mouth and tongue become red and sore, with white patches. The condition often occurs after a course of antibiotics, when the bacteria that normally control levels of *Candida* in the body have been killed. While oral thrush is easily treated and usually clears within a matter of days, recurrent infections can occur in people with diabetes or any long-term illness. Anticandidal creams and tablets can be used to treat oral thrush, and pessaries are available for vaginal thrush.

Bacterial skin infections

SEE ALSO

➤ Bacterial infections, p216

Bacteria are just one of the many groups of micro-organisms that can affect the skin. There are two main types of bacteria – *Streptococcus* and *Staphylococcus*. Bacteria can live on the skin without symptoms but if the skin's protective barrier is breached, infection can result.

CELLULITIS

This infection tends to be found in the feet and calves and can be quite extensive. Many patients need antibiotic injections in the first three to five days in order to control the infection. Once it is under control, this is usually followed by a few weeks of oral antibiotics to clear up the infection.

A type of infective cellulitis that affects only the face – called erysipelas – is caused by a particular *Streptococcus* and clears up with penicillin treatment.

IMPETIGO

This usually affects children. A moist rash develops, often around the mouth or nose, with yellow crusts. Treatment involves antibiotic creams and a course of antibiotics.

FOLLICULITIS

This is usually a mild inflammation of the hair follicles due to infection and requires little, if any, treatment. Antibiotic cream can be used in extensive infections. It usually clears up in a week.

ERYTHEMA NODOSUM

This firm, tender, dark-red rash occurs on the legs and resembles bruising as it settles down. It commonly affects young adults, particularly women, and is caused by:
• Bacteria or fungi.
• Drugs, such as the contraceptive pill or sulphonamide drugs.
• Inflammatory bowel disease, such as Crohn's disease and ulcerative colitis.
Treatment involves bed-rest and non-steroidal anti-inflammatory drugs.

Viral skin infections

SEE ALSO
➤ Causes of infectious disease, p214
➤ Sexually transmitted infections, p163
➤ The roles of blood and lymph, p200

A whole host of viruses give rise to various different skin rashes. These viral rashes include cold sores, warts and molluscum contagiosum. Treatments usually include antiviral creams, although some conditions clear up untreated, given time (in the case of infections such as warts, however, this can be several years). Once you have had certain viral infections, such as the herpes simplex virus that causes cold sores, symptoms are likely to recur. These infections are often contagious and should be treated early to avoid any spread.

COLD SORES

These sores form around the mouth and are caused by the herpes simplex virus. This occurs naturally in most human bodies, but usually it is controlled by the immune system. If the immune system is actively fighting off other viral infections, even those as mild as the common cold, the herpes simplex virus can take hold. The eruption of cold sores is preceded by an itching sensation. This usually develops into groups of small blisters where the skin and the lip membrane meet. Sores can also occur around the nose. They are best treated as soon as the itching develops, with an antiviral cream – a choice of these is available over the counter at your local pharmacy. Cold sores tend to recur.

WARTS AND VERRUCAS

These flat, scaly skin growths are caused by the human papilloma virus. Most people develop immunity to the virus with time and the warts may disappear within three to six months. Most warts will disappear without any treatment.

Verrucas are flat warts on the sole of the foot and require no treatment unless they are painful. However, like other types of wart, they are highly infectious and can be spread easily around the infected area or from person to person. It is recommended that verrucca sufferers should wear protective socks – when swimming, for example, or around the house.

Warts that persist or cause discomfort can be removed. Ways of doing this include destroying the tissue with heat, freezing or laser treatment. Such treatments can usually be performed by your doctor, although several sessions may be needed to clear the warts completely. The best method, however, is applying caustic paints containing salicylic acid.

Warts that affect the genitals need specialist treatment in a genitourinary clinic. Informing/tracing of sexual partners must be carried out.

▽ Cold sores are a common affliction. They usually begin as an itch and develop into small, fluid-filled blisters. As with other viral skin infections, cold sores are highly contagious and can be spread to other areas of the body.

▽ Veruccas are flat warts which appear on the soles of the feet and the toes. The infection is usually contracted from contaminated floors and can be spread easily in public places such as swimming pools.

ERYTHEMA MULTIFORME

In this condition the skin becomes covered with raised red patches. This inflammation is caused by the dilation (opening up) of underlying blood vessels. The centre of each red patch may appear blue, giving the rash a characteristic "target" appearance. The rash has a tendency to affect both sides of the body and in severe cases can cause ulcers on the mouth and genitalia.

The rash is caused by:

➤ Viruses, such as herpes simplex, Epstein-Barr virus, HIV and the weakened virus of BCG vaccination.

➤ Chronic autoimmune diseases, such as systemic lupus erythematosus and sarcoidosis.

➤ Drugs, such as penicillins and barbiturates.

➤ Some cancers, including myeloma, Hodgkin's lymphoma and carcinomas.

The rash settles quickly if treated with steroid creams but tends to recur.

MOLLUSCUM CONTAGIOSUM

These pearl-like lumps, caused by viral infection, are common in children and may occur in multiple clusters around the body. The condition can be caught during contact with an infected person. It usually disappears in six to twelve months, once the child develops immunity to the virus.

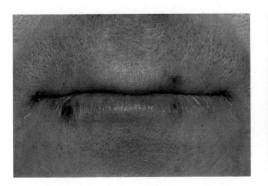

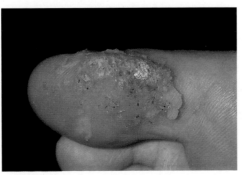

Leg ulcers

These open sores can cause the skin around the ankle or foot to break down. They are common in the West and mainly affect people later in life, when they often cause a long-term problem. About 1 per cent of people over the age of 70 suffer from leg ulcers. People who are bedridden or have reduced mobility are especially at risk. There are different types of leg ulcer: some can be painless but others cause a great deal of discomfort, usually as a result of poor circulation. Treatment ranges from bandaging to amputation in severe cases.

There are several types of leg ulcer, each with its own symptoms and characteristics. Each of these types also responds to different levels of treatment. All ulcers can become unpleasant and problematic if left untreated, so they should be brought to the attention of a medical expert:

- Venous ulcers – These painless ulcers are the most common and are associated with varicose veins that cause the skin around the ankle to become thin and fragile. Early changes to the skin include a brown rash and/or a form of eczema.
- Ischaemic ulcers – These painful ulcers are caused by poor blood supply to the leg (peripheral vascular disease). They are common in smokers and people with a history of high blood pressure, angina and claudication (crampy pain in the legs). This silting up of arteries taking blood to the legs is also a common problem in people with diabetes.

▽ This picture shows an example of a leg ulcer. It formed after a blow to the leg caused severe skin damage. Treatment depends on the type of ulcer, but ulcers like this one would be cleaned, dressed and left to heal. Antibiotics might also be taken to clear up any infection.

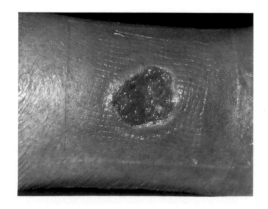

- Diabetic ulcers – People with diabetes are prone to losing the sensation of pain in their feet and so can easily damage the skin without knowing it. Huge infected ulcers can occur and these may be impossible to heal.

WHEN TO SEE YOUR DOCTOR

If you notice unusual skin changes on your legs you should bring them to the attention of your doctor. If your doctor suspects a leg ulcer, you may be referred to a specialist for a Doppler scan – a type of ultrasound scanning – to assess the blood flow in the affected leg.

TREATMENT OPTIONS

Most ulcers are slow to heal and have a tendency to recur. Treatments vary and include the following:

- Venous ulcers – Your doctor will treat your varicose veins in order to prevent ulcers from forming. Once an ulcer has formed, it can take weeks or months of regular high-compression bandaging and leg elevation to ease or heal it. Skin grafts may occasionally be used as a way of healing the ulcer.
- Ischaemic ulcers – An operation to bypass a blockage to the leg arteries may improve the circulation, but these ulcers heal poorly, are prone to infection and can be very painful. To prevent large ulcers developing further the affected leg may be amputated below the knee.
- Diabetic ulcers – If ulcers on the feet are severe, amputation may be the only cure, although this treatment will only be considered as a last resort.

CORNS AND CALLUSES

These patches of thick, hardened skin occur at points of abnormal pressure on the skin and the commonest cause is ill-fitting shoes. Once a corn or callus is formed it is unlikely to settle without treatment, and will probably need to be removed by a chiropodist.

Maintaining good leg and foot health (keeping skin soft and supple, and gentle exercise to improve circulation) is likely to be beneficial for people with diabetes and circulatory disease, in order to prevent the formation of ulcers.

▽ Taking care of your legs and feet can help prevent leg sores and ulcers, and problems such as corns and calluses, especially if you suffer from diabetes or circulatory diseases.

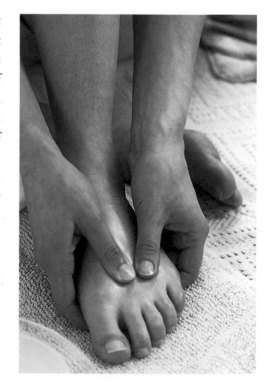

13

BLOOD AND THE IMMUNE SYSTEM

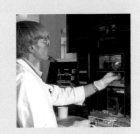

Your blood contains red and white blood cells, plasma and platelets, creating a very efficient system for supplying oxygen and nutrients, getting rid of waste products, fighting infection and healing wounds. The latter two functions mean that the blood is a major component of our immune system – how the body protects itself from illness. Another component of our immunity "machinery" is the network of nodes, vessels and organs that make up the lymphatic system. This system defends the body and also returns our watery tissue fluid to the blood. Closely linked, the blood and lymphatic systems work together to promote optimum health. Problems range from anaemia caused by low red cell counts to cancers of the lymph nodes.

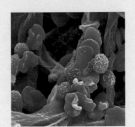

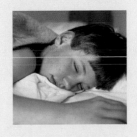

CONTENTS

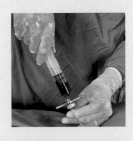

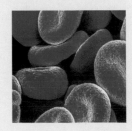

The roles of blood and lymph

Blood is the body's internal transport system. It flows constantly around the body, supplying oxygen and nutrients to the tissues and removing carbon dioxide and waste products. Important signalling chemicals – such as hormones – and dissolved minerals travel in the bloodstream and help to keep the body's internal environment in perfect balance. Vitally important to the circulation is the lymphatic system, which removes excess fluid, or lymph, from the tissues and plays a crucial role in the immune system – the body's defence against foreign invaders.

The average person has 5–6 litres (8½–10½ pints) of blood in their bodies and in a drop of blood the size of a pinhead there are several million red blood cells.

WHAT IS BLOOD?

Blood is a mixture of cells floating in a straw-coloured fluid called plasma. Most blood cells are made in the bone marrow and some white blood cells are made in the spleen and thymus gland.

Plasma is 90 per cent water. Water-soluble substances dissolve in it and are transported to their destination. Substances dissolved in the plasma include:

• Food – Products of digestion such as glucose and fats are taken round the body for use as fuel.

• Waste products – These include carbon dioxide and urea.

• Hormones – These chemical messengers are secreted into the blood and travel to their site of action.

• Proteins – These include the vital clotting factors and antibodies.

• Minerals – Such as sodium, calcium and potassium, vital to body function.

Water-insoluble substances travel around by being bound to a protein called albumin.

FIGHTING FOREIGN INVADERS

Your body is constantly under attack by microbes – potentially harmful invaders. The blood, lymphatic system, specialized cells, antibodies and various organs all work together as an immune system to deal with threats each second of every day.

The lymphatic system includes lymphatic vessels, lymph nodes and lymph fluid. As well as removing excess fluid from the tissues, lymph filters out microbes and triggers the immune response in the lymph nodes – home to disease-fighting white cells called lymphocytes.

RECOGNIZING INVADERS

Special cells and chemicals within the immune system are able to recognize invading microbes:

• You are constantly exposed to infectious agents such as bacteria and viruses. Your immune system deals with the attack, but also remembers the attacker so that it can fight back even more effectively next time.

• Cell division and growth is not infallible and thousands of abnormal, potentially cancerous cells are made every day. The immune system usually recognizes and destroys these cells.

HOW BLOOD CLOTS TO HEAL A WOUND

▽ Your body has an elaborate clotting system that plugs any leaks in the blood vessels. Small leaks are plugged by clumps of platelets. For leaks that are too large to plug, the platelets initiate a cascade of chemical reactions so that a clot is formed to seal the injury. Sometimes the clotting system fails (as in haemophilia), or it may work too well, blocking healthy blood vessels and causing possible heart attacks.

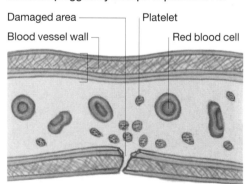

Damaged area — Platelet
Blood vessel wall — Red blood cell

1 As soon as a blood vessel is damaged, it narrows to reduce blood flow. Platelets nearby are activated to become sticky and clump together to plug the damaged area.

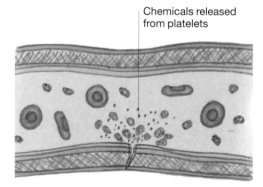

Chemicals released from platelets

2 Chemicals are released from damaged tissue and clumped platelets. These set off a chain reaction involving the blood's clotting factors, each one setting off the next.

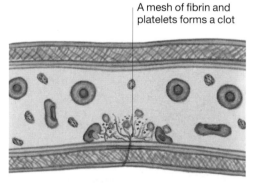

A mesh of fibrin and platelets forms a clot

3 Plasma contains a dissolved protein called fibrinogen. Clotting factors cause fibrinogen to form strands of fibrin, which mesh and trap blood cells to form a clot.

THE LYMPHATIC SYSTEM

▷ This system comprises a network of nodes connected by vessels, plus other organs and tissues. One role of the system is to fight infection, via white blood cells. The other is to return any of the watery fluid (lymph) that has drained into the lymphatic vessels back to the bloodstream. The nodes contain concentrations of white cells, and the major collections of nodes lie at the neck, armpits and groin.

Axillary (armpit) nodes
All the nodes filtering lymph from the arms and breast are concentrated here.

Heart

Liver
This organ plays a crucial role by acting as a "sieve" for toxins entering the body via the digestive tract, which it then destroys. It also produces many of the blood-borne chemicals controlling the destruction of foreign particles.

Inguinal (groin) nodes
This large collection of nodes filters lymph from the legs and pelvis.

Bone marrow
Antibodies made here by white cells stick to foreign proteins (antigens) on the surface of invading organisms and label them for destruction. (Note that red blood cells are also made in the bone marrow.)

Lymph vessels
Lymph circulates through a network of vessels. It passes from the body's tissues into small lymphatic capillaries and from there into larger vessels called lymphatics.

This artwork has been designed to show the different elements of the lymphatic system clearly, and it is therefore not to scale.

Cervical (neck) nodes
These lymph nodes can often be felt as they enlarge to fight infection. A protective ring of lymph nodes around the throat comprises the tonsils and adenoids.

Subclavian veins
Lymph from the whole body drains into the heart via these veins, and so returns to the bloodstream.

Thymus gland
This produces mature T-cell lymphocytes, which fight viruses and parasites.

Spleen
This large, fragile organ produces all types of lymphocytes and nestles under the lower ribs on the left. It is home to many white cells that produce antibodies. People who have had their spleen removed need particular vaccines and antibiotics to protect them from infections.

Intestines
This collection of lymph tissue is in an area exposed to the outside world – the digestive tract – and so is more prone to attack by bacteria.

BLOOD CELLS

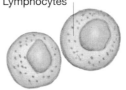

Red blood cells
These doughnut-shaped cells are full of the chemical haemoglobin, which carries oxygen to cells around the body. Haemoglobin gives cells their red colour.

Lymphocytes

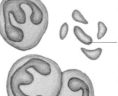

White blood cells
These cells play a vital role in your immune system. Some – the lymphocytes – produce antibodies to alert your body to foreign invaders while others – the phagocytes – destroy debris and bacteria.

Platelets
These tiny blood cells are vital for blood-clotting and for repairing injuries.

Phagocytes

PROBLEMS WITH THE SYSTEM

Sometimes, the immune system over-reacts, producing allergies. "Immunodeficiency" diseases arise when the immune system fails in some way. The system may also attack the body's tissues, such as joints, giving rise to "autoimmune" diseases. Problems can often arise with organ transplantation, as the immune system may see the organ as an "invader" and attack it.

ENLARGED LYMPH NODES

You may notice your glands (especially in the neck) are enlarged, this may be due to:
• Most commonly, a response to infection.
• Invasion by cancerous cells; as part of the body's drainage system, lymph nodes receive fluid from all parts of the body and are a common place for cancers.
• Development of cancers of the lymphatic system (lymphoma).

BOOSTING IMMUNITY
Vaccination is a way of protecting people against infectious diseases. Vaccines, which are usually given by injection, are weakened or dead micro-organisms that prompt the immune system to produce antibodies to fight a disease. People may also be given ready-made antibodies.

Anaemia

SEE ALSO

➤ Haemolytic anaemia, below

➤ Macrocytic and Microcytic anaemia, p203

➤ Sickle cell anaemia, p204

Anaemia describes a group of conditions in which there is a lower-than-normal count of red blood cells (and so less of the oxygen-carrying pigment haemoglobin) in the blood. Anaemia is classified by the size and appearance of the red blood cells. The common types of anaemia are haemolytic, macrocytic and microcytic, and they share similar symptoms, including fatigue and weakness. People suffering from illnesses such as angina may find they are more likely to have attacks if they are also anaemic. A good supply of oxygen in the blood is essential to good health.

SIGNS AND SYMPTOMS

Symptoms include the following:

➤ Tiredness.

➤ Headaches.

➤ Faintness.

➤ Pale skin.

➤ Breathlessness following exercise.

➤ Palpitations (patients with anaemia often have high heart rates).

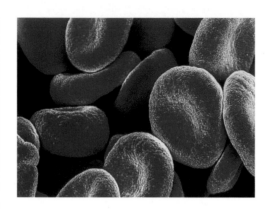

△ Red blood cells get their colour from haemoglobin, an oxygen-carrying protein. Anaemic people have a shortage of these cells.

INVESTIGATING ANAEMIA

Several routine investigations are used to diagnose anaemia:

➤ Full blood count check, which gives numbers of all the cell types.

➤ A blood film test, which examines the red blood cells' colour and shape.

➤ A test to check for low levels of vitamin B_{12} and folic acid.

➤ A test to estimate the body's stores of iron.

➤ A reticulocyte count to measure how many young cells the bone marrow is producing.

There are three main causes of anaemia:
1 Not enough red blood cells being made.
2 Red blood cells being lost from the body at an abnormal rate by slow, chronic bleeding, as with heavy menstrual periods or gastrointestinal bleeding.
3 Red blood cells being destroyed faster than they can be produced.

Haemolytic anaemia

SEE ALSO

➤ Anaemia, p202

The normal lifespan of a red blood cell is 120 days. In haemolytic anaemia, this lifespan is severely shortened as red blood cells are destroyed faster than normal. There are several reasons for this, and the condition can be inherited.

SIGNS AND SYMPTOMS

As well as the common symptoms of anaemia, the patient may be jaundiced, due to abnormally high levels of bilirubin, the breakdown product of haemoglobin. The spleen may enlarge as it is the main site of red cell destruction and in this condition is working harder than usual.

CAUSES OF HAEMOLYTIC ANAEMIA

• Inherited disorders of the cell surface membrane; and disorders of cell contents e.g haemoglobin in sickle cell disease.
• Other inherited disease (see box, right).
• Reactions to blood transfusions.
• Drugs, for example antimalarial drugs.
• Burns.
• Infections such as malaria.
• Mechanical heart valves.

SPHEROCYTOSIS

Hereditary spherocytosis is the commonest inherited haemolytic anaemia. A defect in the red blood cell membrane means that, as the cells pass through the spleen, part of the cell membrane is lost and they become spherical rather than doughnut-shaped. The cells can no longer travel through the spleen and so die.

Macrocytic anaemia

SEE ALSO

➤ Eat healthily, p14
➤ Anaemia and Haemolytic anaemia, p202
➤ Microcytic anaemia, below

In macrocytic anaemia, the red blood cells are larger and paler than normal. These defective red cells are known as macrocytes and they most commonly arise because of a vitamin deficiency – of either vitamin B_{12} or folic acid. Both of these vitamins are essential for the efficient formation of red blood cells in the bone marrow. There may be number of reasons for these deficiencies and these include a poorly balanced diet, too much alcohol, or intestinal problems that mean nutrients are not absorbed properly by the body.

SIGNS AND SYMPTOMS
As well as general anaemia symptoms, this may produce signs such as nervous system dysfunction (B_{12} deficiency) or a sore tongue (folic acid deficiency).

VITAMIN B_{12} DEFICIENCY
The main cause of vitamin B_{12} deficiency is a disease known as pernicious anaemia, in which the cells of the stomach, where B_{12} is absorbed, are destroyed (an autoimmune disease). Pernicious anaemia is more commonly found in people over 60, and in women. It is important that it is treated because it can result in irreversible degeneration of the brain and the spinal cord. B_{12} deficiency can also occur in patients who have undergone a gastrectomy (removal of part or all of the stomach).

FOLIC ACID DEFICIENCY
A lack of folic acid (also known as folate) can result in macrocytic anaemia. Folate deficiency can be caused by:

• A diet low in fresh vegetables.
• Alcohol abuse, because it interferes with folic acid absorption.
• Pregnancy, because larger quantities are needed for the healthy development of the fetus.
• Drugs, such as anticancer and anti-convulsant drugs.

TREATMENT OPTIONS
If anaemia is due to B_{12} deficiency, injections of B_{12} are given. Folic acid deficiency is treated with folic acid tablets.

Microcytic anaemia

SEE ALSO

➤ Anaemia, p202

This form of anaemia is characterized by small, pale red cells. The most common cause is a deficiency of iron, an essential component of haemoglobin. Unfortunately, diets are often deficient in iron. Certain foodstuffs can also interfere with absorption.

SIGNS AND SYMPTOMS
As well as the general symptoms of anaemia, microcytic anaemia can cause brittle, spoon-shaped nails, a smooth, painful tongue and brittle hair.

CAUSES OF IRON DEFICIENCY
• Blood loss – In women this is commonly due to heavy menstrual periods, made worse by the fact that iron-rich red meat is now less popular. Iron deficiency in men is also due to blood loss, usually caused by diseases in the gut or kidney.

• Increased demand for iron – this occurs most commonly while the body is still growing and developing, and during pregnancy.
• Eating iron-poor foods; a problem with some vegetarians and vegans.
• Decreased iron absorption from the intestine.

WHAT MIGHT YOUR DOCTOR DO?
Test results confirm microcytic anaemia when they reveal red cells that are small and pale, and levels of iron that are lower than normal. Your doctor will investigate causes of blood loss and ask about your diet.

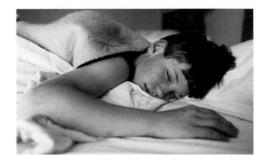

△ In most forms of anaemia, tiredness can be one of the symptoms.

Most people with anaemia can correct the condition by taking an iron supplement, although in very severe cases a blood transfusion may be required.

Sickle cell anaemia

Normal haemoglobin – the substance that carries oxygen around the body inside red blood cells – comprises a haem unit within four globin chains (two alpha and two beta). If the globin structure is abnormal, it can affect the oxygen-carrying capacity of the blood and cause this serious form of anaemia. An inherited condition, sickle cell may first appear very early in life and occurs most commonly in the populations of Africa, India, southern Europe and the Middle East. Sufferers have episodic "crises", where even a simple infection can bring on a life-threatening illness.

THE GENETICS OF SICKLE CELL ANAEMIA

Hb A is the gene responsible for normal haemoglobin; the abnormal haemoglobin gene is Hb S. All is well if an individual inherits an Hb A gene from both parents. Someone inheriting two Hb S genes, one from each parent, will have sickle cell anaemia. Inheriting an Hb S gene from one parent and an Hb A from the other means that you are a carrier of sickle cell trait but do not have the full-blown condition.

Sickle cell anaemia sufferers may feel fine most of the time, but are prone to serious health "crises". In general, these episodes start suddenly and last from a few hours to several days. They may come on seemingly for no reason or be prompted by a variety of factors, such as:

SICKLE CELL ANAEMIA AND MALARIA

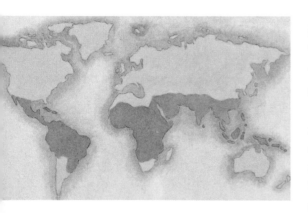

△ The sickle cell condition has one advantage: it protects against the malaria parasite. This means that it is much more common where malaria is endemic (red on the map above).

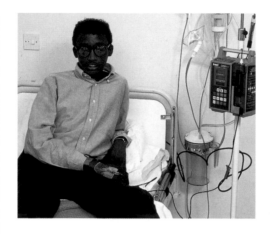

△ In severe sickle cell anaemia, regular blood transfusions are carried out to boost the levels of normal haemoglobin in the blood.

• Cold.

• Dehydration.

• Lack of oxygen (e.g. if at high altitudes).

• Infections.

These factors can cause red blood cells to change from their normal doughnut shape to a sickle shape and clump up, causing a range of severe symptoms (see box, right).

DIAGNOSIS AND TREATMENT

To confirm a diagnosis, you may have blood tests – a full blood count, a blood smear analysis and haemoglobin electrophoresis.

Avoiding the triggering factors is the main method of preventing a sickle cell crisis. A blood transfusion may be given to correct anaemia and may be carried out before major surgery so that the level of abnormal Hb S is reduced. Drugs to boost levels of Hb F, another form of haemoglobin that resists sickling, can be useful, although these are not yet widely available. Transplants of normal red cell-producing cells from the bone marrow of close relatives are another alternative. In the future, gene therapy may be possible, to replace the abnormal haemoglobin gene.

SIGNS AND SYMPTOMS

The abnormal red blood cells are destroyed by the spleen, and this can lead to the development of anaemia – causing fatigue, pale skin and shortness of breath on exertion. Sickle-shaped cells are inflexible and may block small blood vessels. This leads to symptoms including the following:

➤ Bone pain – the most common symptom.

➤ Breathing difficulties.

➤ Priapism in men, a painful persistent erection of the penis that can destroy the penis if left untreated.

➤ Abdominal pain, due to spleen and liver damage.

➤ Strokes and fits if vessels in the brain are blocked.

➤ Blood in the urine, due to kidney damage.

THE OUTLOOK

In the long term, people with sickle cell anaemia can suffer from recurrent infections, leg ulcers, gallstones, bone destruction (particularly of the femur) and blindness. Sufferers and carriers are also advised to seek counselling if they are thinking about having children.

Thalassaemias

SEE ALSO

➤ Anaemia, p202
➤ Sickle cell anaemia, p204

In this condition, production of the globin element of haemoglobin is abnormal. Instead of producing alpha and beta globin chains in equal amounts, someone with thalassaemia fails to make enough of one of these chains. Too few alpha chains causes alpha-thalassaemia, but the most common form is beta-thalassaemia, in which there are few or no beta chains. As with sickle cell anaemia, the signs and symptoms may be evident from childhood. Some forms need little or no treatment, but others may require blood transfusions.

SIGNS AND SYMPTOMS

In mild forms of the disease there may be few symptoms. In more severe cases, signs appear from the age of four to six months. Symptoms may include:

➤ Severe anaemia, causing pale skin, shortness of breath and abdominal swelling due to an enlarged spleen and liver.

➤ Susceptibility to infections.

➤ Bony deformities, particularly of the face, develop as the bone marrow expands to try to produce enough haemoglobin.

TREATMENT OPTIONS

Mild forms need no treatment. Severe cases require lifelong regular blood transfusions, which unfortunately overload sufferers' bodies with iron. To get rid of this excess, drugs are given that bind to the iron, so that it passes out in the urine and doesn't damage the liver, pancreas and heart.

THE STRUCTURE OF HAEMOGLOBIN

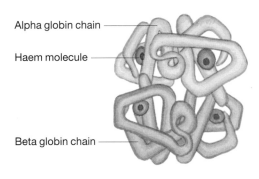

Alpha globin chain
Haem molecule
Beta globin chain

△ Normal haemoglobin has two alpha and two beta globin chains around a haem molecule.

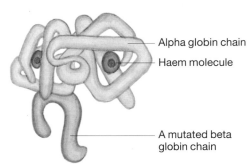

Alpha globin chain
Haem molecule
A mutated beta globin chain

△ Beta-thalassaemia haemoglobin looks very different and causes symptoms of this disease.

Haemophilia

SEE ALSO

➤ How blood clots, p200

Someone with this condition lacks an essential clotting factor in their blood. There is usually a family history of this rare disease. Abnormally severe bleeding can occur after injury or surgery, or spontaneous bleeding may even occur during ordinary daily activities.

SIGNS AND SYMPTOMS

Symptoms depend on the individual and the severity of the condition, but include:

➤ High susceptibility to bruising.

➤ Painful swelling of muscles and joints, due to internal bleeding.

➤ Prolonged bleeding after minor injury.

➤ Blood in the urine.

Haemophilia is a bleeding disorder caused by a deficiency in clotting factor VIII. The condition most commonly affects men, and women are carriers of the condition.

In order to confirm a diagnosis of haemophilia, your doctor will take a sample of blood to send to a laboratory for tests which will include a full blood count, blood film and blood clotting tests.

People with haemophilia are treated with injections of factor VIII. This used to be obtained from donated blood plasma but is now produced using genetically modified yeasts and is known as recombinant factor VIII. Those with mild haemophilia can have levels of their own factor VIII boosted using a drug called DDAVP.

Other rare bleeding disorders include Christmas disease, that is caused by a lack of factor IX, and von Willebrand's disease, in which a factor, that carries clotting factor VIII, called von Willebrand's is missing.

Acute leukaemias

These rare cancers of the white blood cells fall into two types. Acute lymphoblastic leukaemia (ALL) involves lymphocytes and tends to affect children. Acute myelogenous leukaemia (AML) affects a white blood cell called a myeloblast and occurs more often in adults. Acute leukaemia generally develops quickly, whereas chronic leukaemia tends to progress fairly slowly. People suffering from acute leukaemias may find they need regular blood and platelet transfusions. A bone marrow transplant will be considered if chemotherapy alone is unlikely to lead to cure.

SIGNS AND SYMPTOMS

The symptoms of leukaemia are caused by bone marrow failure, where normal marrow is infiltrated and replaced by cancerous cells, and include:

➤ Symptoms of anaemia – pale skin, shortness of breath, fatigue.

➤ Repeated infections.

➤ Bruising or bleeding.

➤ Occasionally, lymph node, liver and/or spleen enlargement.

In leukaemia, blood test results show low numbers of normal red blood cells, white blood cells and platelets, and may also show the presence of characteristic cancerous white blood cells. The blood tests carried out will include:
• A full blood count.

▽ Leukaemia treatment reduces the effectiveness of the immune system; here, a mother wears a mask to protect her child against infection.

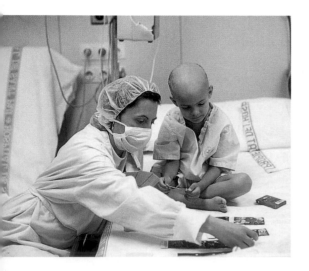

• Bone marrow biopsy (taking a sample of bone marrow tissue).

TREATING ACUTE LEUKAEMIAS

The treatment of these conditions is divided into general treatments and treatment specific to the type of leukaemia. General treatments include:
• Blood and platelet transfusions.
• Rapid treatment of any infection with intravenous antibiotics.

Specific treatments for each form of leukaemia are evolving and improving all the time. The mainstay approaches are chemotherapy (drug treatment to kill the cancerous cells) and bone marrow transplantation. Specific treatments for each form include:
• Acute myelogenous leukemia (AML) – This potentially curable disease can be treated with multidrug chemotherapy. Recurrences of the disease are also managed with chemotherapy, but usually with less success.
• Acute lymphoblastic leukaemia (ALL) – This most commonly affects children. It is also potentially curable through the use of a variety of chemotherapy drugs. Ninety per cent of patients respond to this treatment and 50 to 60 per cent are cured by it. Treatment is usually continued for two to three years. If ALL recurs, it tends to do so in the bone marrow, in which case a bone marrow transplant can be life-saving. Particular drugs can be injected into the spinal fluid to reduce the effects on the nervous system.

BONE MARROW TRANSPLANT

First, the patient's cancerous bone marrow is destroyed using high doses of radiation or chemotherapy and is then replaced by bone marrow from either a close relative or a matched donor. The patient receives bone marrow as an infusion into the bloodstream. Destroying the bone marrow leaves patients vulnerable to infection, bleeding and anaemia, so they are isolated until they start to produce new bone marrow. After the transplant, the patient has to take powerful immunosuppressant drugs, to control rejection of the bone marrow and also to prevent graft-versus-host disease, in which the new bone marrow attacks the recipient's body tissues.

▼ A bone marrow transplant may be the best treatment for a leukaemia sufferer. Here, a doctor harvests genetically compatible bone marrow from a donor; the bone marrow will then be filtered and infused into the recipient's bloodstream.

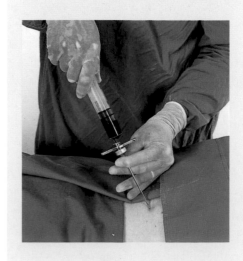

Chronic leukaemias

These white blood cell cancers usually affect adults and, as with acute leukaemias, there are two types – chronic lymphocytic leukaemia (CLL) and chronic myeloid leukaemia (CML). CLL is the most common leukaemia in the world. Chronic leukaemias can be slow to show any symptoms, beginning only with fatigue but gradually showing more definite signs. The exact cause of the chronic types of leukaemia is not yet known, although radiation, some viruses and industrial chemicals have all been connected with the disease.

SIGNS AND SYMPTOMS

Most people with chronic leukaemias have no symptoms, and this may be the case for several decades with CLL. Symptoms can include:

➤ Signs of anaemia – pale skin, shortness of breath, fatigue.

➤ Recurrent infections.

➤ Bleeding.

➤ Enlarged lymph nodes.

➤ Abdominal swelling, due to an enlarged liver and spleen.

➤ Fever and night sweats.

In chronic leukaemia, too many white blood cells are made in the bone marrow. The two different forms of chronic leukaemia reflect the different types of white cell that are affected. In CLL, too many lymphocytes are produced; in CML, it is granulocyte cells.

The first sign for many sufferers is simply feeling tired. However, over a period of time, the spleen gradually enlarges and eventually begins to cause pain in the abdomen. The patient may notice that they have lost weight and begin suffering from nose bleeds or aching in the bones. They may also find they sweat a great deal and are more sensitive to hot conditions than usual.

MAKING THE DIAGNOSIS

All types of leukaemia are progressive, and chronic leukaemias show signs only very gradually. Elderly people – who form the majority of those affected – should seek medical advice as soon as symptoms are apparent. As with acute leukaemias, your doctor will diagnose the condition by undertaking a full blood count to check the levels of red and white cells in the blood.

TREATMENT OPTIONS

There are several treatments, depending on the type of chronic leukaemia, including:

• Chronic lymphocytic leukaemia (CLL) – Most patients are asymptomatic for many years and only require treatment if they develop symptoms. Many patients are treated with supportive measures, such as blood transfusions, and may survive for over ten years after diagnosis. Infection is the commonest eventual cause of death.

• Chronic myeloid leukaemia (CML) – The disease often starts in a mild form that produces few symptoms for three or four years. It may develop into an acute

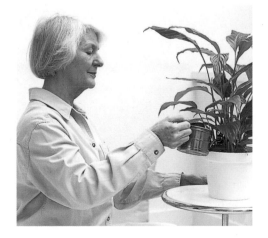
▽ Chronic leukaemias are most common in elderly people.

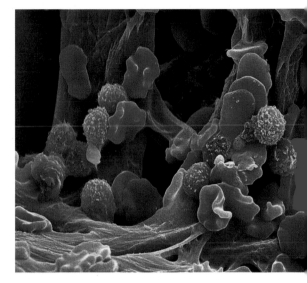
△ These are blood cells taken from a patient with chronic lymphocytic leukaemia. In this condition, too many white blood cells known as lymphocytes (shown here in purple) build up in the body. No one understands why this occurs.

leukaemia, which can be difficult to treat. Life expectancy used to be approximately five years but advances in drug therapy have increased survival times for this disease, and bone marrow transplants may be curative in younger patients.

HAIRY CELL LEUKAEMIA

Occurring most often in middle age, this rare leukaemia causes bone marrow failure. Its name relates to the appearance of the cells on a blood film. Symptoms include those of anaemia, recurrent infection and abdominal pain (due to an enlarged spleen). Hairy cell leukaemia responds well to, and is often cured by, a drug called 2-CDA.

Myeloma

This bone-marrow cancer involves a type of antibody producing white blood cell known as a plasma cell. In this condition, these cells produce large amounts of an abnormal antibody known as paraprotein, some of which (Bence-Jones protein) may be excreted in the urine.

Myeloma is a disease that affects elderly people; the average age of sufferers is about 60. The disease can systematically destroy the bone marrow and bones. Treatment options vary but they are aimed at minimizing symptoms rather than effecting a cure and survival rates are poor.

SIGNS AND SYMPTOMS

Common symptoms include:

➤ Bone pain – most commonly backache.

➤ Anaemia – pale skin, fatigue and shortness of breath.

➤ Kidney failure – feeling unwell, infrequent urination and jaundice.

➤ Bleeding – due to low platelet levels.

Myeloma has several characteristics:
• Bone destruction – The bones of the spine are often affected, leading to collapse and fractures. This may compress the spinal cord and so trap nerves, causing weakness of various parts

▽ As myeloma systematically destroys the bones, one of its most common symptoms is bone pain, often in the form of backache.

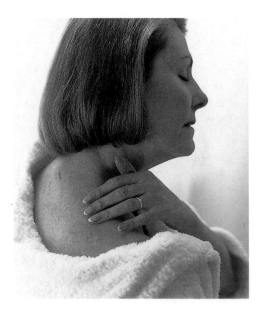

of the body, depending on which nerves are compressed.
• Raised blood calcium levels – The destruction of the bone releases calcium into the bloodstream (hypercalcaemia).
• Bone-marrow destruction – This leads to anaemia and low levels of platelets and white blood cells.
• Kidney damage – This is due partly to excretion of excess antibodies, and partly due to hypercalcaemia.

Patients with myeloma are also susceptible to recurrent infections.

WHAT MIGHT YOUR DOCTOR DO?

Your doctor will arrange a series of tests to confirm the diagnosis and help decide on suitable treatment. Tests include:
• Full blood count – Myeloma is suggested if the results reveal anaemia, low white blood cell count or low levels of platelets.
• Kidney function tests – The results may be abnormal and may show high blood calcium or uric acid levels.
• Electrophoresis – The Bence-Jones protein can be detected through a process called electrophoresis, which is where blood proteins are separated in a gel by using electricity.
• X-rays – Various X-rays may show bony deposits that point to myeloma; these are most easily detected in the skull.
• Urine tests – These are often able to detect the fragments of antibody called Bence-Jones protein.
• Bone marrow biopsy – The tissue sample taken in a biopsy may show infiltration by cancerous cells.

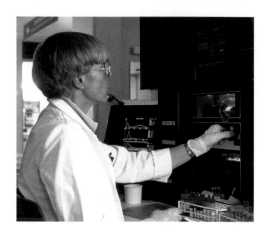

△ A full blood count test is one of the ways of diagnosing myeloma. Here, a technician uses a Coulter counter to measure the sizes of red, white and platelet cells in a blood sample.

TREATMENT OPTIONS

All symptoms are treated appropriately. For example, bone pain usually responds well to radiotherapy, and research shows that raised calcium levels can be reduced using drugs called bisphosphonates. Steroid drugs are also used to relieve the symptoms of bone deposits. Kidney dialysis may be the only treatment option for patients who suffer from kidney failure.

Certain chemotherapy agents have increased the long-term survival of myeloma patients, and new drug regimens show signs of further improvements.

WHAT IS THE OUTLOOK?

Until recently, few people diagnosed with myeloma lived much longer than six or seven months, and for a shorter time if they had complications such as anaemia and kidney failure. Now, myeloma sufferers without complications may survive up to two to three years and possibly longer.

Bone marrow disorders

SEE ALSO

➤ Heart disease, p34
➤ Anaemia, p202
➤ Acute leukaemias, p206
➤ Chronic leukaemias, p207

Bone marrow fills the inside of many of the bones of the body – those of the arms and legs, sternum (breastbone), shoulderblades, pelvis and ribs. Bone marrow produces stem cells that become red blood cells, white blood cells and platelets. When the bone marrow fails to perform this essential task, severe problems may arise, as the correct balance of these cells is vital for efficient functioning of the blood system. The bone marrow disorders covered here include: aplastic anaemia, polycythaemia, myelofibrosis and myelodysplasia.

APLASTIC ANAEMIA

This causes symptoms of anaemia, recurrent infections and bleeding. All cells made by the bone marrow are reduced in number. In half the cases no cause is found, but other common causes include:

• Chemotherapy drugs and occasionally sulphonamide drugs.
• Radiotherapy.
• Pregnancy.
• Chemicals such as benzene.
• Infections, such as measles, tuberculosis and hepatitis.

The outlook for aplastic anaemia is poor. Some patients' bone marrow will recover over time, but recurrent infections can prove life-threatening. Blood transfusions and antibiotics may be used to prevent and treat anaemia and infection. When the bone marrow fails to recover, a bone marrow transplant may correct the problem.

POLYCYTHAEMIA

In this condition there are too many red cells in the blood. The blood becomes significantly thicker, which may cause

BONE MARROW BIOPSY

Bone marrow diseases can be confirmed by taking a sample of bone marrow tissue (biopsy) and analysing it under a microscope. A sample is usually taken from the posterior iliac crest of the pelvis or the sternum (breastbone). Biopsies are carried out to diagnose leukaemias and are swift, safe procedures.

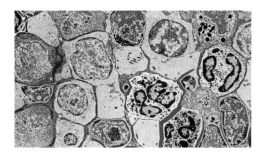

▷ This coloured micrograph shows the three different types of blood cell that are produced in the bone marrow: red blood cells, platelets and some white blood cells.

blood clots and thus strokes, and so some patients have blood removed from their circulation every week until red cell levels return to normal.

NATURAL ADAPTATIONS

Polycythaemia occurs naturally in people who live at high altitudes, in order to compensate for lower levels of oxygen in the air. It can also arise in people with chronic lung or heart diseases, as their bodies try to increase the amount of oxygen in their blood. Smoking is a common cause.

Symptoms of polycythaemia include:
• Ruddy complexion and bloodshot eyes.
• Headache.
• Ringing in the ears.
• Blurred vision.

MYELOFIBROSIS

Here, the bone marrow is replaced by scar tissue. Anaemia and bleeding disorders may develop, as the marrow fails to make enough red cells and platelets. Tiredness and weakness are common symptoms. The cause is unknown, and blood transfusions and drugs are used to control the symptoms.

MYELODYSPLASIA

This failure of the stem cells that produce red cells causes severe anaemia. About 30 per cent of sufferers eventually develop acute myelogenous leukaemia. Myelodysplasia usually affects the elderly and is treated with

blood transfusions and/or chemotherapy. In young patients, a bone marrow transplant can be a successful treatment.

BONE MARROW LOCATIONS

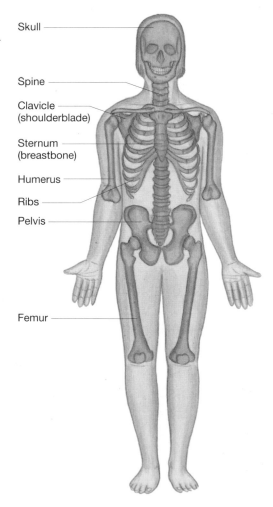

Skull
Spine
Clavicle (shoulderblade)
Sternum (breastbone)
Humerus
Ribs
Pelvis
Femur

Lymphomas

SEE ALSO
➤ Heart disease, p34
➤ Disorders of the liver, p54
➤ The roles of blood and lymph, p200

This general term refers to any cancer of the immune system's lymphoid tissues – principally the lymph nodes and spleen. These tissues produce the white cells that help protect our bodies against invading organisms. There are two main kinds of lymphoma. The type that displays classic abnormalities is called Hodgkin's lymphoma. All other kinds are grouped together under the term "non-Hodgkin's lymphoma". Most lymphomas cause enlargement of the lymph nodes. Rarely, cancer may develop in an organ, such as the thyroid gland, testis or breast.

SIGNS AND SYMPTOMS OF HODGKIN'S LYMPHOMA

➤ Pain-free swelling of lymph nodes in the neck or armpits.

➤ General malaise, fever, night sweats, poor appetite and weight loss.

➤ General itchiness.

➤ Pain after drinking alcohol (rare).

Lymphomas are divided into low- and high-grade, according to how fast they divide and grow. Paradoxically, the aggressive high-grade lymphomas are all potentially curable while the low-grade diseases often resist treatment.

INVESTIGATING LYMPHOMAS

You may undergo the following tests:
• Full blood count – The results may show anaemia, high white blood cell counts and low platelet levels.
• Kidney and liver function tests – Affected lymph tissue within these organs can affect their function.
• Chest or abdominal X-rays or CT scans – Abnormal masses may be seen.

▽ A surgeon carries out a lymph-node biopsy. The sample is then tested for cancerous cells.

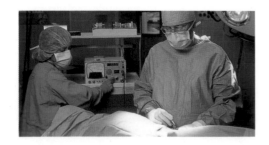

• Lymph node biopsy – This can detect cancerous cells in a sample of tissue.
• Uric acid test to reveal significantly raised levels in the blood.

HODGKIN'S LYMPHOMA (HODGKIN'S DISEASE)

This is a rare condition, affecting men more than women. Usually seen between the ages of 15 and 30 and 55 and 75, it is especially common in later life. Modern treatment has made this condition curable in most cases. The cause is unknown, though the Epstein-Barr virus is a possible link.

TREATMENT OPTIONS

Treatment consists of radiotherapy and/or chemotherapy, repeated over several sessions. The therapy will depend on the distribution and extent of the disease.

NON-HODGKIN'S LYMPHOMAS

This refers to a family of lymphomas – basically any lymphoma that is not Hodgkin's disease. These cancers usually affect those over 50. Each lymphoma in this family represents a cancer of one particular type of B- or T-type white blood cell.

BURKITT'S LYMPHOMA

First identified in West African children, this non-Hodgkin's lymphoma usually affects the jaw. The vast majority of people affected by this lymphoma, particularly children, can be treated successfully with chemotherapy.

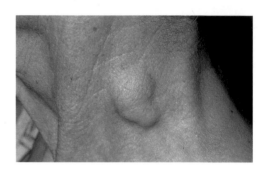

△ This swelling in a patient's neck is caused by an enlarged cancerous lymph node – in this case from a non-Hodgkin's lymphoma.

Again, the exact cause of these conditions has not yet been established, although it is possibly the result of a malfunctioning immune system, and various viruses, including the Epstein-Barr virus, have also been implicated.

TREATMENT OPTIONS

Lymphomas may be slowed by radiotherapy. Powerful anti-cancer drugs are used – chemotherapy – if the cancer has spread. A bone marrow transplant may be necessary.

SIGNS AND SYMPTOMS OF NON-HODGKIN'S LYMPHOMAS

➤ Pain-free swelling of lymph nodes in the neck or groin.

➤ Fever, night sweats, fatigue, weight loss, poor appetite.

➤ Abdominal swelling, enlarged spleen, or enlarged liver.

There may be different symptoms, if the cancer spreads to other organs.

Autoimmune diseases

Rheumatoid arthritis and diabetes are common examples of autoimmune diseases, in which the body's immune system attacks normal body tissue for reasons as yet unknown. Autoimmune conditions are often seen in young adults and it seems that women are more commonly affected than men. Symptoms for the different types of autoimmune disease can vary, but any and all should be investigated as early as possible. The severity of the symptoms and the outlook also varies greatly depending on which parts of the body are affected.

The term autoimmune disease covers a range of conditions in which areas of tissue become inflamed, causing a variety of problems. The inflammation arises when autoantibodies attack the tissue, seeing it as "foreign" matter that must be destroyed.

LUPUS ERYTHEMATOSUS

This condition, often called simply lupus, causes inflammation in various parts of the body. One form, discoid lupus, usually attacks the skin only. A more severe type – systemic lupus erythematosus, or SLE – may strike just about any part of the body, from the skin and joints to internal organs and membranes ("systemic" conditions are those that affect the whole body). In most sufferers, a few organs are affected at the same time.

Lupus is characterised by the production of autoantibodies that target genetic material, but why this occurs is unknown. The general outlook for sufferers is good

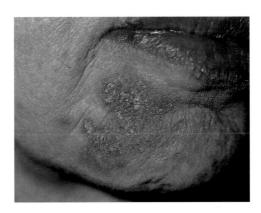

△ The skin rash associated with lupus erythematosus often appears on the face and neck and consists typically of red patches with grey-brown scales.

and symptoms can be controlled by taking corticosteroid drugs for joint inflammation and painkillers. Symptom-free periods do occur. There is usually a family history of the disease and it is rarely found in people outside the 12 to 55 age bracket.

SYSTEMIC SCLEROSIS

Also known as scleroderma, which means "hard skin", systemic sclerosis affects the body's connective tissue (any type of tissue that helps to hold together the body's form and organs). Affected tissues become inflamed, thickened and hardened, and also tighten up. Symptoms may be confined to the skin and joints but the condition can also affect internal organs. Signs of systemic sclerosis may be mistaken for other conditions – for example the joint discomfort is often thought to be rheumatoid arthritis. The disease is most commonly found in people between the ages of 20 and 50, and affects four times more women than men.

SIGNS AND SYMPTOMS OF SYSTEMIC LUPUS ERYTHEMATOSUS

Symptoms vary greatly from one person to another, and depend on which organs are affected, but they may include:

➤ Joint pain.

➤ Fever.

➤ Fatigue.

➤ Skin rashes, often a butterfly-shaped rash on the face.

SIGNS AND SYMPTOMS OF SYSTEMIC SCLEROSIS

Symptoms depend on the severity and spread of the condition and include:

➤ Fingers that are particularly sensitive to the cold (as in Raynaud's phenomenon).

➤ Small areas of hardened skin on the fingers.

➤ Swollen, painful joints.

➤ Muscle weakness.

➤ Difficulty swallowing, due to stiffening of the oesophagus.

There is as yet no cure. The outlook can be good if the skin alone is affected, but is harder to tackle if organs such as the heart, lungs or kidneys are implicated. However, in many people – thankfully – the disease progresses very slowly.

▽ In systemic sclerosis, the immune system turns against the body, causing a hardening of connective tissue. It may affect just one or several parts of the body.

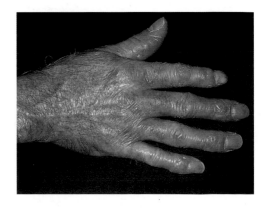

POLYMYOSITIS

This is a rare condition where the skeletal muscles become inflamed and painful. Other characteristics can include a red rash on the skin (usually on the face, chest and the backs of the hands), and if this occurs it is known as dermatomyositis.

Polymyositis usually settles down well following treatment with steroid drugs, but unfortunately it can be associated with certain cancers, including those of the lung, ovary, breast and stomach.

The outlook is much more hopeful for children with this disease than it is for adults, with 70 per cent of children recovering in around two years.

SIGNS AND SYMPTOMS OF POLYMYOSITIS

➤ Weak muscles.

➤ Fatigue.

➤ Difficulty swallowing and speaking, due to the oesophagus being affected.

➤ Shortness of breath, as the chest muscles become affected.

POLYMYALGIA RHEUMATICA

Another relatively rare condition, this inflammation of tissues causes aching and stiffness in the neck, shoulders, hips and lumbar spine. Symptoms of polymyalgia rheumatica tend to be worst first thing in the morning but usually wear off after a few

SIGNS AND SYMPTOMS OF POLYMYALGIA RHEUMATICA

➤ Aching and morning stiffness in the muscles of the neck, shoulders and hips. The torso and lower back can sometimes be affected too.

➤ Fatigue.

hours. There may also be tiredness, fever and weight loss. It almost always affects people over 50.

Diagnosis can be fairly straightforward because a blood test will show signs of inflammation. The condition often occurs together with temporal arteritis. Steroid treatment is usually successful in reducing inflammation, although steroids may need to be taken for several months. The condition tends to recur.

TEMPORAL ARTERITIS

This condition most commonly affects elderly people and causes an inflammation of the arteries in the temples at the sides of the head. It often develops in association with polymyalgia rheumatica.

As with polymyalgia rheumatica, diagnosis will usually be confirmed with a simple blood test, and sometimes by testing a sample taken from one of the temporal arteries. Treatment usually involves high-dose steroid drugs in the first instance; once the symptoms start to subside, the dose is gradually reduced over a period of months. However, this condition does have a tendency to recur.

▽ Many autoimmune disorders, such as polymyalgia rheumatica and temporal arteritis, are common in elderly people. They generally affect more women than men.

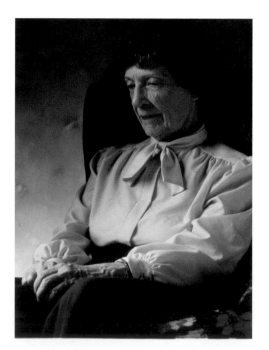

SJÖGREN'S SYNDROME

This chronic condition damages the glands that produce tears and saliva, causing dry eyes and a dry mouth. Nine times more women suffer from this condition than men and it affects people in the 40–60 age group. It is very commonly associated with rheumatoid arthritis. There is no cure but people with this condition use artificial tears, and drinking plenty of fluids can be helpful. A dry mouth may lead to dental problems, so regular check-ups are recommended.

▽ In Sjögren's syndrome, the salivary glands are unable to produce saliva, causing a dry tongue.

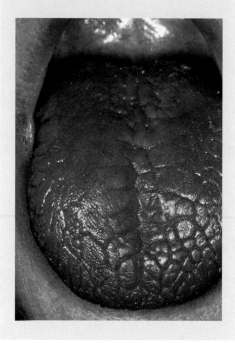

SIGNS AND SYMPTOMS OF TEMPORAL ARTERITIS

➤ Localized headache usually over the temple, which may be very tender to the touch.

➤ Fatigue.

Any visual disturbance, whether temporary or permanent, should be reported to your doctor as a matter of urgency because if this condition is left untreated, it can cause blindness.

14

INFECTIOUS DISEASES

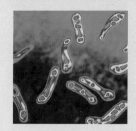

Humans pick up, incubate and pass on infectious diseases every day. Many infections are caught from droplets in the air produced by coughing and sneezing and so are difficult to avoid – just think how many people suffer from the common cold every year. However, your immune system is designed to deal effectively with infections – viral or bacterial – and they often pass with little more than a cough, sneezing, a runny nose and general malaise. Some infectious diseases, however, can be highly dangerous, particularly for very young children or the elderly, so an understanding of the different types and the issues involved can prove invaluable.

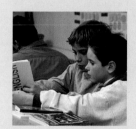

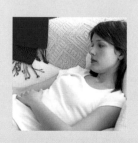

CONTENTS

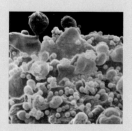

Causes of infectious disease

A vast range of tiny pathogens – disease-causing micro-organisms – are able to infect your body and cause all kinds of problems, from a mild cold to life-threatening malaria. An infection may be localized, where it affects only one part of your body, or systemic, which means that it affects the whole body. Infections can be spread in water or food, through touch or sexual contact, in the air and by insects. These micro-organisms also have the ability to change and adapt in order to outwit medication, so controlling them is a constant battle.

Invading micro-organisms, commonly called "germs", can be classified broadly into several distinct groups – bacteria, viruses, protozoa, and fungi and yeasts. Your body can also be invaded by larger, more complex organisms, such as worms and lice; these are often referred to as "infestations" rather than infections.

BACTERIA

Bacteria are microscopic organisms consisting of one cell. They are able to multiply (by division) very rapidly and are found everywhere – all around us and inside our bodies. There are, in fact, more bacterial cells inside us than body cells. Most bacteria are harmless and many are beneficial – bacteria in our large intestine help us to

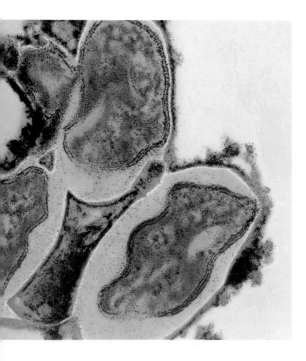

▽ *Mycobacterium tuberculosis* is the rod-shaped bacteria that causes tuberculosis in humans. It has become resistant to many drugs.

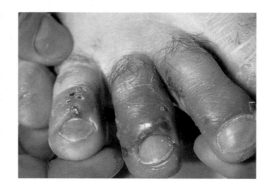

△ Athlete's foot is a fungal infection that causes irritation and inflammation of skin on the feet – typically between and on the toes.

digest and absorb certain food substances, for example. Of the thousands of different types of bacteria that exist, only a handful cause disease in humans. In some cases bacteria disrupt the normal working of cells themselves, while in others they release toxins that do the damage. Bacteria come in various shapes, which can be broadly grouped as:
• Cocci (spheres).
• Bacilli (rods).
• Spirochaetes (curved or twisted forms).

Common bacterial infections can include tuberculosis, pneumonia, meningitis and urinary tract infections.

FUNGI AND YEASTS

Fungi that cause disease tend to fall into two groups – filamentous fungi and single-celled yeasts. Yeasts resemble human cells (which is why they are used in genetic engineering, to produce copies of human substances such as insulin). They tend to cause only mild diseases such as skin infections but they can prove deadly in

people with a reduced immune system, such as people suffering from AIDS or those receiving a transplant.

Fungal infections include thrush (candidiasis), which can be vaginal or oral and can be treated with antifungal medication.

VIRUSES

These powerful organisms are made up of simple protein packets containing a few strands of genetic material. They are so tiny that millions of viruses could fit inside one human cell. Viruses bind to animal and plant cells and use these cells' own machinery to replicate themselves. In this process the host cell is destroyed, resulting in disease. Because viruses interfere with the

▽ The common cold is the most frequent, and usually one of the mildest, viral infections. Avoid spreading the virus through the air by covering your mouth as you cough or sneeze.

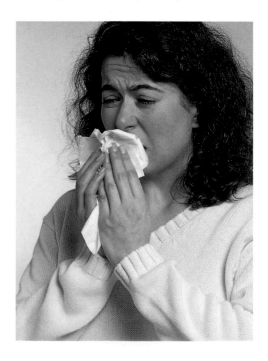

genetic structure of cells, many viruses have been implicated as factors that may lead to cancer. They have a great ability to dodge the defences of the immune system and can lie dormant for years.

Viruses cause diseases that range from relatively mild problems – the common cold or an upset stomach – to very severe and often fatal conditions, which include ebola, rabies and HIV.

PROTOZOA

A protozoan is a single-celled organism that scavenges food from other micro-organisms. They live mainly in moist environments such as soil and water but some can live inside creatures, such as the parasitic protozoan that causes malaria, which is found inside mosquitoes.

Common protozoal infections include malaria, sleeping sickness and toxoplas-mosis.

PARASITIC WORMS, MITES AND LICE

These creatures live in close contact with one another and cannot live without their hosts. This is why the most advanced parasites do not kill their host.

Common parasitic worm and lice infestations are tapeworm, pinworm, scabies and head lice.

▽ Head lice are a common problem in schools as they are easily spread when an infested child is in close contact with other children.

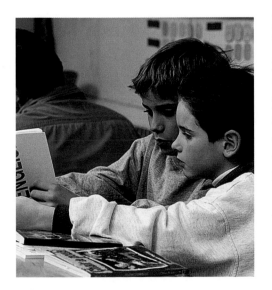

CONTROLLING INFECTION

Until the last 60 or so years, infectious diseases killed huge numbers of people all over the world; the very young and the elderly being particularly vulnerable. The spread of infectious diseases has been greatly controlled in recent times, thanks to better hygiene, cleaner water and pest control. Other vital factors that have made a significant difference to fighting infectious disease are widespread vaccination programmes and the use of drugs – antibiotics, antivirals and antifungals.

➤ Immunization – For many infectious diseases, especially viral ones, this is the only treatment available. Vaccines work by prompting and boosting the immune system to deal with a specific pathogen so that, next time around, it can deal with the infection more effectively.

➤ Antibiotics – The treatment of bacterial infections was revolutionized by the discovery of penicillin. This antibiotic was first made generally available to allied troops in the Second World War. Other antibiotics quickly followed and their ability to deal with infectious disease was dramatic – formerly fatal diseases were cured in a few days. Unfortunately, some bacteria have developed resistance to certain antibiotics. New drugs continue to be developed, but doctors are concerned that they won't always be able to keep a

step ahead in the battle against bacteria, and many are now more cautious in prescribing antibiotics for routine illnesses.

➤ Antiviral drugs – A few viral infections, such as herpes or HIV, can be controlled by drugs, but on the whole there is no treatment for viral illness other than trying to support the patient as they fight off the infection. Vaccines are still the best weapons against viral disease.

➤ Other drugs – These are used against pathogens such as parasites, fungi and yeasts. Unlike an antibiotic, which may defeat a range of bacteria, each of these drugs is usually efffective against just one particular pathogen.

▽ Immunization is one of the most effective ways to prevent infection, by boosting the immune system to fight specific pathogens.

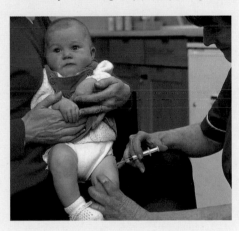

PRIONS

These unusual pathogens are protein particles without any DNA or RNA (genetic material). For reasons that are presently unknown, prions are able to replicate themselves rapidly, damaging surrounding body cells in the process. The term prion stands for proteinaceous infectious particle, and was suggested by Stanley Prusiner – who isolated the particle – to demonstrate that this was not a virus.

Prions are responsible for many diseases of the brain. The most notable being the new variant Creutzfeldt-Jakob disease

(vCJD) in humans, which is the equivalent of bovine spongiform encephalopathy (BSE) in cows.

Other diseases assigned to prions include fatal familial insomnia, which usually starts to affect people in middle age and causes worsening insomnia, memory loss, speech defects, muscle spasms and general physical and mental deterioration.

Prions are resistant to heat and all forms of sterilization and so can be passed around in contaminated food. Currently, there is no treatment available for diseases caused by prions.

Bacterial infections

SEE ALSO

➤ Meningitis, p84

➤ Urinary tract infections, p142

➤ Bacterial skin infections, p196

In the past, bacterial infections were a major cause of death all over the world. Since the advent of antibiotics, however, even the most serious bacterial infections can often be dealt with quickly and effectively. There are numerous bacterial infections that can attack the body, including tetanus, diphtheria and tuberculosis, most of which are now rare in developed countries because of long-standing and effective vaccination programmes. If a bacterium causes disease by releasing a powerful toxin, specific antitoxins can be prescribed.

PERTUSSIS

Also known as whooping cough, pertussis is caused by the bacterium *Bordetella pertussis*. It is highly contagious and is spread through the air in droplets formed by coughing and sneezing. It tends to occur in epidemics every few years, although most children under two are now vaccinated and so cases are rare.

Pertussis can occur at any age, although it is mainly found in children under the age of five. As with many bacterial and viral infections, its occurrence in adulthood can be much more severe.

The incubation period for the infection is seven to ten days, and in the initial catarrhal stage the patient is highly infectious. The early symptoms are tiredness, lack of appetite, a runny nose and

▽ Pertussis, or whooping cough, most commonly affects young children. It is highly contagious and can be very distressing.

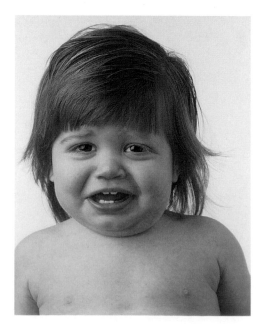

SIGNS AND SYMPTOMS OF PERTUSSIS

➤ Tiredness and loss of appetite.

➤ Symptoms as for the common cold.

➤ Severe and prolonged coughing, followed by a sharp intake of breath.

➤ Vomiting.

streaming eyes – symptoms very similar to those of the common cold.

As the infection progresses, however, it reaches a paroxysmal stage, so-called because of the paroxysms (bouts) of coughing that characterize this disease. A run of coughing as the child breathes out is followed by a large intake of breath, often causing the typical whooping sound. Vomiting may follow. This distressing stage can last for two weeks and may lead to serious complications as it affects the ability to breathe properly.

If caught in the first stage, an antibiotic can abort or reduce the severity of the disease. There is no effective treatment, however, once the cough starts, and often the only thing to do is wait for the infection to run its course.

TETANUS

In this disease, a powerful neurotoxin made by the bacterium *Clostridium tetani* attacks the nerves and causes muscle spasm. It occurs when these bacteria (which live in soil and in the intestines of humans and animals) contaminate a wound. In

DIPHTHERIA

A toxin made by the bacterium *Corynebacterium diphtheriae* causes diphtheria. Typical symptoms are:

➤ A sore throat.

➤ Fever.

➤ Swelling of the throat and larynx, which can block the airway.

Diphtheria may also affect the heart, causing inflammation of the heart muscle (myocarditis), and the brain, again causing inflammation (encephalitis).

Most people recover completely if treated promptly with antibiotics and antitoxin injections. Prevention is the best approach, however, via vaccination.

It is thanks to vaccination that diphtheria is now uncommon in developed countries, although it is on the increase in Eastern Europe and Russia. It is vital to keep vaccination levels up to prevent recurrence of this serious disease.

▽ The bacteria *Corynebacterium diphtheriae* – the cause of the dangerous condition diphtheria. Fortunately it is now uncommon in the developed world.

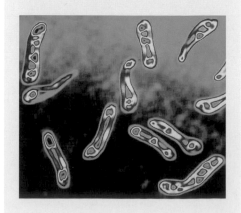

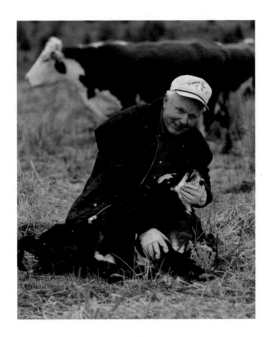

△ Tetanus bacteria thrive in soil and animal intestines, so farmers are particularly at risk – these bacteria are easily passed to humans.

developed countries, tetanus often occurs in elderly people who have injured themselves while gardening.

The toxin causes muscle spasm, particularly of the jaw muscles, hence tetanus's familiar name of "lockjaw". Other symptoms of the disease may include a high fever and headache, along with a characteristic grinning facial expression called *risus sardonicus*. The muscle spasm can also affect the muscles of the larynx, bladder and chest, which can be extremely dangerous because it affects the efficient functioning of these organs.

Occurrences of the disease used to be far more common than they are now, and 60 per cent of cases were fatal. This has been massively reduced to 20 per cent with the widespread use of antibiotics, antitoxins and, most importantly, good nursing care.

Immunization is the key to preventing cases of tetanus. All children in developed countries now have a course of three tetanus injections followed by regular boosters. Adults need a booster at least every ten years, but those most at risk, such as farmers, should have boosters every five years.

TUBERCULOSIS

This disease is caused by *Mycobacterium tuberculosis*, which is a slow-growing bacterium that causes a chronic infection. Tuberculosis is often rife among people who live in substandard social conditions in poorer parts of the world. In the world's richer countries, improvements in food, sanitation and housing over the past 50 years or so have led to significant reductions of tuberculosis cases. However, since 1985 there has been an increase in cases of tuberculosis worldwide, and this is possibly because the disease is becoming resistant to antibiotics, and may also be due to the rising prevalence of HIV and AIDS because so many more people are vulnerable to this type of infection.

Infection with *Mycobacterium tuberculosis* often causes only a mild illness with fever and cough, although this may persist for many weeks and produce a greenish-yellow sputum, but more severe cases can be dangerous. Tuberculosis bacteria are spread from person to person in airborne droplets in coughs and sneezes. Once a case has been detected, it is vital to trace and screen any contacts the patient may have had, in order to prevent the start of an epidemic. The infection can lie dormant for many years and reactivate itself long after the initial illness.

Fortunately, tuberculosis is readily treated nowadays, although it often needs treatment with multiple antibiotics for many months. It is also partially prevented with the BCG vaccine, which many people receive during adolescence. The efficiency of this vaccine depends on latitude – with 94 per cent protection in higher latitudes of

SCARLET FEVER

Scarlet fever bacteria (*Streptococcus pyogenes*) are spread by airborne droplets in coughs and sneezes. The red rash, which often develops after a throat infection, mainly affects the face and hands. It spreads rapidly and skin layers may peel away. The tongue may have a white coating with red spots (strawberry tongue). One week of antibiotic treatment usually clears it up.

▽ Scarlet fever rash is caused by toxins produced by the offending bacteria. The rash may spread all over the body.

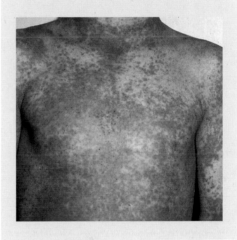

the globe to 0–20 per cent of the population near the equator.

Tuberculosis usually focuses on the lungs but it can spread to affect many different parts of the body, including the brain, the bones, the digestive tract and the skin.

Doctors use a chest X-ray to diagnose the disease but may also take a sputum sample to culture the bacterium.

SIGNS AND SYMPTOMS OF TETANUS

➤ Fever.

➤ Headache.

➤ Muscle spasms, particularly in the jaw.

➤ A grinning facial expression.

➤ Stiffness of the limbs.

SIGNS AND SYMPTOMS OF TUBERCULOSIS

➤ Fever.

➤ Persistent cough.

➤ Greenish-yellow sputum, or sputum streaked with blood.

➤ Night sweats.

➤ Weight loss.

Viral infections

SEE ALSO
➤ Viral encephalitis, p85
➤ Hepatitis, p163
➤ Sore throat and tonsillitis, p175
➤ Viral skin infections, p197

Most of the everyday infections you pick up will be viral – from a cough and cold to bouts of diarrhoea. Treatment for such conditions is usually supportive, which means it is aimed at managing the symptoms while your immune system conquers the viral attackers. Supportive treatment involves painkillers, bedrest and plenty of fluids. Sometimes, an antiviral drug is available to kill a particular virus, but on the whole your body's immune system does all the work. Common viral infections include chickenpox and measles.

CHICKENPOX

The virus *Varicella zoster* causes chickenpox. It is spread through the air and by contact with the characteristic skin blisters. The infection usually occurs in childhood and confers lifelong immunity. The disease is much more severe in adults who did not have it as children, and so it is important to

▽ A chickenpox rash is made up of small, itchy red spots which turn into fluid-filled blisters. Calamine lotion can be used to soothe irritation.

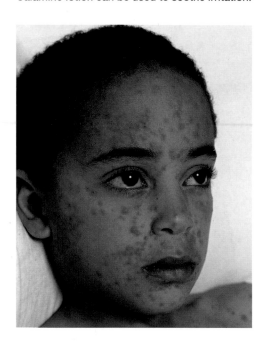

SIGNS AND SYMPTOMS OF CHICKENPOX

➤ Headache.

➤ Fever.

➤ Malaise.

➤ Itchy red rash all over the body, which develops into fluid-filled spots.

SHINGLES

Shingles is caused by the chickenpox virus. Most people have chickenpox in childhold, and then the virus usually lies dormant in the nerves of the spinal cord. Sometimes it reactivates to produce shingles – pain along a nerve and a skin rash following the line of the nerve. There may be fever, headache and malaise too.

keep infected children away from public places. Pregnant women are vulnerable to chickenpox, which could damage the fetus, and so should seek medical help if they may have been exposed to the virus.

The course of the disease takes two to three weeks from incubation to recovery. It often begins with fever, malaise and headache. A red blistering rash develops all over, even inside the mouth in many cases, and the red spots quickly fill with fluid and crust over. Children must be kept isolated until all the blisters have dried up.

Rarely, chickenpox can cause a severe form of pneumonia and viral encephalitis. Children usually require no specific treatment, but in people over 16 and in those with a reduced immune system, antiviral drugs may be used.

RUBELLA

Also known as German measles, this viral infection produces a mild illness in children. In adults, the disease can be more serious.

▷ A rubella rash consists of tiny red spots. Rubella is most dangerous if it affects pregnant women in the first four months of pregnancy.

SIGNS AND SYMPTOMS OF RUBELLA

➤ Fever.

➤ Mild malaise.

➤ A fine red rash all over the body.

There are rarely any complications in children but unimmunized pregnant women are particularly vulnerable to this infection. Rubella can cause congenital rubella syndrome in a woman's developing baby, resulting in various complications including heart malformations, cataracts, mental retardation and deafness. There is no treatment for these malformations once the infection has developed, so it is vital to prevent outbreaks of this disease via vaccination. Rubella vaccine is now combined with those for measles and mumps in the MMR vaccine.

It can be spread through airborne droplets produced while sneezing or coughing. The incubation period (the time after infection before symptoms develop) of the rubella virus is two to three weeks.

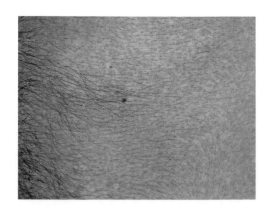

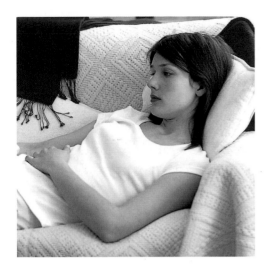

△ Listlessness and fatigue are often the longest lasting symptoms of glandular fever.

GLANDULAR FEVER

Also known as infectious mononucleosis, this disease is common worldwide among adolescents and young adults. It is caused by the Epstein-Barr virus and is transmitted by saliva (hence its nickname, "kissing disease") and via small droplets in the air.

Infection causes swollen lymph nodes (commonly known as glands) and a sore throat (making it difficult to swallow), along with fever, headache and malaise. These symptoms appear weeks after the initial infection and develop over several days. Once established, symptoms last for a few weeks.

Glandular fever may produce a rash and an enlarged spleen. Furthermore, the person may have a poor appetite and lose weight. Some people can be debilitated for months and become depressed. To confirm the disease, your doctor tests a blood sample for the presence of antibodies against the virus.

△ A measles rash appears first on the face and then spreads over the body.

There is no specific treatment for glandular fever and supportive treatments are usually all that is required. Almost everyone makes a full recovery and one attack provides lifelong protection. However, a lengthy illness can prove disastrous for some, especially young athletes and those about to sit examinations.

MEASLES

The measles virus causes a serious infection in children. One child in 500 with the disease will die. In developed countries, occurrence is rare due to vaccination, but the number of cases rises when parents stop getting their children vaccinated after scares about the vaccine leading to various illnesses.

The virus passes from person to person in the air, carried in droplets of water, and is contagious from four days before until two days after the rash develops. In the initial phase the symptoms include fever, malaise and a cough. Characteristic grey patches with a red base (known as Koplick's spots) may appear in the mouth. A widespread, non-itchy red rash then develops, initially on the face but spreading to other parts of the body.

In healthy children there are usually no complications, but serious complications can occur in those with other diseases, including pneumonia, infection of the heart muscle (myocarditis) and inflammation of the brain (encephalitis). The measles virus does not cause fetal malformations but it can cause premature labour and abortion.

There is no specific treatment for measles. The best way is to avoid it altogether via vaccination.

MUMPS

This viral infection is now rarer, due to vaccination. The mumps virus is spread by sneezing and coughing and by skin contact, and affects mainly schoolchildren and young adults. Early symptoms of fever, malaise and headache are followed by painful swelling of one or both parotid salivary glands in the cheeks, causing a hamster-like appearance. Symptoms usually subside after two or three weeks. Mumps can have serious complications, including inflammation of the brain (encephalitis) and painful swelling of the testicles (epididymo-orchitis), which can cause sterility.

▽ The mumps virus causes swelling of the parotid glands in the angle of the jaws, resulting in red, swollen cheeks.

SIGNS AND SYMPTOMS OF GLANDULAR FEVER

➤ Swollen lymph nodes.

➤ Listlessness and fatigue.

➤ Headache.

➤ Fever.

➤ Rash.

➤ Sore throat.

SIGNS AND SYMPTOMS OF MEASLES

➤ Cold and fever.

➤ An angry red rash.

➤ Malaise.

➤ A cough.

➤ Conjunctivitis.

➤ Sneezing.

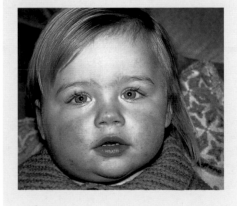

HIV and AIDS

The first cases of human immunodeficiency virus (HIV) infection were identified on the west coast of the US in 1981. The World Health Organization now estimates that there are about 40 million people worldwide infected with HIV. The parts of the globe that have been particularly affected are sub-Saharan Africa and the Indian subcontinent. The source of the virus is still not fully understood but, like many tropical viral illnesses, it is believed to have developed first in apes and then to have been transmitted to humans.

It took some years after the first cases of this new and aggressive disease before the virus was identified and medical experts began working on treatments and possible cures. In that time, before many people were even aware of it, the number of cases rose dramatically. Today, awareness of the disease and how it is contracted is so widespread that the incidence should have dropped, but this appears not to be the case. Precautions should always be taken when having sexual intercourse with any partner who has not been tested for HIV or AIDS.

In the US, Canada and the UK, HIV is most commonly transmitted during sex between homosexual men and via shared needles in intravenous drug-users. There are, however, increasing reports of new cases among heterosexual men and women, which may be due to changes in the virus and to increases in sexual promiscuity amongst younger people. In sub-Saharan Africa and India, where HIV has reached epidemic proportions, the patterns of transmission are different and it is most commonly transmitted via heterosexual sex.

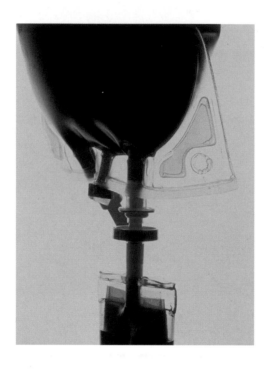

△ Blood that is used for transfusions is screened for HIV, among other things, to ensure there is no danger of the virus being transmitted.

HOW IS HIV TRANSMITTED?

The HIV virus can be found in blood, semen, vaginal secretions and breast milk. The known modes of transmission for the HIV virus are:

• Sexual intercourse (vaginal, anal and oral) – The most common mode of transmission worldwide is vaginal intercourse but in the US, Canada and the UK, HIV is more commonly spread among gay men.

• Contaminated blood and blood products – Before compulsory screening was introduced for donated blood, after the virus had been identified in 1981, thousands of people with haemophilia became infected with HIV. Routine screening in many countries has made this much rarer.

• From mother to child – Transmission can occur either in the womb via the placenta, during birth or through breastfeeding.

• Contaminated needles – Intravenous drug-users often share needles; this route to infection is a common one in the US and Europe.

• Needlestick injuries – Healthcare workers can become infected with HIV if they accidentally injure themselves on a needle contaminated with HIV-positive blood from a patient.

There are a number of less common ways of becoming infected. For example, some cases are believed to have been contracted when a tattooist used the same needle for several customers.

SIGNS AND SYMPTOMS OF THE ONSET OF AIDS

Deterioration of the immune system causes symptoms that vary in each case and which may signal AIDS:

➤ Oral thrush.

➤ Recurrent vaginal thrush.

➤ Recurrent herpes infections.

➤ Intermittent fever.

➤ Weight loss.

➤ Diarrhoea.

➤ Muscular aches and pains.

SIGNS AND SYMPTOMS OF HIV

Initial infection may cause minor illness or none at all. These early symptoms can typically include:

➤ Flu-like symptoms.

➤ Generalized lymph node enlargement.

➤ Fatigue and dizziness.

WHAT HIV DOES TO THE BODY

HIV infects and eventually destroys particular white blood cells, which reduces the efficiency of the body's immune system. Once the virus starts to destroy these white blood cells, then the door to illness opens.

HIV infection typically progresses through three stages. In the first stage, when a person has just been infected, the virus starts to reproduce rapidly. Some people experience flu-like symptoms for a week or two at this time; others have no symptoms at all. During this early phase, blood tests may well not reveal the presence of antibodies to HIV – which is how doctors can tell whether someone is HIV-positive. It usually takes some weeks (in a few cases, up to a year) after infection before the antibodies reach a detectable

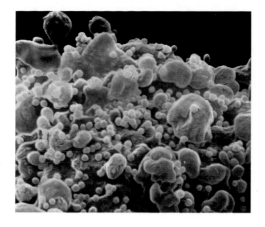

△ This electron micrograph shows white blood cells that have been infected with the HIV virus – the virus is shown in green.

level. At this stage, the immune system is still generally effective but there may be an increasing susceptibility to infections.

In stage two of the HIV cycle, there is an asymptomatic (showing no symptoms) period. This may last for around ten years. Further deterioration in the immune system generally follows, due to falling levels of white blood cells. This increases the chance of developing more serious and potentially life-threatening illnesses, often called "AIDS-defining conditions". An HIV-positive person who develops any of these conditions has reached the third stage – full-blown AIDS (acquired immunodeficiency syndrome). At present, most HIV-positive people go on to develop AIDS, but a few do not, and they may provide clues as to how the disease can be beaten in the future.

MANAGEMENT OF HIV AND AIDS

Although there is no cure for HIV infection or AIDS, treatment has been transformed over the past ten years by the development of a number of antiviral drugs capable of significantly delaying the progression of this condition. Anyone who is diagnosed with the HIV virus will usually be prescribed these HIV-protease inhibitor drugs. They reduce the ability of the virus to replicate itself in human cells and slow down the process of deterioration. Several have been proven to work and others are currently being investigated and tested.

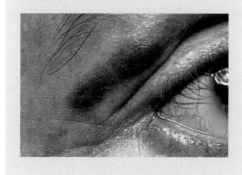

These drugs are usually administered in combinations of three drugs on an indefinite basis. A number of other medications may also be taken – in order to prevent various bacterial, fungal and viral infections from taking hold and causing complications. Someone suffering from HIV will probably need to take these drugs for the rest of their life, but we have seen that life-expectancy can be greatly extended through their use.

Drug treatment and public health programmes have decreased the number of HIV-related deaths in the US, Canada and parts of Europe, but in countries that are unable to afford such treatments, the number of deaths continues to rise rapidly.

Awareness and understanding of HIV and AIDS has grown as people realize that it cannot be transmitted through the air or via normal contact with infected people. However, many still seem unaware of the real dangers of this disease and do not take preventative measures seriously. Educating people is key to preventing the worldwide spread of this virus.

Malaria

SEE ALSO

➤ Travel health and safety, p26

➤ Anaemia, p202

➤ Sickle cell anaemia, p204

Malaria is a disease that is widespread throughout the tropics, and it is caused by a group of parasites that colonize the red blood cells and the liver. These parasites (protozoa) belong to the *plasmodium* group and there are four subtypes that infect humans – *p. falciparum*, *p. malariae*, *p. ovale* and *p. vivax*. Each causes a slightly different illness and needs particular treatment. The most serious form of the disease is *falciparum* malaria. The parasites are carried by mosquitoes, which pass them on to humans when they bite them to suck their blood.

SIGNS AND SYMPTOMS

The symptoms are caused by the parasite multiplying inside red blood cells, often destroying them in the process. Symptoms usually start ten days to six weeks after being bitten and infected. The symptoms include:

➤ Intermittent high fever.

➤ Anaemia – with fatigue, pale skin and headache.

➤ An enlarged liver or spleen, with abdominal pain.

Malaria is a common disease in tropical countries and cases are increasingly found amongst travellers. It currently affects 250 million people and is fatal in around 1 per cent of cases. It is endemic in India, parts of Africa and Central and South America.

▽ This magnified image shows a red blood cell infected with the malaria parasite, which will eventually destroy it.

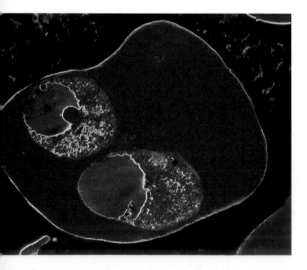

MALARIAL FEVER

The fever characteristically goes through three phases:

1 The "cold stage" – The patient feels cold and shivery despite having a high fever.

2 The "hot stage" – The patient feels very hot and may be delirious.

3 The "sweating stage" – The bedclothes may be drenched, but the patient feels better, although they will be very tired and may sleep for large parts of the day.

In most forms of malaria, the fever occurs every other day, can last for several weeks and has a tendency to recur.

In the most serious form – *falciparum* – the malarial fever is more severe and is usually continuous. During this time, the parasite kills large numbers of red blood cells. This form of the disease can be fatal within 48 hours. It can also damage the kidneys, liver, brain and gut, and may leave the patient permanently debilitated if they survive at all. In addition, it causes two unique complications:

• Cerebral (brain) malaria – This causes convulsions, coma and death.

• Blackwater fever – The large number of dead red blood cells causes the urine to become dark brown-black and can lead to kidney failure.

WHEN TO SEE YOUR DOCTOR

If you have recently visited a malarial zone and develop a fever shortly after returning home, see your doctor immediately.

Your doctor may suspect malaria if you have recently returned from a tropical country and have a fever. The diagnosis can be confirmed by laboratory examination of a blood sample, which will identify the presence of the malarial parasite.

The mainstay of treatment of this very serious illness is antimalarial drugs. Painkillers and drugs to reduce fever are also helpful. In severe cases, urgent hospitalization may be needed in order to treat the disease effectively.

PREVENTING MALARIA

One of the most effective ways to prevent malaria is antimalarial drugs. Seek medical advice on the most up-to-date recommendations for the country you intend to visit. It is also important to avoid being bitten (remember that mosquitoes are more active at night):

➤ Apply insect repellents at dusk.

➤ Sleep under a mosquito net.

➤ Wear light-coloured long-sleeved shirts and trousers in the evening.

▽ When travelling to countries where malaria is endemic, it is advisable to sleep under a protective net to avoid being bitten by mosquitoes.

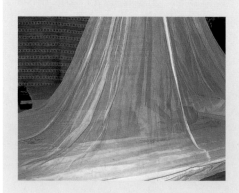

15

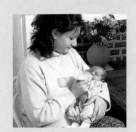

CHILDREN'S HEALTH

Children are vulnerable to infections and certain illnesses because their immune systems, along with all their other body systems, are still developing. They are also more likely than adults to suffer complications from diseases such as pneumonia. It is therefore important that parents monitor their child's illness, and consult a doctor if there are any unusual, severe or persistent symptoms. However, most children have an ability to bounce back to health with enviable speed, and many recurrent childhood problems – such as eczema and asthma – improve as a child gets older.

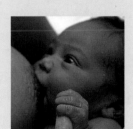

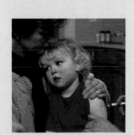

CONTENTS

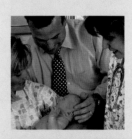

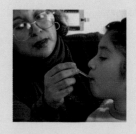

Protection against infection

Infectious diseases used to be the most common cause of death in children and young adults. However, since doctors started using immunization – injecting vaccines, for example – to help our immune systems fight harmful invaders, infections such as meningitis, measles and tetanus are no longer widespread killers. A range of methods have been developed to boost the immune system, and if immunized early in life a child can be protected even before they are at risk from infection. Most immunizations are very safe and produce few side effects.

"Immunization" is a general term for the ways in which medicine can help the body prepare in advance to fight disease. Immunization is achieved by giving vaccines, typically by injection. These may be dead or weakened forms of disease-causing micro-organisms (bacteria or viruses), which stimulate the body to produce disease-fighting antibodies against that illness. In this way, the immune system is primed to recognize and defeat the micro-organism if the child encounters it at a later date. This method is also known as vaccination. (The other immunization method involves giving people actual antibodies, which provides shorter-term protection.) Vaccination can give your child

WHAT VACCINATIONS ARE CURRENTLY AVAILABLE?

National vaccination programmes may vary slightly but they tend to follow the schedule outlined below. Your doctor will advise you on the best specific schedule for your child.

Age	Vaccination
2 months	DTP, Hib, polio, meningitis C
3 months	DTP, Hib, polio, meningitis C
4 months	DTP, Hib, polio, meningitis C
12–15 months	MMR
4–5 years	DT, MMR
10–13 years	BCG

Key: D = Diphtheria; T = Tetanus; P = Pertussis; Hib = *Haemophilus influenzae* B;
MMR = Measles, mumps and rubella; BCG = bacillus Calmette-Guérin for tuberculosis.

HOW ANTIBODIES FIGHT INFECTION

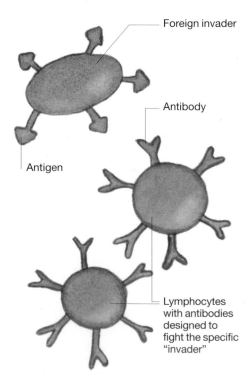

Foreign invader

Antibody

Antigen

Lymphocytes with antibodies designed to fight the specific "invader"

◁ ▽ Lymphocytes (a type of white blood cell) produce antibodies that fight infection. Specific antibodies "recognize" specific antigens (substances that form part of disease-causing micro-organisms) and so can destroy invaders.

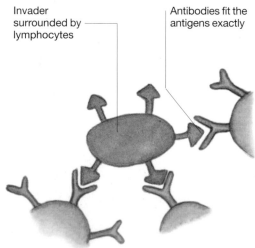

Invader surrounded by lymphocytes

Antibodies fit the antigens exactly

long-term protection from a range of infectious diseases that either cannot be treated or that spread so rapidly that treatment is inadequate.

A different vaccine is given for each disease, because the immune system produces specific antibodies to kill each invader. For most infections, several vaccinations are needed so that the immune system builds up and maintains a protective level of antibodies.

WHY VACCINATE?

Vaccination gives a significant level of protection against potentially fatal diseases. Many of these diseases still do not have an effective treatment, so vaccination may be the only way to protect your child.

Immunization can also help to eradicate the virus or bacterium from circulation. This is because, when the majority of

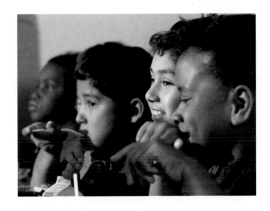

△ Immunization effectively protects your child against disease-causing micro-organisms, even if they come into close contact with a child who has already been infected.

children in a population are fully immunized, there are fewer potential carriers – if the virus or bacterium cannot spread it will gradually die out.

Smallpox, the first disease for which there was a vaccine, has been eradicated worldwide, and vaccination is no longer necessary. By contrast, cases of measles are becoming more common, because concerns over possible side effects cause some parents to decide against vaccinating their children.

SIDE EFFECTS OF VACCINATION
Most vaccines produce few side effects – the polio, diphtheria and tetanus vaccines are all extremely safe. Others – notably the MMR vaccine – are capable of causing very mild forms of the diseases they are designed to fight. Common side effects for all forms of immunization include the following:
• A mild fever for 24–48 hours after the immunization. This may be relieved by giving the child paracetomol syrup.
• A localized allergic reaction, causing redness, swelling and pain at the site of the injection. This usually subsides within days and has no lasting effect.

The MMR vaccine may cause the following side effects:
• A fever and a measles-like rash, which may occur one week after the vaccination.
• Swelling in salivary glands (the parotid glands which are just in front of the ears) up to three weeks after vaccination.

• Sore joints two to three weeks following the vaccination.

If a child falls ill after receiving a vaccination, it is worth remembering that the two events are not necessarily linked. Babies and children succumb to a large number of minor infections in the first years of life, and it is inevitable that some of these will coincide with a vaccination.

WHAT IS THE RISK OF SERIOUS SIDE EFFECTS?
Serious side effects are rare and are thought to occur in about one out of every 100,000 vaccinations. Severe reactions can take several different forms:
• A local allergic reaction may occur, in which an extensive area of redness and swelling spreads out from the site of the original injection.
• General reactions may include a high fever (39.5°C/103°F or above) that develops within 48 hours of the vaccination, severe irritability and/or convulsions.
• Rarely, a child may suffer a severe allergic reaction that can lead to anaphylactic shock. This can be fatal if emergency medical treatment is not provided.

The pertussis (whooping cough) vaccine carries a minimal risk of brain damage. However, the disease is more likely to

▽ This two-year-old girl is receiving her MMR vaccination, which will protect her against measles, mumps and rubella.

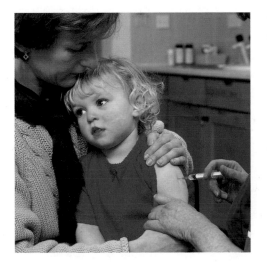

cause damage than the vaccine. Some people have suggested a link between MMR and autism, but this is not proven. Generally it is safer for a child to be vaccinated than not, and most people decide that the advantages of vaccination outweigh the risks. However, if you are worried, you should discuss your concerns with your health visitor or doctor. If your child develops any serious side effects after a vaccination, you should seek medical help immediately.

IS THERE AN ALTERNATIVE?
There are no proven and effective alternatives to the vaccination programme available now. Homeopathic medicines have been developed but there is no evidence that they provide children with significant levels of protection.

Colds and sore throats

SEE ALSO

➤ Colds and flu, p128

➤ The function of the ears, nose and throat, p166

➤ Hayfever, p172

➤ Sinusitis, p173

All children suffer from frequent colds and sore throats. A normal, healthy child may have at least five or six colds in a year, and more if he or she attends a nursery or has older brothers and sisters. Most colds and sore throats are caused by viruses and result in a relatively short episode of illness from which your child quickly recovers. Usually all that is needed is simple treatment to reduce fever and relieve other symptoms. Only if the child has a very high fever, symptoms such as a rash on the skin, or a headache is there usually any cause for concern.

SIGNS AND SYMPTOMS

A child with a cold or sore throat may feel reasonably well or they may have:

➤ Fever.

➤ Tired, heavy, aching feeling.

➤ Runny nose.

➤ Earache.

Colds and sore throats generally get better with supportive treatment such as:

• Painkilling syrup, such as paracetamol, to help to bring down a fever.

• Simple decongestants in the form of liquid drops for the pillow or a rub for the chest to relieve a blocked nose.

• Plenty of fluids to prevent the child from becoming dehydrated.

▷ Sponging with tepid water is a possible way to reduce a fever.

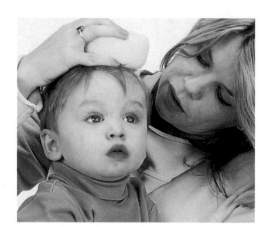

Earache in children

SEE ALSO

➤ Earache, p168

One of the most common childhood health problems is earache, which is usually the result of teething or an infection. Most earaches get better by themselves, but painkilling syrup can relieve discomfort. If the cause is a bacterial infection, antibiotics may be necessary.

Ear infections can damage hearing, so it is important that you take your child to the doctor if they have a persistent earache.

Most ear infections start in the throat and then travel via the Eustachian tube to the middle ear chamber. This condition, known as otitis media, is the most common ear infection suffered by children.

TYPES OF OTITIS MEDIA

In acute otitis media, the middle ear can become filled with infected secretions. The eardrum turns red and bulges out. It may rupture, which is a defensive reaction to allow the infection to drain, and there may a small amount of blood too. The earache often improves once the eardrum has burst and any perforation usually heals very quickly. Painkilling syrup relieves the pain.

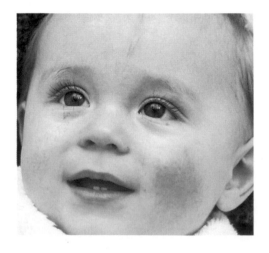

◁ Babies often develop earache when teething. Fever and vomiting may be the only symptoms.

Otitis media with effusion (glue ear) is a common cause of earache, but many children with this condition have no pain. The ear becomes filled with a thick, sticky secretion or "glue", often as a result of repeated viral infections. This fluid fails to drain via the Eustachian tube, which leads to temporary deafness. Repeated bouts of deafness can affect a child's speech.

Most cases of glue ear settle on their own, but an operation to drain the glue may be required. This operation consists of making a small hole in the eardrum and inserting a plastic tube – which is known as a grommet – to keep the hole open.

If a child suffers recurrent and severe earache, antibiotics are usually advised.

Bronchiolitis

SEE ALSO
➤ Smoking and your
  health, p20
➤ The breathing
  process, p126
➤ Viral infections, p218

Bronchiolitis is an infection of the tiny airways (the bronchioles) in the lungs. It is usually caused by the respiratory syncytial virus (RSV), which is spread via coughing and sneezing. Bronchiolitis most commonly affects children during the first year of their lives, and may occur in epidemics during winter. Children living in overcrowded conditions or whose parents smoke are at greater risk. The condition can be serious: the airways may become inflamed, restricting breathing. If your child has difficulty breathing, urgent hospital treatment is required.

SIGNS AND SYMPTOMS

The typical symptoms of bronchiolitis include:

➤ An initial cold or sore throat.

➤ A dry cough.

➤ Wheezing.

➤ Rapid breathing.

➤ Difficulty in breathing.

➤ Difficulty in feeding.

You should consult a doctor if your child develops the symptoms of bronchiolitis. Mild cases can be managed at home with regular doses of painkilling syrup to control fever; sitting your child in a steamy bathroom can help to ease breathing. More serious cases need to be admitted to hospital for intravenous fluids, inhaled bronchodilator drugs and oxygen.

Many infants are prone to recurrent episodes of wheezing for a year or two after developing bronchiolitis. These usually occur when they have a cough or cold.

CROUP

This viral infection of the windpipe most often affects children of six months to three years. Typical symptoms are:

➤ A barking cough.

➤ Rapid, harsh and noisy breathing.

➤ Fever.

Sitting the child in a steam-filled bathroom often helps to relieve symptoms, but severe attacks require hospital treatment.

Pneumonia

SEE ALSO
➤ The breathing
  process, p126

Pneumonia is an inflammation of the air sacs (alveoli) within the lungs. It is caused by a viral or bacterial infection. The alveoli become inflamed and fill with white blood cells, which makes it harder for oxygen to cross into the blood vessels and circulation.

SIGNS AND SYMPTOMS

Pneumonia is a serious condition which causes the child to:

➤ Feel severely unwell.

➤ Look flushed and have a high fever.

➤ Have a persistent cough.

➤ Wheeze.

➤ Breathe rapidly.

➤ Breathe in so strongly that the spaces between the ribs are sucked in.

Young children are at greater risk of developing pneumonia than adults because their immune systems are not fully developed. They are also more likely to suffer life-threatening complications.

You should take a child with the symptoms of pneumonia to see a doctor immediately. Most children with pneumonia require hospital admission to treat the infection. They will usually start to improve rapidly once treatment with oxygen, intravenous antibiotics and fluids has been started.

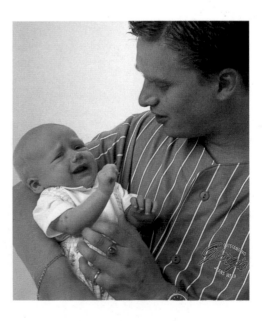

▷ A baby or child with pneumonia will usually appear flushed and will develop a fever.

Diarrhoea, vomiting and constipation

Children frequently suffer from bouts of diarrhoea and vomiting (often caused by gastroenteritis), and may also suffer from constipation. Most cases are straightforward and clear up in a matter of days. However, children suffering from vomiting or diarrhoea are at risk of dehydration because it is difficult for them to replace lost fluids quickly enough. It is therefore important that you encourage a child to drink during an illness. You should take your child to visit a doctor if the symptoms are particularly severe or last longer than a few days.

In general terms, the number and consistency of bowel motions passed by children is variable, especially during infancy. Breastfed babies often pass yellow, very loose stools several times a day while bottle-fed babies usually pass firmer stools less frequently. Many older children continue to have three or four bowel motions a day. This is not usually a cause for concern, unless a child is also failing to gain weight normally. Children of any age may also be prone to occasional episodes of constipation.

DIARRHOEA

Bouts of diarrhoea may have a simple cause such as the introduction of a new food into a baby's diet, or excitement or anxiety in a child. However, they can also be due to conditions such as:

• Infection of the gastrointestinal tract by a virus or, less commonly, a bacterium. This condition, known as gastroenteritis, is the most common cause of diarrhoea in

▽ The bowel habits of babies can vary widely, and may depend on whether they are fed from a bottle or the breast.

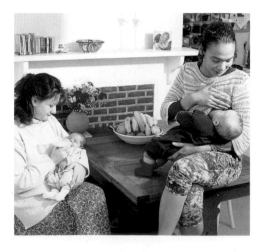

VOMITING WARNING

If your child is suffering from any of the following symptoms in addition to vomiting, you should seek urgent medical attention.

➤ Bloody or black stools.

➤ Purple spots on the skin that do not fade after being pressed with the side of a glass.

➤ Prolonged abdominal pain.

➤ Unusual drowsiness.

➤ Signs of dehydration (see box).

children and infants. It can also cause bouts of vomiting.

• Difficulty in absorbing certain foods. This can be due to coeliac disease, in which there is a sensitivity to gluten in wheat and other foods.

• An allergy to cow's milk, which occurs in 1 in 25 babies. It is caused by sensitivity to proteins in cow's milk or ordinary formula milks.

VOMITING

Vomiting is a distressing symptom. It is an unpleasant experience for a child and can also be very upsetting for the parents. The causes of vomiting are many and varied, and they include:

• Infection – gastroenteritis is a common cause of vomiting, but almost every childhood infection – including ear, urinary and respiratory infections – can make a child sick.

• Difficulty in absorbing certain substances – for example, a sensitivity to gluten.

• An allergy to cow's milk.

• Emotional problems. Stress or anxiety can lead to vomiting in children.

• Digestive disorders such as a weakness in the muscles around the entrance to the stomach (gastro-oesophageal reflux), or an abnormality in the outlet of the stomach (pyloric stenosis).

• Rarely, vomiting can be the result of a head injury.

WHAT SHOULD I DO?

Vomiting is commonly the result of gastroenteritis, which clears up by itself. The main supportive treatment is to ensure that your child drinks plenty of fluids (see the entry on gastroenteritis).

You should always seek medical help if a child seems particularly unwell, if they have had abdominal pain for longer than four hours, or if the vomiting is persistent.

DEHYDRATION WARNING

If a child becomes dehydrated, they may develop the following symptoms:

➤ Drowsiness and listlessness.

➤ Dry tongue and lips.

➤ Sunken eyes.

➤ Passing a small amount of dark urine.

➤ In infants, a sunken fontanelle (the soft spot on the crown of the head).

Seek immediate medical help if your child develops any of these symptoms.

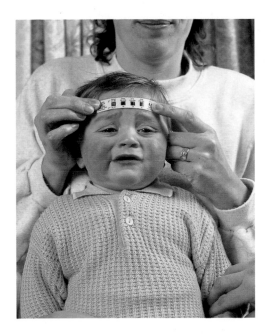

△ A high fever can indicate gastroenteritis. When checking a temperature, bear in mind that strip thermometers such as this one are easier to use on small children, but are not epecially accurate or reliable – you may want to double-check with a conventional thermometer.

Unexplained vomiting in babies or small children requires medical assessment.

GASTROENTERITIS

Most cases of gastroenteritis are mild. They usually clear up by themselves after a few days or perhaps a week. The focus of treatment should be to ensure that your child remains well hydrated.

Doctors usually tell you to give a child plenty of clear liquids and to avoid giving

SIGNS AND SYMPTOMS OF GASTROENTERITIS

The symptoms of gastroenteritis often develop quite quickly over the course of one or two days. Your child may have any combination of the following symptoms:

➤ Vomiting.

➤ Abdominal pain.

➤ Diarrhoea.

➤ High temperature.

➤ A cough and/or runny nose.

milk unless you are breastfeeding. Milk and the lactose it contains are difficult to digest effectively during such an infection, and it may cause more diarrhoea. Antidiarrhoeal drugs are too toxic for small children and should never be given.

HOW TO AID RECOVERY

• Encourage your child to drink small amounts of fluid at frequent intervals. This should be a glucose and electrolyte mixture for small children or clear fluids for older children (water, diluted fruit juice or lemonade).
• Breastfed babies should continue to breastfeed throughout their illness, even though this may provoke more diarrhoea.
• Infants on bottled formulas should be given clear fluids to drink. They can also be given half-strength milk (milk that is made up with half the normal number of scoops of milk powder).
• Once your child has started to recover, reintroduce a very light diet and upgrade to full-strength milk where appropriate.

CONSTIPATION

Many children have difficulty in passing hard faeces at some point. Constipation in childhood is usually a temporary complaint and rarely indicates a more serious problem.

Constipation is often related to diet. It may occur when an infant changes from breast to bottle milk, or if an older child is not eating enough fibre. A healthy, varied diet – that contains plenty of fruit and vegetables and does not rely on convenience and fast foods – will help both to prevent and ease constipation. It is also important that your child drinks plenty of clear fluids such as water or diluted juice. Regular exercise and sport will also be helpful.

Constipation may indicate that a child is distressed. For example, a small child can become constipated if their parents are going through a stressful time at home. If this is the case, more attention to a child's

▷ Children usually make a quick recovery from stomach upsets, but persistent abdominal pain or vomiting should be investigated.

COLIC

Colic is a common problem in small babies. It usually starts at two or three weeks of age and may last until the child is about four months old. The usual symptoms, which are often worse in the evening, may include:

➤ Prolonged crying at roughly the same time each day, with the baby proving to be inconsolable.

➤ Drawing the legs up.

Colic can be distressing but is harmless and not an indication of any serious condition. The cause is not known, but doctors no longer think that it is connected with wind or abdominal pain. There are some over-the-counter preparations that may help and painkilling syrups will help to make a child more comfortable.

emotional needs may be necessary. Some toddlers develop constipation when they are being toilet-trained. The problem usually resolves itself, given time and patience.

Consult a doctor if a child's constipation persists for longer than a week. The doctor may examine the child's rectum by inserting a gloved finger into it. Mild laxatives may be prescribed in persistent cases or if straining to pass hard faeces has caused a tear in the anal tissue.

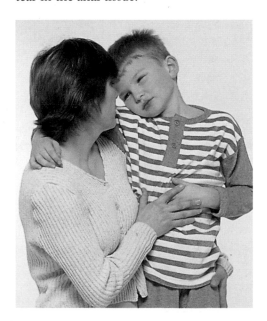

Migraines in children

SEE ALSO
➤ Headaches and migraines, p76
➤ Meningitis, p84
➤ Anxiety, p94

A migraine can be a very distressing and debilitating condition, and it can affect children as well as adults. The symptoms of childhood migraine may be different to the adult form – the main symptom is usually abdominal pain, although headaches and other adult symptoms may occur as the child gets older. Migraines can affect children as young as two and will usually recur. The cause is not fully understood, and there will often be a history of migraines in the family. Statistically, more girls than boys suffer from migraines.

SIGNS AND SYMPTOMS

A young child with a migraine may demonstrate quite different symptoms to those experienced by adults. They may suffer from:

➤ Abdominal pain.

➤ Nausea and vomiting.

➤ Dizzy spells.

➤ Pale skin.

Older children usually develop more typical adult symptoms:

➤ One-sided headache.

➤ Nausea and vomiting.

➤ Visual disturbance, such as seeing flashing or shimmering lights.

➤ Aversion to bright lights.

➤ Occasionally, weakness in an arm or a leg.

There may be a warning period during which the child feels unwell and in time they may be able to recognize that a migraine is about to start.

About 1 in every 20 children has suffered a migraine by the age of 15, and children as young as 2 have been affected. The exact cause of migraines is not fully understood but may be connected to changes in blood flow inside the skull. Temporary alterations in brain chemicals may also be a factor, causing symptoms elsewhere in the body.

Migraine attacks may be triggered by stress and anxiety, or by particular food

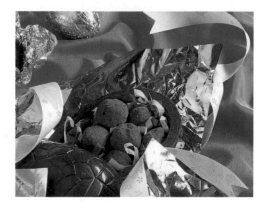

△ If your child suffers from migraines, it is often worth looking at their diet. Chocolate is one of the common food triggers.

substances – some of the most common food triggers are bananas, chocolate, citrus fruits and cheese. Perfume, petrol, tobacco smoke and other inhaled substances may also trigger an attack.

As with adult migraines, the symptoms usually develop gradually over several hours, and an attack can last for several days. In most cases, the child will suffer from recurrent attacks.

WHAT MIGHT YOUR DOCTOR DO?

Doctors can usually diagnose migraine from the child's symptoms, and further hospital investigations are rarely necessary. Occasionally, a CT scan or an MRI of the head may be arranged to discount other possible causes. Young children may be sent for ultrasound scanning of the abdomen.

If the attacks are short-lived, simple painkillers may be all that is needed to relieve symptoms. These are best given during the very early stages of an attack. It can also be helpful for the child to lie down in a darkened, quiet room.

For children who suffer from frequent attacks, your doctor will be able to recommend a number of effective antimigraine drugs that can be used on a regular preventative basis.

Since dietary factors may be significant in approximately 10 per cent of cases, your doctor may arrange for the child and parents to see a dietician. This is often helpful because it can pinpoint any dietary triggers for the attacks, and these foods can then simply be avoided.

The migraines often disappear once a child reaches adulthood, however, in some cases migraine episodes will continue throughout life.

▽ A simple painkilling syrup can help to relieve the symptoms, and is most effective if given in the early stages of a migraine.

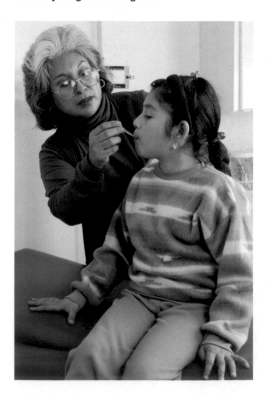

Febrile convulsions

SEE ALSO
➤ The breathing process, p126
➤ Protection against infection, p224

A febrile convulsion is a fit that has been induced by a high fever. This fairly common condition affects about 5 per cent of children between the ages of six months and five years, and is more likely to affect boys than girls. Febrile convulsions often run in families, and about one-third of children that have had one fit are likely to have another. Although frightening to witness, febrile convulsions are rarely serious. They are usually due to an infection in the body, and do not indicate a brain disorder or epilepsy, as is often feared by parents.

SIGNS AND SYMPTOMS

Febrile convulsions often occur in association with an upper respiratory tract infection, such as a runny nose or sore throat. The symptoms include:

➤ Loss of consciousness.

➤ Stiffness of limbs.

➤ Jerking of limbs.

➤ Abnormal eye movements such as the eyes rolling upwards.

A febrile convulsion normally lasts for between two and four minutes. The basic first-aid procedure is as follows:

• Lie your child on his or her side.
• Make sure the child is safe by placing cushions all around him or her, and by clearing the area of any objects that could cause injury. Do not try to restrain the child in any way.
• If this is the first time that your child has had a fit, call the emergency services immediately.
• Sponge your child down with tepid water to bring the fever down.
• Give painkilling syrup once your child comes round, to help to reduce the fever.

AFTER A FIT

The child usually falls asleep after a fit. Contact your doctor if you have not already done so. Where minor infection is diagnosed, keeping the child cool and giving painkilling syrup to bring down the fever are all that is needed. Where there is uncertainty about the cause, the child will usually be admitted to hospital for further investigations, such as antibody tests, tests on blood and urine, and a lumbar puncture.

Balanitis

SEE ALSO
➤ Causes of infectious disease, p214

Balanitis is an infection of the tip of the penis and the foreskin. It is a common childhood infection and may be caused by a bacterium or, more rarely, by a fungus. This type of infection is less likely by the age of five when in ninety per cent of boys the foreskin can be retracted.

In balanitis, the tip of the boy's penis and his foreskin become sore and itchy. There may also be some discharge or a rash.

As soon as you notice any symptoms take the child to your doctor who will examine the area and may take a swab to check for infection. The problem may clear up on its own, but antibiotics may be given. Some doctors use steroid ointment which has been shown to be effective in some studies. Further treatment is not usually necessary unless the child has phimosis, in which case balanitis may recur. Surgery may be recommended in some severe cases.

PHIMOSIS

Phimosis is a contraction of the foreskin. It occurs when the foreskin is too tight or the opening too narrow. It may:

➤ Make a child more vulnerable to balanitis.

➤ Cause difficulty passing urine.

➤ Result in ballooning of the foreskin when urine is passed.

➤ Cause recurrent infections.

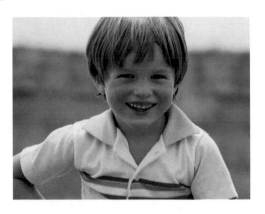

▽ Until they are about five, boys are prone to balanitis because cleaning under the foreskin is difficult as it does not always retract (pull back).

Nappy rash

SEE ALSO

➤ Causes of infectious
  disease, p214

➤ Bacterial infections
  p216

Nappy rash is an almost inevitable consequence of wearing nappies. A nappy allows urine and faeces, which have irritant effects, to come into contact with the skin. Eventually the skin becomes red and sore, sometimes causing the baby distress. Nappy rash usually clears up in a matter of days if soothing cream is applied and air is allowed to reach the area. If the problem remains after a few days and the rash seems especially sore, contact your doctor for advice. The baby may have a fungal or bacterial infection that needs medical attention.

Nappy rash is more likely to occur if the baby's nappy is not changed regularly or if the area is not cleaned thoroughly. However, almost every baby will develop it at some point. Simple nappy rash can easily be treated at home. Emollients such as aqueous cream are usually sufficient to clear up the problem in less than a week.

WHEN TO VISIT THE DOCTOR

Take the baby to the doctor if the rash is severe, if it persists longer than a week or if you are worried. The doctor will check for signs of fungal infection and may prescribe antifungal creams or oral drops, to reduce the amount of the *Candida* fungus in the digestive tract. Oral antibiotics may be necessary if a bacterial infection is suspected.

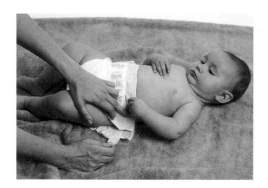

◁ Changing your baby's nappy regularly will reduce the risk of nappy rash.

HELPING TO PREVENT NAPPY RASH

➤ Change your baby's nappies frequently.

➤ Wash the nappy area at each change and allow the skin to dry thoroughly.

➤ Use a simple barrier cream at the earliest sign of irritation.

➤ Avoid perfumed skin products.

➤ Have nappy-free periods during each day.

Eczema in children

SEE ALSO

➤ Asthma, p130

This common skin condition affects as many as 20 per cent of children under the age of five. The cause is not well understood but there may be a genetic link as the condition often runs in families. Diet, such as sensitivity to cow's milk, is a possible causative factor.

SIGNS AND SYMPTOMS

➤ Intense itching and inflammation of the skin.

➤ In infants, a red, scaly rash on the face, neck, elbows and knees.

➤ In older children, a red, scaly rash in creases of the skin.

Children with eczema may also suffer from asthma and hayfever.

Childhood eczema can last several years, but it may clear up as the child gets older. Scratching the skin can cause it to become infected and make the problem worse.

MANAGING ECZEMA

If your child has eczema, they should avoid perfumed skin products, and should use skin moisturizers and moisturizing soaps. A doctor may prescribe corticosteroid creams for persistent rashes, and steroid-antibiotic creams for up to two weeks at a time to clear infected eczema.

OTHER ITCHING CONDITIONS

Scabies – Caused by a mite burrowing into the skin. Typical symptoms include intense itching, raised pink spots and brown lines between fingers and toes. Anti-parasitic lotion clears the condition.

Head lice – Tiny insects infest the scalp, causing intense itching. Spread by close contact and sharing combs and hats, poor hygiene is not a cause. Wet combing and special shampoo cures the problem.

Urinary tract infection in children

SEE ALSO
➤ The urinary organs, p138
➤ Urinary tract infections, p142
➤ Febrile convulsions, p231

Infections of the urinary tract often occur when bacteria around the anus find their way up the urethra, which empties the bladder. An abnormality in the tube (ureter) that connects the bladder to the kidneys can also make infection more likely. A urinary infection is not always easy to spot, especially in young children. However, prompt treatment is vital. If the infection is missed, it could damage the kidneys. This may make the child more prone to further infections and will also increase the likelihood of kidney disease in later life.

SIGNS AND SYMPTOMS

In babies or young children, the symptoms of urinary infection can be hard to distinguish from those of other conditions. They may include:

➤ Fever.

➤ Vomiting.

➤ General ill-health.

➤ Failure to thrive.

➤ Febrile convulsions.

In older children, symptoms may be similar to those experienced by an adult.

➤ A frequent need to pass urine.

➤ A painful, burning sensation when urine is passed.

➤ Discomfort or pain in the side or the lower abdomen.

➤ Wetting during the day or night after a period of being dry.

▽ A simple test using a dipstick can determine whether or not your child has a urinary infection.

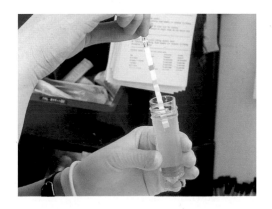

Urinary infections are easily treatable with antibiotics, as long as they are caught at an early stage. If you suspect that your child has a urinary infection, you should visit your doctor immediately.

WHAT MIGHT A DOCTOR DO?

The child will need to provide a urine sample, and the doctor will test this for the presence of any protein and/or red and white blood cells, which indicate infection. If infection is shown, a course of antibiotics will be prescribed. A sample of urine should also be sent to a laboratory so that the specific bacteria responsible can be identified. Once the doctor knows the cause of the infection, the antibiotic treatment may be changed.

If the infection has reached the kidneys – a condition known as pyelonephritis – the child may need to be treated in hospital with intravenous antibiotics. Babies and very young children may also be referred to hospital for treatment. Most children make a full recovery from an infection in the urinary tract. However, the infection may recur, so you should ensure that they always drink plenty of fluids.

FURTHER INVESTIGATION

Your child may need to undergo further investigation in hospital in order to identify abnormalities in the urinary tract or to check for kidney damage.

DMSA scanning is carried out to look for scarring in the kidneys. In this procedure, a dye is injected into the child's arm. A photograph of the kidneys is then taken using a special camera (a gamma

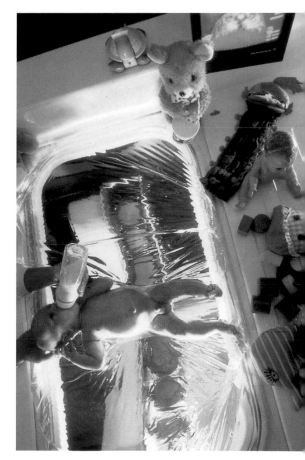

△ This infant is having his kidneys scanned on a special "water bed" scanner. A clear ultrasound image is recorded on the nearby screen.

camera). Ultrasound scanning of the kidneys may also be performed.

Other tests include a special X-ray to examine the urinary tract. This involves a dye being introduced into the bladder, and then X-rays being taken as the child passes urine. This test will identify whether the child has urinary reflux, in which urine flows back towards the kidneys rather than being passed out of the body. In this case, the child may be given low-dose antibiotics until the risk of infection has diminished.

Cystic fibrosis

SEE ALSO
➤ The process of digestion, p44
➤ The breathing process, p126

Cystic fibrosis is the most common inherited condition in the Western world, affecting about 1 in every 1000 babies. This disease affects the mucus-producing glands in the pancreas and in the lungs, causing extra-thick secretions to be produced. As a result, children with the condition experience recurrent chest infections and have problems absorbing nutrients from their food. Current treatments have extended the life expectancy of those affected well into adulthood, and researchers hope that gene therapy will soon be used to treat the disease.

Cystic fibrosis is caused by an abnormal gene carried by both parents. The parents may be "carriers" of the gene and need not necessarily have the disease themselves.

The symptoms usually appear within the first few weeks of life. The baby is fretful and fails to thrive, has a swollen abdomen and passes greasy stools (faeces) that float and have an offensive smell.

WHAT MIGHT YOUR DOCTOR DO?

The earlier the diagnosis, the better the outcome. A diagnosis can be confirmed by a sweat test – high levels of salt in the sweat indicate cystic fibrosis. Treatment involves daily physiotherapy to clear excess mucus from the lungs. The baby is given pancreatic enzyme granules before food, along with a high-calorie diet, to maximize digestion and nutrition. Antibiotic treatment is necessary if a chest infection occurs.

Heart problems

SEE ALSO
➤ The cardiovascular system, p28

A congenital heart disease is one that is present from birth. They affect about 1 in every 100 babies and are usually diagnosed during the very early stages of life. Most problems are mild and disappear as the baby grows, although some can be life-threatening.

Many heart problems cause no symptoms, and are picked up only during routine examinations. A doctor may hear a heart murmur – caused by turbulent blood flow – when listening to the heart with a stethoscope. If a congenital heart defect is suspected the child is referred to a specialist for tests, such as an electrocardiogram (ECG) and an echocardiogram (ultrasound). In approximately two-thirds of cases, the problem clears up by itself, but one in three children may need surgery.

COMMON CONGENITAL HEART PROBLEMS

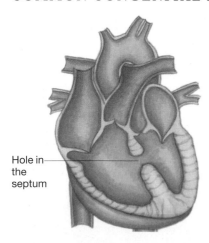

Hole in the septum

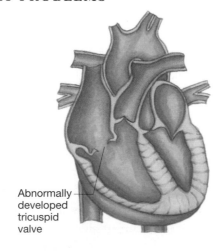

Abnormally developed tricuspid valve

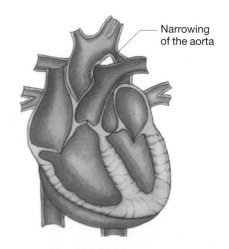

Narrowing of the aorta

△ A septal defect, also known as a hole in the heart, is where there is a hole in the septum (the part of the heart that divides it in two).

△ A valve defect is when a heart valve develops abnormally, and any of the heart's four valves can be affected in this way.

△ Coarctation of the aorta is a narrowing of the main artery. This restricts blood flow to the lower body, which places strain on the heart muscle.

Congenital hip dysplasia

SEE ALSO
➤ The musculoskeletal system, p106
➤ Osteoarthritis, p112

This condition affects newborn babies and is much more common in girls than in boys. It often affects babies who are born by breech delivery, which puts excessive strain on their hip joints. In mild cases, there is a looseness of the ligaments around the hip joint, which results in excessive flexibility. In very severe cases, the hip joint is permanently dislocated. Hip dysplasia may correct itself within weeks of the baby's birth, but a plaster cast might need to be worn for up to six months. Corrective surgery may be necessary in some cases.

SIGNS AND SYMPTOMS

Mild cases may show no symptoms at all, but babies with severe hip dysplasia often have the following:

➤ Asymmetrical skin creases on the backs of the legs.

➤ Shortening of the affected leg.

An older child may have a limp if congenital hip dysplasia has not been picked up by doctors during development tests. This condition is most effectively treated early on, and if treatment is delayed, a child is at risk of developing osteoarthritis at a young age, and may also suffer permanent damage to the hip joint.

Congenital hip dysplasia may be due to weakness of the hip joint ligaments or, in more severe cases, to an abnormality in the hip socket.

If the problem does not right itself within the first few weeks, it is vital that the

▽ Babies are examined in the first weeks of life to check the stability and range of movement of their hips. Any problem is then fully investigated.

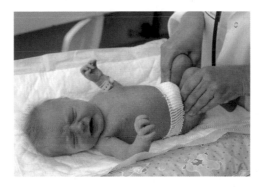

ROUTINE HIP EXAMINATION

All babies are examined during the first day or two of life by a paediatrician or family doctor, and this examination is repeated at the age of six weeks. If there is any suspicion of hip looseness or dislocation, the baby will be referred immediately to a paediatric orthopaedic specialist. An ultrasound scan can be done to confirm or refute the diagnosis.

affected head of the femur is correctly positioned in the hip socket, so that the hip can develop normally. The orthopaedic specialist will use a harness or a plaster cast to keep the hip in correct alignment, and this may need to be worn for six months.

Perthes' disease

SEE ALSO
➤ Osteoarthritis, p112

Perthes' disease is a rare condition in which the head of the femur (thigh bone) breaks down and gradually reforms over about two years. The condition tends to occur in boys between the ages of four and eight. Typical symptoms are limping and pain in the hip or knee.

Doctors do not know why children develop Perthes' disease, but it may be due to disrupted blood supply to the femur. If your child has an unexplained limp, you should arrange to see your doctor about it.

WHAT A DOCTOR MIGHT DO

X-rays or MRI scans of the affected hip will be done to confirm the diagnosis. The condition usually responds to bed-rest but sometimes a child's legs may need to be put in plaster to relieve pressure on the bone. In severe cases, surgery may be needed. Most children make a full recovery, but some may develop osteoarthritis in later life.

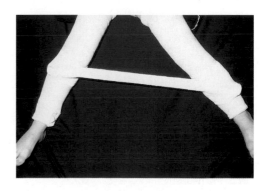

▷ This is a broomstick plaster, which may be used to treat Perthes' disease. It holds the child's legs apart, reducing friction on the bone.

Sudden infant death syndrome

SEE ALSO

➤ Smoking and your health, p20

➤ Addictive behaviours, p102

➤ The grieving process, p242

The death of a child is a tragic event and one of the most distressing aspects of sudden infant death syndrome (SIDS) is that it happens without warning, usually in the place where a baby should be safest – at home. We still do not know what causes SIDS, but doctors have identified certain risk factors. Since new advice based on this research has been made known to parents, the incidence of SIDS has fallen and there are a number of measures that you can take to minimize the risk. Babies between one and six months old are most at risk from SIDS.

Despite much research, the causes of sudden infant death syndrome are still not fully known. However, doctors believe that it may be related to unusual breathing patterns. SIDS is more common in premature babies who were born before 37 weeks gestation. Statistically, siblings of children who have died of SIDS are slightly more at risk.

KNOW THE RISK FACTORS

The risk factors that increase the likelihood of SIDS include:

- Parental smoking.
- Parental drug abuse.
- Recent upper respiratory tract infection such as a cold.
- Putting babies to sleep on their fronts.
- Putting babies to sleep in an overheated room or overwrapping them, particularly during illness, so that they overheat.
- Bottle-feeding rather than breastfeeding your baby.

▽ Health visitors will advise parents on ways to protect their baby from SIDS and provide the best possible chance of good health.

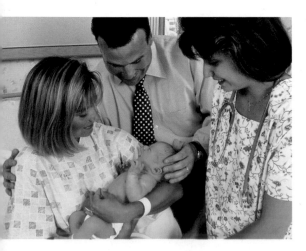

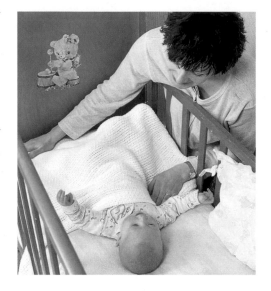

△ Placing your baby on his or her back to sleep is one of the most important steps that you can take to reduce the risk of SIDS.

PREVENTING SIDS

Research has identified many risk factors for SIDS. There are a number of ways in which you can reduce the risk, and these include the following:

- Putting your baby down to sleep on his or her back at the foot of the cot.
- Using a firm mattress in the cot.
- Not using a pillow until your baby has reached the age of one year.
- Not using too many blankets, as there is a danger that your baby may overheat.
- Not smoking at home, or allowing visitors to smoke in your house. Avoiding taking your baby anywhere where people are smoking.
- Breastfeeding for the first few months of your baby's life, because this can boost his or her immune system and may help to make SIDS less likely.

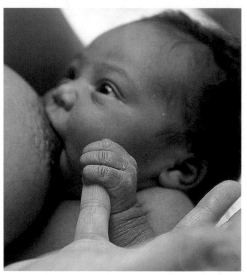

△ Research suggests that babies who are breastfed have a slightly lower risk of SIDS than those who are bottle-ted.

Although many parents use baby monitors to check on their baby's breathing, there is no research to suggest that these devices reduce the likelihood of a baby being affected by SIDS. Often they can heighten the parents' anxiety rather than alleviate it.

Some parents learn cardiopulmonary resuscitation so that they feel able to deal with the situation more confidently. In the unlikely event that SIDS affects your baby, ring the emergency services – or send a helper to do so – and start resuscitation while you wait for them to arrive. Doctors will try to resuscitate a baby on its arrival at hospital, but this is rarely successful.

If a baby dies from SIDS, parents will need support and help. Specialist counselling can be helpful in coming to terms with such a loss and support groups can provide valuable long-term help.

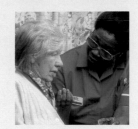

CARING FOR THE TERMINALLY ILL

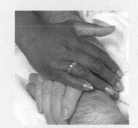

16

Coping with an advanced disease can be traumatic for both the patient and for family, friends and carers. Under these circumstances it is important that everyone knows and understands the patient's wishes and that they in turn have someone they trust who can make decisions on their behalf if they find themselves unable to do so. There is a confusing range of decisions to be made when it comes to making choices about caring for the terminally ill, and an understanding of the practical issues will help family and friends deal with the situation as well as facing the emotional repercussions and, eventually, the grieving process.

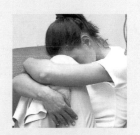

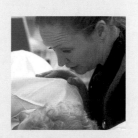

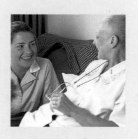

Coping with terminal illness

SEE ALSO
➤ The grieving process, p242
➤ Acupuncture, p245

During the more advanced stages of a terminal illness, the focus of medical treatment often shifts. Although treatments will continue for as long as possible, an increasing emphasis may be placed on quality of life. To this end, your doctor or carers will increasingly involve the patient and/or his or her family in decisions about how to manage the illness. It is important that everyone concerned starts to think through the many issues associated with an impending death, both emotionally and practically, and how they want to deal with them.

Treatment of terminal illness involves weighing up a huge number of medical, physical, psychological and emotional issues. These issues are often difficult to tackle and are often best resolved if the patient, their family and doctors or health workers discuss them carefully together.

MAKING CHOICES

Some people may need, or want, to stay in a hospital, while for others hospice care is the better option. If there is a strong family network to provide care, the patient may even be able to go home.

If particular medicines are unlikely to prolong life, or if they are doing so at considerable personal cost, for example by causing unpleasant side effects, it may be appropriate to stop them. This may apply

WHAT IS A LIVING WILL?

A "living will" (also called an advance statement) outlines your beliefs, wishes and values specifically related to medical treatment during the course of a terminal illness. If you or someone you know wishes to write a living will, it may be helpful to do so with your doctor. Such documents usually include some of the following issues:

➤ Nominating a person who understands what you would like to happen in different situations and who will be able to make decisions for you if you are unable to do so.

➤ Setting out clear guidelines about whether you would like a specific treatment up until a particular time or whether you want to refuse certain treatments, such as tube feeding, up until the time of death.

➤ Deciding that you do not want to receive life-sustaining or reviving treatment, such as resuscitation, if it becomes necessary.

➤ Making it clear whether or not you would like to donate any of your body organs to be used after your death.

to medicines that have previously been taken to prevent or delay disease progression. This is inevitably a difficult decision to make and should ideally be taken by the affected person in close consultation with those most involved in his or her care, and with the full support of relevant healthcare professionals.

It may also be appropriate to plan ahead and consider what to do in the event of further deterioration. A terminally ill person is often prone to acute episodes of infection, and much thought needs to be given to whether this should be actively treated or whether it is preferable to refrain from treating these further diseases or infections.

The situation, which places an incredible strain on family and friends, becomes more difficult if the dying person is confused or not fully conscious. Some time may be needed for appropriate courses of action to become clearer to all concerned. Some

patients will have already discussed these issues and may have made a "living will" (see box) that explains what they would like to happen under such circumstances.

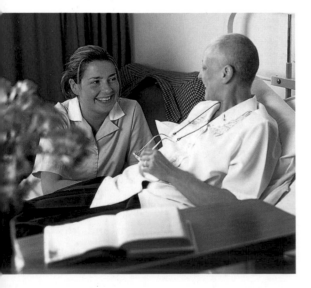

▽ Open and honest discussion with family members may not be possible, so relationships with carers can often provide invaluable understanding and advice, and the chance to talk in-depth about feelings and anxieties.

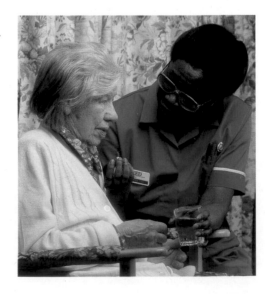

▽ Healthcare professionals are trained to provide care and support for patients who are confused and anxious about their situation.

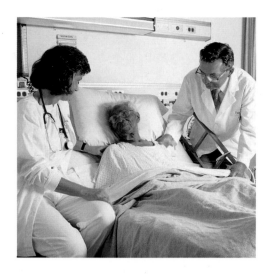

△ Doctors should consult with the patient at every stage about pain relief and life-sustaining treatments, and about what to do if the patient becomes unable to make such decisions.

Where someone chooses to spend their last days or weeks is very important. Many people choose to die at home if they are asked but some choose hospice care instead if it is offered. This wish should be honoured wherever possible, although practical considerations may sometimes make this difficult.

AN EMOTIONAL TIME

For a patient, the process of acknowledging and accepting terminal illness involves a very complex mix of emotions, and will often result in severe mood swings. The range of feelings may include:
• Shock, disbelief and denial.
• Anger and frustration.
• Fear, anxiety and depression.
• Resignation and acceptance.

It is important to remember that a similar range of emotions will also be experienced by those closest to the dying person.

Generally, it is more common to be honest and open about the reality of the situation and prognosis. Many terminally ill patients find that they experience less depression and anxiety once they have had the opportunity to discuss all their fears with both loved ones and healthcare professionals. However, each case should be considered individually, and openness and honesty are not always appropriate. Each person should be offered understanding and support to enable them to cope with the

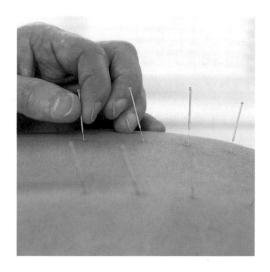

△ Acupuncture is thought to stimulate endorphins, the body's natural painkillers. It is offered to some terminally ill patients as an alternative to drugs that have unpleasant side effects such as nausea or constipation.

situation in their own way. Carers and friends and family may well need to be perceptive and intuitive in order to gauge accurately how a patient feels, because in many cases they are simply not able to make their wishes clear, and do not want to face the reality of their situation.

CONTROLLING PAIN

Pain can be an important factor in advanced and terminal illness, and fear of pain can cause great anxiety and agitation for many patients. Most physical pain can be effectively relieved by the use of strong painkilling drugs. Opiates such as morphine can be administered orally or via a subcutaneously sited infusion (which delivers drugs into the fatty tissue below the skin to disperse slowly) if it is too difficult to swallow. Opiate drugs tend to have an anxiety-reducing effect but also induce constipation and a degree of nausea, particularly for a few days after they have been started. Fentanyl (similar in potency to morphine) can be administered via a patch applied to the skin every 72 hours and is a useful alternative.

Many patients find acupuncture is effective for relieving pain and this treatment is available in some hospices as an alternative to prescribed drugs.

HOSPICE CARE

Hospices provide a range of nursing and medical services. Nurses, carers and doctors provide specialized palliative care for patients with advanced diseases such as cancer, neurological disease and cardiorespiratory disease. Palliative care is designed to provide appropriate treatments and support for patients in the weeks and months following a terminal diagnosis, and generally focuses on dealing with symptoms, and controlling pain and anxiety throughout the course of a terminal illness.

Hospices also offer respite care, which provides a break for patients and carers. Individuals are often admitted to a hospice for two or three weeks at a time.

A range of other services is often available, for example physiotherapy, occupational therapy, various complementary therapies and access to counsellors and spiritual care.

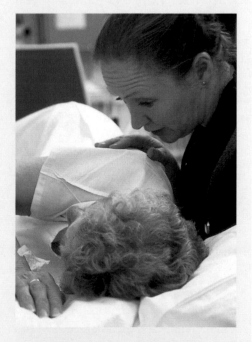

△ A hospice can offer specialized care for terminally ill patients, focusing on quality of life and offering respite to relatives.

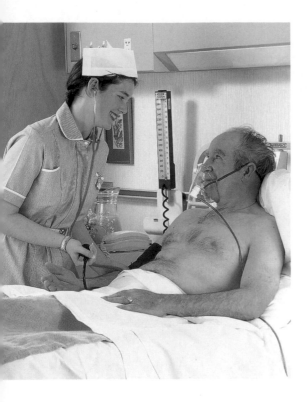

△ Regular blood pressure checks and sessions with an oxygen mask may be vital for a patient's care, but relying on others in this way can cause feelings of powerlessness and frustration.

CONTROLLING NAUSEA AND VOMITING

Nausea and vomiting are common symptoms of terminal illness and can be distressing. This may be a result of disease or a side effect of certain drugs, notably those used to control pain. Antisickness or antiemetic drugs are usually effective and may be administered orally, by suppository or by subcutaneous infusion.

RELIEVING CONSTIPATION AND DIARRHOEA

Constipation is a common symptom in people who are confined to bed and whose movements are limited. It may be caused by lack of fluid (dehydration) and food, and it can be aggravated by deteriorating health and the use of strong opiates. Constipation usually responds to extra fluids where this is possible and to the use of simple laxatives.

Diarrhoea is more common in people dying from advanced HIV infection and usually responds to a range of antidiarrhoeal medicines, including opiate painkillers.

Both diarrhoea and constipation can be distressing for the patient, who may also feel humiliated if they are unable to relieve themselves without assistance. Drugs can alleviate these symptoms, but it is important that carers understand the feelings of frustration that this dependence can cause, and help the patient to feel as normal and capable as possible.

TREATING SHORTNESS OF BREATH

Difficulty with breathing sometimes affects terminally ill patients, especially those with advanced heart or lung disease, and can be very distressing – both for sufferers and for onlookers. It may trigger panic attacks and serious anxiety, which makes breathlessness even worse. Morphine is often an effective treatment, but if the underlying cause is a lung infection, the breathlessness may be relieved by antibiotics, which can help to clear any infection. A person may receive oxygen therapy if it helps to improve symptoms of breathlessness, and this can be particularly useful for those dying from progressive cardiorespiratory disease. Oxygen tents are sometimes used, but in most cases an oxygen mask over the nose and mouth, or oxygen tubes fitted into the nostrils, is more appropriate.

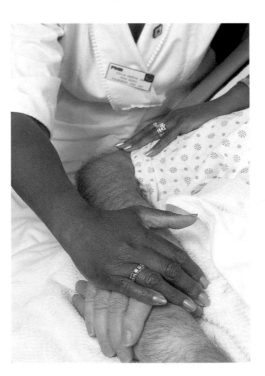

CALMING ANXIETY AND AGITATION

Terminally ill patients are often anxious and agitated. It may be helpful to talk things through to make sure that they are as fully informed as they want to be. This will hopefully reduce feelings of powerlessness and frustration by making the patient feel more in control.

Opiate drugs tend to have an anxiety-reducing effect. There are also a number of other anxiety-reducing and mildly sedating drugs that can be used orally or via an infusion if necessary.

Certain complementary therapies, such as massage and aromatherapy, and the use of touch in general, may be invaluable in relieving anxiety. Simply holding someone's hand can be soothing and comforting, helping the patient to feel less alone and alleviating feelings of panic and agitation.

For many people, dying with dignity is very important and one of their greatest fears is of becoming increasingly dependent on others and being unable to make their own decisions. This can cause anxiety and frustration and it is usually helpful for

▽ Patients who are confined to bed and are more or less immobile require special nursing care to keep their skin clean and healthy, and free from pressure sores.

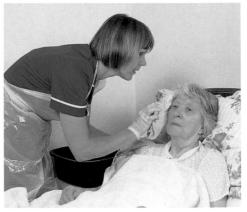

◁ The prospect of dying can be terrifying, and this can cause more anxiety than the pain or symptoms of the terminal disease itself. Talking things through and offering a comforting touch can help people to work through their fears. Touch can be remarkably calming and makes the patient feel less alone.

someone close to the patient – whether family or carer – to calm these fears by talking through every eventuality and making it clear that their wishes have been understood and will be followed.

Another cause of anxiety is being in a strange environment. Many people do not want to die in a hospital and may feel the need to be in their own homes, surrounded by their possessions and loved ones. If possible, this desire should be respected and the patient allowed to return home. However, this is often not practical and indeed many people choose to remain in hospital, or to move to a hospice, where they can be given the best medical treatment and specialized care and support.

INTAKE OF FOOD AND FLUID

People naturally tend to eat less and less as they become more ill. This can be very distressing for those closest to the dying person. Emphasis should always be placed on the needs of the patient and they should not be forced to eat if they do not want to – it may be uncomfortable for them to do so. Usually a lack of appetite and calories in the last stages of an illness does not cause any specific problems.

As the dying person's condition deteriorates, there comes a point when he or she cannot drink much fluid, if any at all. Once again, in the later stages of terminal illness this will not cause specific problems. The sensation of thirst can be prevented by keeping the mouth, lips and gums moist and clean. Tiny sips of water may suffice for this process.

Fluids will often be taken for some time after food has been rejected, but eventually even fluids cannot be tolerated. Again, this is a natural progression and is not usually a specific problem. As long as care is taken to maintain oral hygiene, and the mouth is kept moist, the sensation of thirst is often not apparent. This rejection of food and drink comes towards the end of a terminal illness and, although it is upsetting for family and friends, it is a normal process and should not be a cause of concern.

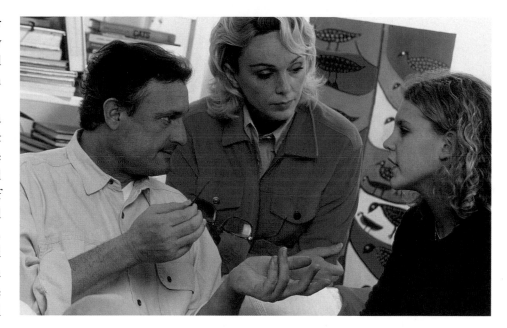

PREVENTING PRESSURE SORES

When a person is in bed all day or is for the most part immobile, he or she can develop aches, pains and sores on the skin. Special beds and mattresses are available that cushion the body and enable carers to wash and move patients more easily and so prevent the development of pressure sores. Specialized nursing care is essential for all-round patient comfort and skin health.

MAKING PLANS

Although many terminal patients can make a "living will", giving directions about their treatment (see earlier box), planning what will happen after death can be too distressing for many to contemplate and this should be respected. In some cases, sufferers may turn to their religion or beliefs to help them, and representatives of their faith can help to make plans and will be the most comforting figures at the end.

The question of whether or not healthy organs should be removed for donation after the patient has died is an issue that many people do not want to discuss with the dying, but the idea of helping someone else live after their death can be a comforting thought. Many people carry donor cards or they may broach the subject themselves. Some patients feel they need to discuss how organ donation works with a medical expert before they make a decision.

△ Discussing funeral plans or organ donation as a family is very important. It is often difficult to make these decisions alone, and sharing the responsibility is usually helpful.

As with many other aspects of dealing with the terminally ill, making plans about matters such as these may help them feel they are still in control.

Another matter that family and friends often avoid when dealing with terminal illness is the arrangement of the funeral. Once again, many patients may not want to discuss this, but others may welcome the opportunity to make some of these decisions for themselves. Planning the funeral, or at least making certain stipulations, can help the patient come to terms with the situation. It can also relieve some of the pressure on family and friends, who are often too grief-stricken after the death of a loved one to think through what they might have wanted. Many people, for example, request that there should be no flowers at their funeral and that the money should be donated to a charity. They may also have a preference for certain music or readings, or feel strongly about whether people should be dressed in black.

It is often a comfort to all concerned that the wishes of the patient in such matters are respected, and making these plans can help the dying person and their friends and family.

The grieving process

SEE ALSO

➤ Learn to manage stress, p12

➤ Depression, p98

Coming to terms with the death of someone close to you is a difficult and traumatic issue, and it can be particularly difficult if you have been taking care of someone during a prolonged illness. The situation is emotionally exhausting and life-changing, and most people find that they seriously reconsider their own lives as a result. Grief manifests itself in many different ways and the grieving process is unique to each individual. It may, however, be both possible and helpful to identify certain stages during the grieving process.

FACING LOSS

Anticipating grief may be helpful before an inevitable loss. Where a loved one is dying from a terminal illness, this can at least give relatives and friends the opportunity to take stock of the situation and to start dealing with the loss before it actually happens. This may result in a greater feeling of strength and acceptance when death actually occurs. The chance to say goodbye to a loved one can help enormously.

▽ Initially, in the first hours or days after the death of a loved one, the overpowering emotions are those of shock, confusion and numbness.

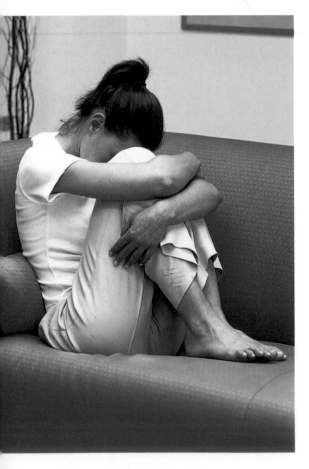

INITIAL REACTIONS

Feelings of numbness and detachment are common after death has occurred, and the emotions one may have anticipated may not arrive for some time. There is usually shock and an overwhelming sense of loss, along with feelings of emptiness, despair and helplessness. Your pattern of life will probably be disrupted for some time, and you may experience a lack of appetite and difficulty in sleeping.

DEPRESSION AND SADNESS

Initial numbness will at some point give way to a range of emotions that tends to include depression and sadness. There may be a feeling of isolation and incredible loneliness. There may also be frustration and anger. Anger might be directed at other people or at yourself. There may be terrible guilt and self-reproach for not having been more available, or for failing to say enough before it was too late. Helplessness and frustration are two key emotions that people feel after someone they know has died.

These are all natural reactions and most will be present to greater or lesser degrees and for different lengths of time in everyone experiencing grief. It is often helpful to know that during this confusing and difficult time others will be going through similar emotions to you. They too will be reproaching themselves and feeling lonely. Often talking to other people who knew the loved one can help. As with most types of trauma or grief, bottling it up can make it worse, and talking can often be a relief and a comfort.

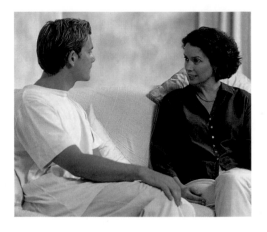

△ At first, most people simply feel numb when someone close dies. This usually develops into a wide range of emotions that can be difficult to deal with. Specialist grief counsellors can help you through this difficult time.

While it may be a comfort to talk thoughts and feelings through with your family and friends, it may also be helpful to seek specialist advice from your doctor or from a counsellor.

RESOLUTION

At some point, life starts to return to some semblance of normality. The timing of the recovery process is different for everyone – it can take from six months to several years. You will find that you start to have more energy and are able to reorganize your life and adjust to your loss. There will often be feelings of guilt for having moved on; the process of recovery may be slow and all the emotions can come flooding back at any time. Birthdays and anniversaries are difficult and you will often relive many of the feelings of initial grief. Eventually, however, you will feel able to start making plans and decisions about your future.

17

COMPLEMENTARY THERAPIES

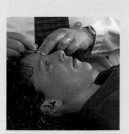

Therapies such as acupuncture and aromatherapy were first used by some of the most ancient civilizations in the world, many thousands of years ago. Until recently, they have been regarded with suspicion by many practitioners of Western medicine. Nowadays, however, increasing numbers of people are turning to these less invasive and more natural forms of treatment for a wide variety of conditions. More doctors accept the effectiveness of various complementary therapies and many incorporate them into their treatment programmes or suggest them as alternative methods of diagnosis and relief.

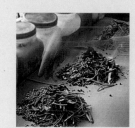

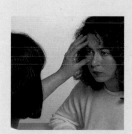

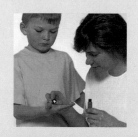

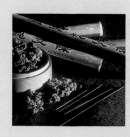

Complementary therapies and their uses

There has been a considerable growth of interest in complementary therapies in recent years – it is not that long ago that such therapies were viewed with suspicion and hostility in the West. This trend has been accompanied by a shift in attitude by some members of the medical and allied professions. Over the last few decades, there have been attempts to integrate some therapies into mainstream medical settings. It is now not uncommon, for example, to find massage and aromatherapy available on some hospital wards.

Many complementary therapies have evolved from ancient traditions and represent systems of medicine that were first practised many thousands of years ago. All complementary therapies take a holistic approach to health rather than simply treating physical symptoms.

General practitioners regularly refer patients to osteopaths, and a small but growing number of doctors are undertaking some training in homeopathy and acupuncture for example.

CHOOSING A THERAPY

Complementary medicine covers a wide range of therapies and the therapy that you choose will depend upon a number of factors. You may already have had experience of one or more therapies. Sometimes it may be necessary to try a range of approaches before deciding on the right one for you.

Evidence of the effectiveness and safety of any therapy is also important. Osteopathy and chiropractic and traditional Chinese medicines such as acupuncture all have a growing evidence base that testifies to the effectiveness of treatment in a variety of situations. There is a wide range of other specialities, for example reflexology and shiatsu, that have been less vigorously and objectively examined. This does not mean, however, that a less researched therapy is not effective. There are usually many people who are prepared to testify that these therapies have worked for them.

FINDING A THERAPIST

Most complementary therapists practise alone or in one of a growing number of complementary medicine or natural health centres. A fee is usually charged at the end of each session. People with private healthcare insurance may be covered for a

BE WISE, BE SAFE

It is advisable to consult your doctor before trying out any complementary therapy, especially if you have a particular medical condition. Your doctor may advise against therapies that interfere with prescription medicines you are taking on a regular basis. Chinese herbalism, for example, often uses powerful ingredients that could interact with certain drugs and cause serious side-effects. Aromatherapy oils must also be used carefully, as many are very potent and are not advised if you have certain conditions, and especially if you are pregnant. Most oils should be diluted in carrier oil before being applied to the skin. If you are regularly having any type of complementary therapy, tell your doctor when you next visit.

limited number of treatments by a specified range of therapists (most commonly osteopaths and acupuncturists).

The best way to find a therapist is via personal recommendation – from a friend, relative or doctor – and it is a good idea to check that any therapist that you consult is well qualified and a member of the appropriate professional body (remember that anyone can set themselves up in practice as a complementary therapist, so tread carefully). Contact details for the Institute of Complementary Medicine are in the Useful Addresses listing at the back of this book. The Internet is another valuable source of information about professional bodies.

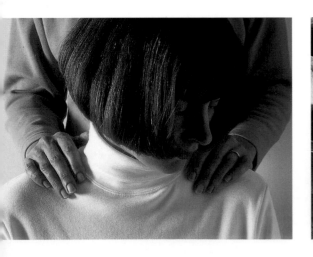

▽ Many complementary therapies use the concept of the soothing and comforting power of healing hands.

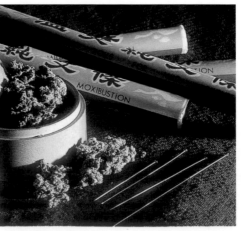

▽ Acupuncture points are also stimulated by "moxibustion": burning of herbs over the skin, using acupuncture needles or special sticks.

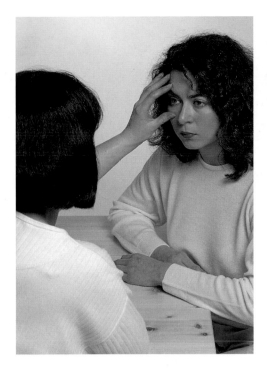

△ As with any treatment, your practitioner will begin by taking a full history of your symptoms and medical problems.

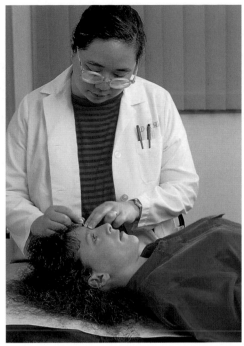

△ An acupuncturist inserts fine needles into the skin in order to correct imbalances in the flow of energy around the body.

WHAT TO EXPECT

Most therapists, like other medical practitioners, will start by taking a formal history. This is followed in most therapies by a physical examination. The therapist will explain the treatment to be used and give you your first session. The length of treatment depends on the nature of your problem. An acute back problem may require one or two sessions with an osteopath, whereas a chronic condition may require a much longer course of treatment.

ACUPUNCTURE

Acupuncture originated about 5000 years ago as one component of traditional Chinese medicine. The system is based upon the belief that there is an energy system within the body and that imbalances within this system result in different forms of illness. The ancient Chinese identified 14 "meridians" in the body, through which they believed a strong energy flowed. The meridians link a series of points where energy and blood flow converge. There are 365 of these acupuncture points. Each point or group of points is believed to be associated with a specific organ or bodily system. An acupuncturist tries to diagnose such energy imbalances by taking a history, examining the tongue and feeling the range of pulses (six at each wrist). Once the imbalances have been identified, fine, sterile needles are inserted at various points to restore the body's equilibrium.

Western medicine does not generally accept the system of Chinese medicine, although there is some acknowledgement that acupuncture is an effective treatment for certain conditions, notably pain relief. Western medicine explains the effects of acupuncture by asserting that any detectable effect is the result of stimulating the production of endorphins (the body's natural painkillers, produced in the brain).

AROMATHERAPY

The therapeutic properties of aromatic oils have been understood for thousands of years and ancient records describe their widespread use. The use of essential oils which became known as aromatherapy was developed in Europe during the early 20th century by doctors in France.

During treatment, an essential oil is either applied to the skin in a diluted form or inhaled. Each oil has certain properties and is used alone or in combination for a specific condition or ailment. Aromatherapy can treat a wide range of physical and emotional problems. There is a growing interest in administering essential oils orally (medical aromatherapy) – never do this unsupervised as it can be very dangerous.

▽ In aromatherapy, essential oils (usually diluted in carrier oil) are placed on the skin, or a few drops are placed on a tissue and inhaled.

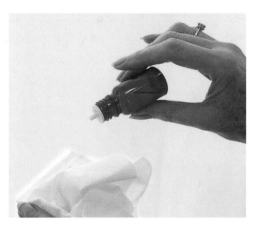

ACUPUNCTURE/MAIN USES
➤ Arthritis.

➤ Digestive disorders.

➤ Hayfever.

➤ High blood pressure.

➤ Migraines.

➤ Pain relief.

AROMATHERAPY/MAIN USES
➤ Colds.

➤ Asthma.

➤ Skin disorders, e.g. acne and ezcema.

➤ Stress-related illnesses.

➤ Urinary tract infections.

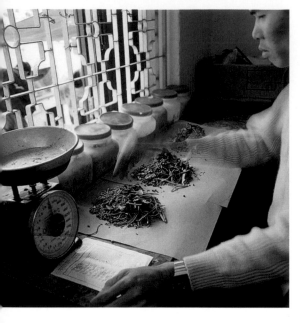

△ This herbalist is using scales to weigh out remedies. This must be done with the utmost precision, according to stringent rules.

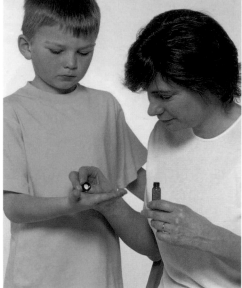

△ Homeopathic remedies can be given in the form of ointments, powders, tinctures or pills, to treat a variety of ailments.

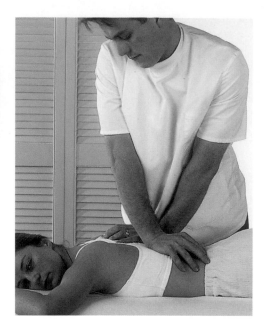

△ This chiropractor is manipulating the spine to ease pain and correct faulty alignment caused by an injury.

HERBALISM

Herbalism is an ancient therapy which makes use of the medicinal properties of plants. Most cultures throughout the world have a history of using plants to heal and to maintain health.

The majority of herbal therapies use a holistic approach based on the idea that an emotional and physical balance is required for overall health and wellbeing.

Herbal remedies are usually taken in the form of infusions, powders, tinctures, ointments and capsules. Some nausea or diarrhoea may be experienced when starting to take these remedies, and it is always advisable to consult both your doctor and a recognized herbalist about your treatment.

HOMEOPATHY

In homeopathy, a practitioner works on the principle of treating "like with like". Homeopathy stimulates the body's self-healing abilities by exposing it to tiny amounts of a substance that produces similar symptoms to those of the illness.

In the 5th century BC, the Greek physician Hippocrates was the first person to recognize that like cures like. However, it was not until the late 18th century that the German physician Samuel Hahnemann started to develop homeopathy.

Homeopathy can be used to treat most complaints, although some people respond better than others. A wide variety of homeopathic preparations are available

from health food shops and pharmacies, but it is advisable to consult a homeopath for a full and thorough assessment before taking any remedy.

OSTEOPATHY AND CHIROPRACTIC

These therapies evolved during the 19th century and have much in common, although each has its own system of learning and accreditation. Both disciplines aim to prevent and treat health problems, often musculoskeletal pain, by restoring structural balance and function with a combination of counselling, nutritional advice, manipulation of the spine and other joints, and massage of soft tissues.

HERBALISM/MAIN USES
➤ Digestive disorders, such as irritable bowel syndrome.

➤ Eczema, psoriasis and other skin disorders.

➤ Fatigue.

➤ Migraines.

HOMEOPATHY/MAIN USES
➤ Allergies.

➤ Anxiety.

➤ Asthma.

➤ Eczema.

➤ Menstrual and menopausal problems.

OSTEOPATHY AND CHIROPRACTIC/MAIN USES
➤ Asthma.

➤ Back and neck pain and sciatica.

➤ Digestive disorders.

➤ Headaches.

➤ Insomnia.

REFLEXOLOGY

The practice of reflexology is based on the principle that it is possible to influence and affect the functioning of the body by stimulating specific points on the feet and hands. Each area of the foot and hand relates to a different body system.

This belief system is related to that of ancient Chinese medicine, following the idea that energy flows in certain ways around the body. When this energy is disrupted or out of balance, then illness or pain can result.

By stimulating the hands and feet it is possible to interpret energy patterns and redirect the flow of energy. Reflexology is therefore both diagnostic and therapeutic.

REFLEXOLOGY PRESSURE POINTS

▽ The art of reflexology is based on the belief that stimulating different parts of the feet and hands can relieve symptoms or identify problems in related areas of the body. This diagram shows the pressure points on the bottom of the foot.

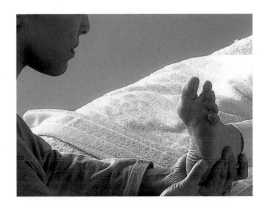

△ A reflexologist manipulates the foot to work out how your body's energy is flowing. If there is blockage, the skin will feel tender or tight, and this can be unblocked using massage.

REFLEXOLOGY/MAIN USES
➤ Anxiety.

➤ Back and neck pain.

➤ Circulation.

➤ Diagnosing other illnesses.

➤ Headaches.

SHIATSU

Shiatsu massage developed in Japan in the early 20th century but has its roots in ancient Chinese medicine. Shiatsu means finger pressure. It follows the principles of meridians and energy flow as in acupuncture. The meridians run through all the body organs and channel energy flow. All meridians, or energy channels, start or end in the fingers and toes. The energy flow maintains your physical body and affects your mind and spirit too. Massage and exercises can stimulate the meridians to maintain wellbeing.

SHIATSU/MAIN USES
➤ Arthritis.

➤ Circulatory problems.

➤ Headache and migraine.

➤ Insomnia.

➤ Stress.

▽ Shiatsu therapy applies pressure to certain points along meridian lines (energy channels in the body) using massage, stretches, holds and supportive touch. This seated position is used by the shiatsu therapist to treat the large intestine and the gall bladder meridians, which cross in the shoulder.

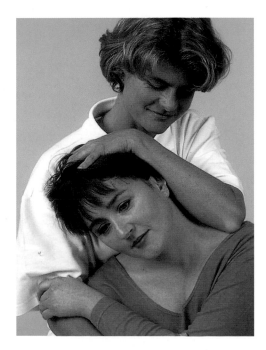

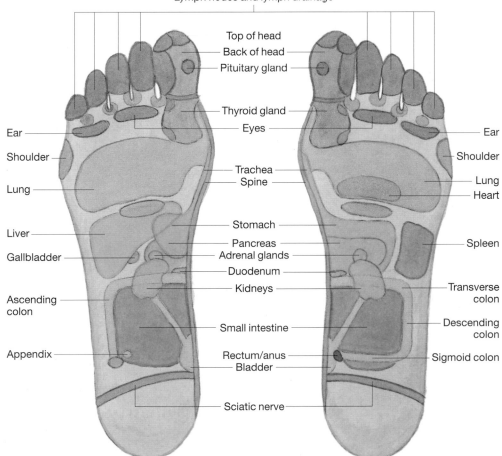

Lymph nodes and lymph drainage

Top of head
Back of head
Pituitary gland

Thyroid gland
Eyes

Ear
Shoulder

Trachea
Spine

Lung

Ear
Shoulder

Lung
Heart

Liver

Stomach
Pancreas
Adrenal glands
Duodenum
Kidneys

Spleen

Gallbladder

Ascending colon

Transverse colon

Small intestine

Descending colon

Appendix

Rectum/anus
Bladder

Sigmoid colon

Sciatic nerve

Glossary

Note: this glossary also includes useful terms that are not used in the book itself.

ACE inhibitors Drugs that block the action of angiotensin, a hormone involved in blood pressure; used in heart failure.

Acute An illness of short duration.

Allergen Substance that induces an abnormal hypersensitive reaction (allergy).

Anaesthetic Drug that is used to numb a particular area of the body (local anaesthetic) or to induce unconsciousness (general anaesthetic).

Analgesics Pain-relieving drugs.

Anaphylaxis An immediate hypersensitive reaction to an allergen, which leads to potentially fatal respiratory distress.

Antacids Substances that neutralize stomach acids, and ease indigestion.

Antibiotics Drugs that kill disease-causing bacteria. Different antibiotics are needed for different bacteria.

Antiemetics Drugs that work on the organs of balance in the ear to reduce sickness.

Antihistamines Drugs that block histamine, a substance involved in the body's allergic reactions.

Antihypertensives Drugs that reduce blood pressure.

Antioxidants Compounds that mop up harmful molecules in the bloodstream. (See Free radicals.)

Antivirals Drugs that fight viruses. Very few effective antivirals have been developed.

Asymptomatic Term used to describe conditions that cause no obvious symptoms.

Beta-blockers Drugs used to control high blood pressure by slowing the heart rate or by reducing the contraction of the arteries.

Biopsy Removal and examination of a tissue sample in order to aid diagnosis.

Blood film Test in which a sample of blood is smeared on to a slide and examined under a microscope.

Blood sugar test Test that measures the concentration of glucose in the blood; a high level may indicate diabetes.

Bronchodilators Drugs that widen the airways. They are used in the treatment of asthma and bronchitis.

Bronchoscopy An examination of the airways where a small, flexible viewing tube is passed through the nose or mouth and into the lungs.

Cardiology Specialist branch of medicine that deals with the heart.

Catheter Thin hollow tube that is inserted into a cavity or organ to allow fluid to drain. A catheter may be used, for example, to drain urine from the bladder.

Chemotherapy Treatment that uses drugs to kill cancerous tissue or harmful micro-organisms. These drugs also destroy some normal cells, so rest periods are needed between treatments.

Chronic An illness of long duration.

Clinical Term used to describe anything that relates to the observation of ill people.

Clinical trial Evaluation of a medicine by studying its effects on a group of patients and comparing them with those of a placebo (inactive substance) given to another group.

Colonoscopy Examination of the colon using a flexible tube which is passed through the anus.

Complementary medicine Therapies that can be used alongside orthodox medicine techniques. Osteopathy and acupuncture are forms of complementary medicine that are gaining wider acceptance by doctors.

Contraindication Condition that makes a particular form of treatment undesirable. For example, high blood pressure is a contraindication for certain drugs.

CT scan A computed tomography scan is an X-ray-based imaging technique in which a computer builds up images of "slices" of the body. CT scanning is routinely used to examine the brain and abdominal organs.

Cystoscopy Examination of the urethra and bladder using a flexible viewing device.

Dermatology Specialist branch of medicine dealing with problems of the skin.

Dialysis Treatment to filter impurities from the blood and remove excess fluid from the body. In healthy people, these processes are carried out by the kidneys; dialysis is needed by people whose kidneys have failed.

Diuretic Substance that increases the excretion of urine. Diuretics are used to treat high blood pressure and heart failure.

Echocardiogram Ultrasound examination of the structure and function of the heart.

Electroencephalogram Known as an EEG for short, this test measures electrical activity within the brain by means of electrodes that are attached to the skin.

Embolus Substance – such as a blood clot, air or foreign body – that lodges in a blood vessel, causing a blockage.

Endemic Used to describe a disease that is established in a region or group of people.

Endocrine glands Organs that produce hormones and secrete them into the blood or lymph. The pancreas, ovaries, testicles adrenal glands and thyroid are all examples of endocrine glands.

Endorphins Natural painkilling substances produced by the body.

Endoscopy Examination of an area of the body by means of a flexible viewing tube.

ENT Specialist branch of medicine that deals with the ear, nose and throat, plus other organs in the neck.

Epidemic Outbreak of an infectious disease that affects many people in one area.

Expectoration The coughing up of mucus from the airways.

Free radicals Unstable molecules that have the potential to harm body cells. They are produced by normal bodily processes such as breathing, and increased by smoking or environmental damage. (See Antioxidants.)

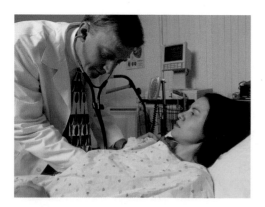

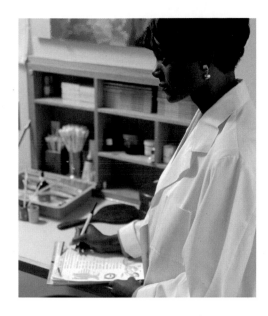

Full blood count Blood test to count the number of different blood cells per litre of blood. Cell size and concentration of haemaglobin are also checked. The test is used to diagnose anaemia and leukaemia.

Gastroenterology Specialist branch of medicine dealing with the digestive system.

Geriatrics Specialist branch of medicine dealing with the health of older people.

Gynaecology Specialist branch of medicine dealing with the female reproductive system.

Haematology Branch of medicine dealing with the blood and blood-producing tissues.

Holistic Term used to describe treatments that consider the whole person rather than simply the diseased part or symptoms.

Hormone Chemical substance produced by one part of the body to create a specific effect elsewhere. For example, insulin is produced by the pancreas and regulates the level of glucose in the blood.

HRT Hormone replacement therapy, in which oestrogen and progesterone are used to alleviate symptoms of the menopause.

Hypertension High blood pressure.

Immune Protected against contracting an infectious disease. People may become immune after an initial infection, as occurs with chickenpox, or after being vaccinated against a certain disease such as rubella.

Immunization Administering antibodies or altered forms of disease-causing micro-organisms in order to stimulate the body's immune system into resisting disease.

Immunosuppressant Substance that suppresses the body's immune responses.

Laparoscopy Inspection of the abdominal cavity using a fibre-optic viewing tube.

Laxative Substance that encourages the bowels to pass faeces or increase the amount of fluid in the bowel, relieving constipation.

Lithotripsy Technique to break up kidney stones using ultrasonic shockwaves.

Neurology Branch of medicine dealing with the nervous system.

Nonsteroidal anti-inflammatory drugs Known as NSAIDs for short, these drugs are used to reduce inflammation and pain.

Metastasis The spread of cancer from one area of the body to another. ("Metastases" are the secondary tumours that result.)

MRI Magnetic resonance imaging: radiation-free scanning technique which produces detailed images of "slices" of the body to examine the content of tissues. The images are created by a computer, using magnets and radiowaves.

Obstetrics Branch of medicine dealing with pregnancy and labour.

Occupational therapy Treatment – both therapeutic and physical exercises – that helps people return to everyday life following a period of ill health.

Oncology Branch of medicine dealing with the treatment of cancer.

Ophthalmology Branch of medicine dealing with the eyes and sight.

Opioids Painkilling drugs that are powerful but potentially addictive.

Orthopaedics Branch of medicine dealing with the bones and joints.

Paediatrics Branch of medicine dealing with children's health.

Palliative medicine Medical care that focuses on symptom relief rather than cure, as in the final stages of terminal illness.

Parasites Organisms that live on or within a host, causing it harm. Worms, fungi, bacteria and viruses are all forms of parasite.

Pathogen Disease-producing substance or micro-organism.

Pathology Branch of medicine dealing with the causes of disease and the changes it effects in the body.

Physiotherapy Hands-on physical therapy used to help people recover from injuries. In the United States, they are called physical therapists.

Psychiatry Branch of medicine dealing with mental health.

Psychology The scientific study of the mind and behaviour. Psychologists, unlike psychiatrists, are not usually medical doctors.

Radiography Photography of the inside of the body by means of X-rays (radiation).

Radiotherapy Cancer treatment involving the use of large doses of X-rays.

Sedatives Drugs that reduce the activity of the brain, and are used to treat anxiety, insomnia or psychiatric disturbance.

Speech therapy Treatment to help people to speak more clearly. It is often used to help people who have suffered a stroke.

Steroids Powerful substances that can be used to reduce inflammation and immune responses. They are used in the treatment of many conditions including asthma.

Swab A specimen (of bodily fluids, for example) taken for examination. Also describes material such as cotton or gauze used to clean wounds or take specimens.

Systemic Term used to describe a disease that affects the body as a whole rather than a particular area or organ.

Ultrasound scan Technique that uses soundwaves to produce images of internal organs.

Urology Branch of medicine dealing with the urinary system in men and women, and with the male genital organs.

Vaccination Administering killed or weakened forms of a disease-causing micro-organism, usually by injection, to help the body fight that disease.

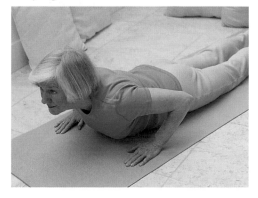

Useful addresses

Note: Health information from a website or helpline must be considered alongside your doctor's advice.

UK

Allergy UK
Deepdene House, 30 Bellegrove Road,
Welling, Kent DA16 3PY
Tel: 020 8303 8583 (helpline)
www.allergyfoundation.com
info@allergyuk.org

Arthritis Research Campaign
Copeman House, St Mary's Gate
Chesterfield, Derbyshire S41 7TD
Tel: 01246 558033
www.arc.org.uk; info@arc.org.uk

British Heart Foundation
14 Fitzharding Street, London
W1H 4DH
Tel: 020 7935 0185
www.bhf.org.uk; internet@bhf.org.uk

British Red Cross Society
9 Grosvenor Crescent
London SW1X 7EJ
Tel: 020 7235 5454
www.redcross.org.uk
information@redcross.org.uk

CancerBACUP
3 Bath Place, Rivington Street
London EC2A 3DR
Tel: 0808 800 1234
www.cancerbacup.org.uk
info@cancerbacup.org.uk

Diabetes UK
10 Parkway, London NW1 7AA
Tel: 020 7424 1000 (helpline)
www.diabetes.org.uk; info@diabetes.org.uk

Eating Disorders Association
Wensum House, 103 Prince of Wales Road
Norwich NR1 1DW
Tel: 01603 621414 (helpline)
www.edauk.com; info@edauk.com

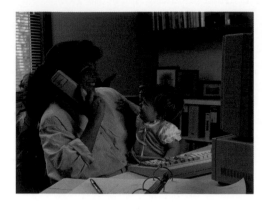

Epilepsy Action/British Epilepsy
Association
New Anstey House, Gate Way Drive
Leeds LS19 7XY
Tel: 0808 800 5050 (helpline)
www.epilepsy.org.uk
helpline@epilepsy.org.uk

Family Planning Association
2–12 Pentonville Road, London N1 9FP
Tel: 0845 310 1334 (helpline)
www.fpa.org.uk

Help the Aged
207–221 Pentonville Road
London N1 9UZ
Tel: 020 7278 1114
www.helptheaged.org.uk
info@helptheaged.org.uk

Institute for Complementary Medicine
PO Box 194, London SE16 1QZ
Tel: 020 7237 5165
www.icmedicine.co.uk
icm@icmedicine.co.uk

National Asthma Campaign
Providence House, Providence Place
London N1 0NT
Tel: 0845 701 0203 (helpline)
www.asthma.org.uk

National Eczema Society
Hill House, Highgate Hill
London N19 5NA
Tel: 0870 241 3604 (helpline)
www.eczema.org

NHS Direct
Tel: 0845 4647
www.nhsdirect.nhs.uk

Royal College of General Practitioners
14 Princess Gate, Hyde Park
London SW7 1PU
www.rcgp.org.uk

The Stroke Association
123 Whitecross Street
London EC1Y 8JJ
Tel: 0845 303 3100 (helpline)
www.stroke.org.uk

USA

American Academy of
Family Physicians
11400 Tomahawk Creek Parkway
Leawood, Kansas 66211-2672
Tel: 1-800-274-2237
www.aafp.org; fp@aafp.org

American Heart Association
7272 Greenville Avenue
Dallas, Texas 75231
Tel: 1-800-242-8721
www.americanheart.org

American Lung Association
61 Broadway, 6th Floor
New York 10006
Tel: 0212-315-8700
www.lungusa.org; info@lungusa.org

American Red Cross
431, 18th Street NW
Washington DC 20006

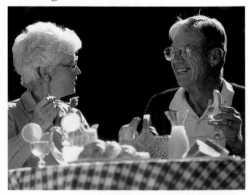

Tel: 0202-639-3520
www.redcross.org

Child Family Health International
953 Mission Street, Suite 220
San Francisco, California 94103
Tel: 0415-957-9000
www.cfhi.org; cfhi@cfhi.org

Canada
Asthma Society of Canada
130 Bridgeland Avenue, Suite 425
Toronto, Ontario M6A 1Z4
Tel: 1-800-787-3880
www.asthma.ca; info@asthma.ca

Canadian Cancer Society
Suite 200, 10 Alcorn Avenue
Toronto, Ontario M4V 3B1
Tel: 0416-961-7223
www.cancer.ca; ccs@cancer.ca

Canadian Red Cross
170 Metcalfe Street, Suite 300
Ottawa, Ontario K2P 2P2
Tel: 0613-740-1900
www.redcross.ca; info@redcross.ca

College of Family Physicians of Canada
2630 Skymark Avenue
Mississauga, Ontario L4W 5A4
Tel: 0905-629-0900
www.cfpc.ca

Heart and Stroke Foundation
of Canada
222 Queen Street, Suite 1402
Ottawa, Ontario K1P 5V9
Tel: 0613-569-4361
ww1.heartandstroke.ca

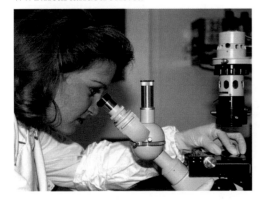

Australia
Australian Red Cross
155 Pelham Street
Carlton, Victoria 3053
Tel: 03 9345 1800
www.redcross.org.au; nat@redcross.org.au

Cancer Council Australia
Level 5, Medical Foundation Building
92–94 Parramatta Road
Camperdown, New South Wales 2050
Tel: 02 9036 3100
www.cancer.org.au; info@cancer.org.au

Children's Health Development Foundation
8th Floor, Samuel Way Building
Women's and Children's Hospital
72 King William Road
North Adelaide, South Australia, 5006
Tel: 08 8161 7777
www.chdf.org.au; chdf@wch.sa.gov.au

National Asthma Council Australia
1 Palmerston Crescent
South Melbourne, Victoria 3205
Tel: 03 9214 1476
www.nationalasthma.org.au
nac@nationalasthma.org.au

National Heart Foundation of Australia
Corner Denison Street and Geils Court
Deakin ACT 2600
Tel: 1300 36 27 87
www.heartfoundation.com.au
heartlinesa@heartfoundation.com.au

New Zealand
Asthma and Respiratory Foundation NZ
Rossmore House, 123 Molesworth St
PO Box 1459, Wellington
Tel: 04 499 4592
www.asthmanz.co.nz; arf@asthma.co.nz

Cancer Society of New Zealand
Molesworth House, Level 2
101 Molesworth St
PO Box 12 145, Wellington
Tel: 04 494 7270
www.cancernz.org.nz
admin@cancernz.org.nz

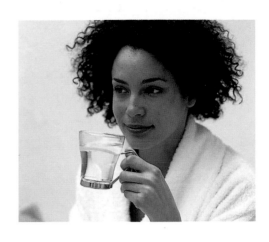

National Heart Foundation NZ
9 Kalmia Street, Ellerslie, PO Box 17160,
Greenlane, Auckland 1130
Tel: 09 571 9191
www.nhf.org.nz; info@nhf.org.nz

New Zealand Red Cross
P.O. Box 12–140
Thorndon, Wellington 6038
Tel: 04 472 3750
www.redcross.org.nz
national@redcross.org.nz

South Africa
Allergy Society of South Africa (ALLSA)
PO Box 88, Observatory 7935
Cape Town
Tel: 021 447 9019
www.allergysa.org

Cancer Association of South Africa
(CANSA)
37A Main Road, Mowbray 7701
Tel: 021 689 5381
www.cansa.org.za; cansainfo@cansa.org.uk

Heart Foundation South Africa
PO Box 15139
Vlaeberg 8018
Tel: 021 447 4222
www.heartfoundation.co.za
heart@heartfoundation.co.za

South African Red Cross Society
PO Box 50696
Waterfront, Cape Town 8002
Tel: 021 418 6640
www.redcross.org.za; info@redcross.org.za

Index

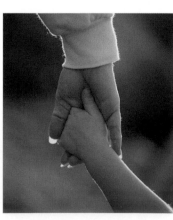
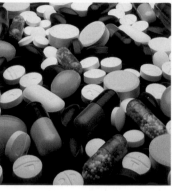

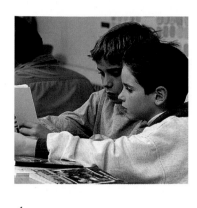

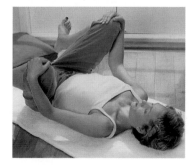

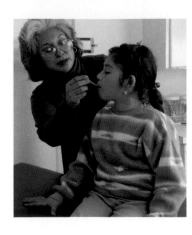

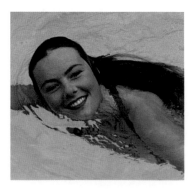

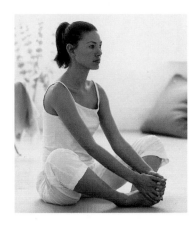

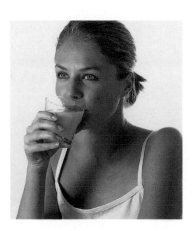

Photographic credits

All photographs other than those listed below are copyrighted to Anness Publishing Ltd.
Key: l=left; r=right; t=top; b=bottom

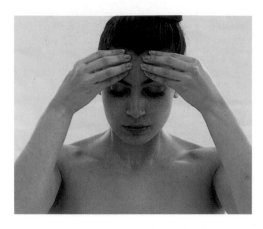

Acknowledgements

The publishers would like to thank:
Everyone at the Royal College of General Practitioners, London, for their patient and scholarly help, from the Chairman of Council, Professor David Haslam FRCGP and Helen Farrelly, Publications Manager, to the team of painstaking verifiers: Dr Rodger Charlton FRCGP, Dr Helen Liley, and Krysia Saul.

Additional verifying and advice: Dr Tim Wallington, consultant immunologist at the National Blood Service, Bristol, and his colleague, haematologist Dr Edwin Massey;

Margaret Hallendorff, Chief Executive, The Royal College of Ophthalmologists, London.

Thanks also to Luci Gosling and Arran Frood at the Science Photo Library for all their cheerful, highly efficient help, and to Pat Coward for compiling the index.

Dr Peter Fermie would like to thank his wife Ellen and daughter Anna for putting up with his long periods spent in front of the computer while working on this book!

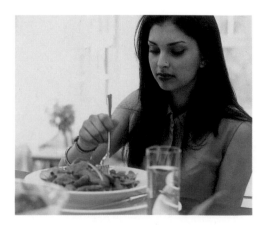

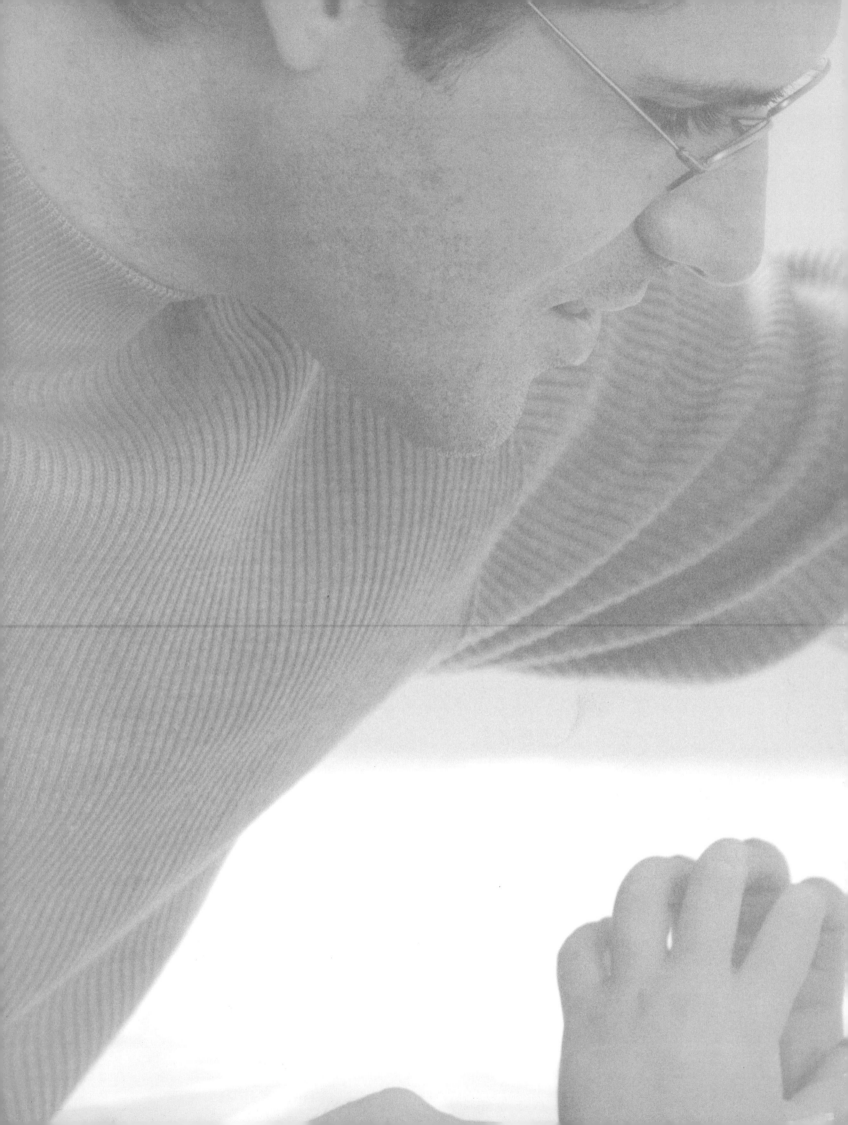